Dental Caries: Assessment and Clinical Management

Dental Caries: Assessment and Clinical Management

Edited by Marcus Ward

hayle
medical

New York

Hayle Medical,
750 Third Avenue, 9th Floor,
New York, NY 10017, USA

Visit us on the World Wide Web at:
www.haylemedical.com

ISBN: 978-1-63241-566-0

Cataloging-in-Publication Data

Dental caries : assessment and clinical management / edited by Marcus Ward.
   p. cm.
Includes bibliographical references and index.
ISBN 978-1-63241-566-0
1. Dental care. 2. Dental hygiene. 3. Dental public health.
4. Mouth--Diseases--Treatment. 5. Dentistry. I. Ward, Marcus.
RK58 .D46 2019
617.600 68--dc23

Table of Contents

Preface

The main aim of this book is to educate learners and enhance their research focus by presenting diverse topics covering this vast field. This is an advanced book which compiles significant studies by distinguished experts in the area of analysis. This book addresses successive solutions to the challenges arising in the area of application, along with it; the book provides scope for future developments.

Dental caries is commonly known as tooth decay. It refers to the decay of teeth caused by bacteria and the acids produced by them. It causes pain while eating. It can also lead to tooth loss, dental abscess and inflammation of the tissues around the teeth. Mutans streptococci, most prominently Streptococcus mutans and Streptococcus sobrinus, and lactobacilli are common types of bacteria that cause dental cavities. X-rays and lasers are used to detect dental caries. It can be prevented by practicing a healthy oral health regime such as regular teeth cleaning and flossing, avoiding a sugar intensive diet and lower intake of fluorides. Dental caries is often classified to represent the severity of tooth decay accurately. It may be classified on the basis of location, rate of progression, etiology and affected hard tissues. This book is a compilation of chapters that discuss the most vital concepts and emerging trends in the assessment and management of dental caries. It includes contributions of experts and dentists, which will provide innovative insights. For all those who are interested in dental caries, this book can prove to be an essential guide.

It was a great honour to edit this book, though there were challenges, as it involved a lot of communication and networking between me and the editorial team. However, the end result was this all-inclusive book covering diverse themes in the field.

Finally, it is important to acknowledge the efforts of the contributors for their excellent chapters, through which a wide variety of issues have been addressed. I would also like to thank my colleagues for their valuable feedback during the making of this book.

Editor

Regeneration and Repair in Endodontics—A Special Issue of the Regenerative Endodontics—A New Era in Clinical Endodontics

Tarek Mohamed A. Saoud [1], Domenico Ricucci [2], Louis M. Lin [3,*] and Peter Gaengler [4]

[1] Department of Conservative Dentistry and Endodontics, Faculty of Dentistry, University of Benghazi, El Salmania, Abn Alathera Street No. 113, Benghazi 00218, Libya; tarek_saoud@yahoo.com

[2] Private practice, Piazza Calvario 7, 87022 Cetraro, Italy; dricucci@libero.it

[3] Department of Endodontics, College of Dentistry, New York University, 345 East 24th Street, New York, NY 10010, USA

[4] Department für Zahn-, Mund- und Kieferheilkunde, Fakultät für Gesundheit, Universität Witten/Herdecke, Alfred-Herrhausen-Strabe 50, 58448 Witten, Germany; peter.gaengler@uni-wh.de

* Correspondence: lml7@nyu.edu;

Academic Editor: George T.-J. Huang

Abstract: Caries is the most common cause of pulp-periapical disease. When the pulp tissue involved in caries becomes irreversibly inflamed and progresses to necrosis, the treatment option is root canal therapy because the infected or non-infected necrotic pulp tissue in the root canal system is not accessible to the host's innate and adaptive immune defense mechanisms and antimicrobial agents. Therefore, the infected or non-infected necrotic pulp tissue must be removed from the canal space by pulpectomy. As our knowledge in pulp biology advances, the concept of treatment of pulpal and periapical disease also changes. Endodontists have been looking for biologically based treatment procedures, which could promote regeneration or repair of the dentin-pulp complex destroyed by infection or trauma for several decades. After a long, extensive search in *in vitro* laboratory and *in vivo* preclinical animal experiments, the dental stem cells capable of regenerating the dentin-pulp complex were discovered. Consequently, the biological concept of 'regenerative endodontics' emerged and has highlighted the paradigm shift in the treatment of immature permanent teeth with necrotic pulps in clinical endodontics. Regenerative endodontics is defined as biologically based procedures designed to physiologically replace damaged tooth structures, including dentin and root structures, as well as the pulp-dentin complex. According to the American Association of Endodontists' Clinical Considerations for a Regenerative Procedure, the primary goal of the regenerative procedure is the elimination of clinical symptoms and the resolution of apical periodontitis. Thickening of canal walls and continued root maturation is the secondary goal. Therefore, the primary goal of regenerative endodontics and traditional non-surgical root canal therapy is the same. The difference between non-surgical root canal therapy and regenerative endodontic therapy is that the disinfected root canals in the former therapy are filled with biocompatible foreign materials and the root canals in the latter therapy are filled with the host's own vital tissue. The purpose of this article is to review the potential of using regenerative endodontic therapy for human immature and mature permanent teeth with necrotic pulps and/or apical periodontitis, teeth with persistent apical periodontitis after root canal therapy, traumatized teeth with external inflammatory root resorption, and avulsed teeth in terms of elimination of clinical symptoms and resolution of apical periodontitis.

Keywords: apical periodontitis; clinical symptom/sign; immature teeth; immunity; innervation; mature teeth; necrotic pulp; periapical healing; pulp tissue regeneration; regenerative endodontics; vital tissue

1. Introduction

Caries is the most common cause of pulp-periapical disease. When the pulp tissue involved in caries becomes irreversibly inflamed and progresses to necrotic, the only treatment option is root canal therapy because the infected necrotic pulp in the root canal system is not accessible to the host's innate and adaptive immune defense mechanisms and antimicrobial agents. Therefore, the infected necrotic pulp tissue must be removed from the canal space by pulpectomy to prevent development or persistence of apical periodontitis.

It was the most acceptable treatment strategy for teeth with infected or non-infected necrotic pulps that the disinfected root canal space should not be left empty and should be filled with biocompatible material to prevent reinfection of the canal space for many decades. The root canal filling was expected to prevent coronal leakage, retard bacterial penetration from the canal space into the periapical tissues, and hopefully entomb bacteria in the canal space. Unfortunately, root canal filling is not able to achieve these desirable expectations in all endodontically treated teeth [1].

As our knowledge in pulp biology advances, the concept of treatment of pulpal and periapical disease appears to change accordingly. Endodontists have been looking for biologically based treatment procedures, which could promote regeneration of the dentin-pulp complex destroyed by infection or trauma, for several decades. After a long, extensive search in *in vitro* laboratory and *in vivo* preclinical animal experiments, multipotent dental stem cells capable of differentiating into odontoblast-like cells, such as dental pulp stem cells [2], stem cells from human exfoliated deciduous teeth [3], and stem cells from apical papilla [4], were discovered. Since then, the pulp biologists have tried to take advantage of these multipotent mesenchymal stem cells to regenerate the dentin-pulp complex. Several preclinical animal studies have demonstrated that it is possible to regenerate the dentin-pulp complex using dental pulp stem cells [5–8]. These preclinical animal studies established the basic concept of application of regenerative endodontics in clinical practice.

Long before the discovery of dental pulp stem cells capable of differentiating into odontoblast-like cells and producing the dentin-pulp complex, Nygaard-Ostby [9] was the pioneer who tried to explore the potential of regenerating tissue in the partially filled canal space of endodontically treated teeth by inducing periapical bleeding in dogs and human beings. It was found that the tissue that formed in the canal spaces was not pulp-like tissue, but fibrous connective tissue and cellular cementum [10]. Subsequently, Nevins *et al.* [11–13] tried to induce hard tissue formation into pulpless immature teeth with open apex using collagen-calcium phosphate gel in rhesus monkeys. These early studies laid the foundation for investigation of regenerative endodontics.

Regenerative endodontics is defined as biologically based procedures designed to physiologically replace damaged tooth structure, including dentin and root structures, as well as the pulp-dentin complex [14]. According to American Association of Endodontists' (AAE) Clinical Considerations for a Regenerative Procedure [15], the primary goal of the regenerative procedure is elimination of clinical symptoms/signs and resolution of apical periodontitis. Thickening of the canal walls and/or continued root maturation is the secondary goal. Therefore, it can be stated that the primary goal of regenerative endodontic procedures and traditional non-surgical root canal therapy is similar. The difference between regenerative endodontic therapy and non-surgical root canal therapy is that the disinfected root canal space in the former therapy is filled with the host's own vital tissue and the canal space in the latter therapy is filled with biocompatible foreign materials.

The purpose of this article is to review the potential of using regenerative endodontic procedures for immature and mature human teeth with necrotic pulps, teeth with persistent apical periodontitis after root canal therapy, traumatized teeth with external inflammatory root resorption, horizontal root fracture, and avulsed teeth in terms of elimination of clinical symptoms/signs and resolution of apical periodontitis and arrest of root resorption.

2. Revascularization and Regenerative Endodontics

The term "revascularization" was used in the studies of pulpal wound healing after replantation of immature permanent teeth [16,17]. Iwaya and associates [18] were the first to coin the term "revascularization" in their endodontic treatment of an immature permanent tooth with apical periodontitis and a sinus tract. The treatment procedures included sodium hypochlorite irrigation and intra-canal antibiotic paste (ciprofloxacin, metronidazole) medication without mechanical debridement. The treatment resulted in elimination of clinical symptoms and resolution of apical periodontitis. In addition, radiographic thickening of the canal walls and continued root development were observed [18]. Therefore, it was thought that the dentin-pulp complex was regenerated, perhaps, by some vital pulp tissue remaining in the apical area of the canal, which might have survived in the tooth clinically diagnosed as having devitalized and infected pulp [18]. Continued root development was also speculated, perhaps, due to survival of the apical papilla in apical periodontitis, because stem cells from the apical papilla were shown to be capable of differentiating into odontoblasts [4] and producing root dentin. Since the report of Iwaya and associates [18], revascularization has been performed in many human immature permanent teeth with necrotic pulps and apical periodontitis [19]. The treatments also achieved similar results as those reported by Iwaya and associates [18,19].

Induction of periapical bleeding into the canal space is a necessary step in regenerative endodontic procedures of immature permanent teeth with necrotic pulps. It was suggested that blood clots in the canal space could serve as a matrix or scaffold to promote pulp tissue wound healing [20]. Subsequently, Lovelace and associates [21] showed that provoked periapical bleeding also brought mesenchymal stem cells from the periapical area into the canal space. Blood contains many platelet-derived growth factors [22,23]. Therefore, induced periapical bleeding brings fibrin scaffold, mesenchymal stem cells, and blood-derived bioactive growth factors into the canal space. In addition, growth factors embedded in the dentin matrix are also released into the canal space after demineralization of dentin with Ethylenediaminetetraacetic acid (EDTA) rinse in regenerative endodontic procedures [24]. Stem cells, growth factors and a scaffold are the essential triad of tissue engineering or tissue regeneration. Therefore, the term "regenerative endodontics" was introduced in clinical endodontics, which also includes revascularization/revitalization to describe the treatment of immature permanent teeth with necrotic pulps.

3. Induction of Periapical Bleeding

Besides growth factors, blood clots, and mesenchymal stem cells, humoral (complement components, immunoglobulins, chemotaxins, antibacterial peptides) and cellular (polymorphonuclear leukocytes, macrophages) components of the innate and adaptive immune defense system are also brought into the canal space during the induction of periapical bleeding. These bioactive peptides and immune cells are contained in the blood [25]. Complement components such as C3b can opsonize bacteria and immunoglobulins can coat and localize bacteria to facilitate phagocytosis by activated polymorphonuclear leukocytes and macrophages through C3b and Fc receptors on these phagocytes. In addition, mesenchymal stem cells can secrete antimicrobial peptide LL-37 [26], up-regulate genes involved in promoting phagocytosis and bacterial killing [27], and augment the antibacterial activity of immune cells and secret large amounts of IL-6, IL-8, and MIF (macrophage migration inhibitory factor) cytokines to recruit and activate polymorphonuclear leukocytes and macrophages [28]. It was also suggested that LL-37 might contribute to regeneration of the dentin-pulp complex in regenerative endodontics [29]. Therefore, induction of periapical bleeding into the canal space during regenerative endodontic therapy may enhance antimicrobial clearance in the canal space. In addition, the possibility that residual bacteria in the canal space after regenerative endodontic therapy might be killed by immune defense mechanisms of regenerated vital tissue cannot be ruled out. This rationale is supported by the high success rate of immature permanent teeth with infected pulps and apical periodontitis after regenerative endodontic therapy [19].

4. Root Canal Fillings

A concern in regenerative endodontic therapy for immature or mature permanent teeth with necrotic pulps is residual bacteria remaining in the canal space after root canal disinfection because bacteria may grow without a root filling. Contemporary root canal infection control protocols, including mechanical instrumentation, sodium hypochlorite irrigation, and intra-canal medication with calcium hydroxide, are not able to eliminate all bacteria in the root canal system because of its anatomic complexity [30,31]. Calcium hydroxide, the most popular intra-canal medication in root canal therapy, has its shortcomings in eliminating intra-canal bacteria, because dentin and hydroxylapatite have inhibitory effects on the anti-microbial activity of calcium hydroxide [32,33]. The triple antibiotic paste (ciprofloxacin, metronidazole and minocycline) used in regenerative endodontic therapy of immature permanent teeth with necrotic pulps may also have limitations in killing intra-canal bacteria. It has been shown that triple antibiotic paste was capable of disinfecting the infected root dentin and eliminating bacteria *in vitro* [34,35]. However, these *in vitro* studies did not exactly simulate the clinical situation in which the teeth indicated for regenerative endodontic therapy usually have had a long-standing history of infection with well-established biofilm on the canal walls and bacteria in the dentinal tubules. An *in vivo* study also showed that triple antibiotic paste was able to eliminate most but not all bacteria in artificially infected root canals in dogs [36]. Ciprofloxacin inhibits DNA gyrase synthesis, metronidazole inhibits DNA synthesis, and minocycline inhibits protein synthesis of microbes [37]. These antibiotics are effective when microbes are in an active state of replication and synthesis of cell walls, proteins, or DNA but not in a stationary state. Therefore, residual bacteria are likely to remain in the canal space of mature or immature permanent teeth with infected necrotic pulps after root canal disinfection using sodium hypochlorite irrigation and intra-canal medication with calcium hydroxide and/or triple antibiotic paste [30,31,38]. Accordingly, it is recommended that the disinfected root canal space should be filled with biocompatible filling materials. The root canal filling is expected to seal the root canal space from communicating with the periapical tissues, prevent coronal leakage, and hopefully entomb residual bacteria in the canal space after root canal therapy. The root canal filling might accomplish one or more of these expectations, but not always all three. Otherwise, teeth with apical periodontitis after non-surgical root canal therapy should be able to achieve complete periapical healing. A systematic review of the outcome of primary root canal therapy does not support this notion [1].

It is not known that how much the root canal filling contributes to the success of non-surgical root canal therapy. Sjogren and associates [39] showed clinically in human teeth with apical periodontitis that if bacteriologic cultures of the canals before root-filling were negative, the success rate of root canal therapy was 94%. In contrast, if bacteriologic cultures were positive, the success rate was 68%. In monkey models, Fabricius and associates [40] also demonstrated that when bacteria remained after endodontic treatment, 79% of root canals showed non-healed periapical lesions, compared with 28% where no bacteria was found. These studies emphasize that control of root canal infection is more important than root-filling. It has also been shown in humans and animals that root canal filling was not necessary if the root canal infection was properly controlled and coronal leakage was prevented [41,42]. The quality of the root filling was found to be less critical for the periapical healing to occur than the presence or absence of bacteria in the canal space [40]. This indicates if the bacterial load in the canal space were able to reduce to the sub-threshold level, which might be determined by negative pre-obturation bacteriologic cultures of the canals, periapical wound healing could take place [39,40]. The host's defense and the number and virulence of microbes determine the infection/inflammation [37]. In regenerative endodontic therapy, although the canal space is not filled with biocompatible foreign materials, induction of periapical bleeding and generation of vital tissue in the canal space may kill the residual bacteria remaining in the canal space as previously mentioned. However, it must be emphasized that effective control of root canal infection is paramount to regenerative endodontic therapy and non-surgical root canal therapy.

5. Size of Apical Foramen

The size of the apical foramen appears to be a major concern in regenerative endodontic therapy. It was suggested that an apical foramen at least 1.1 mm in diameter was necessary for successful revascularization of the pulp tissue in re-implanted human permanent incisors [16]. Therefore, human mature permanent teeth with completely formed root apices having necrotic pulps were considered not suitable for regenerative endodontic therapy. However, a study using an animal model showed that the size of an apical foramen 0.32 mm in diameter did not prevent revascularization and ingrowth of new tissue into canals after transplantation [43].

In studying regeneration of dental-pulp-like tissue by chemotaxis-induced cell homing, the apical foramina of the human mature permanent incisors and canines were not enlarged. Dental-pulp-like tissue was formed in the entire root canal from the root apex to the pulp chamber upon delivery of growth factors into the chemo-mechanically debrided canals of the teeth implanted in mouse dorsum [8]. Complete pulp regeneration in the canals of mature teeth with closed apices was also observed after pulpectomy by transplantation of autologous pulp CD105$^+$ stem cells with stromal cell–derived factor-1 implanted in dogs [7]. Furthermore, it was shown histologically that new tissues could be generated in the canals of mature teeth with necrotic pulps and apical periodontitis after regenerative endodontic therapy when the canals were instrumented to #60 K-file in an animal model [44].

In human regenerative endodontic therapy studies of mature permanent teeth with necrotic pulps and apical periodontitis, Shah and associates [45] enlarged the apical foramen to #30 K-file, Paryani and Kim to #60 K-file [46], and Saoud and associates to #35 K-file [47]. Based on these animal and human studies, it is concluded that the size of the apical foramen does not have to be 1 mm in diameter for new tissue to grow into the canal space after regenerative endodontic therapy. The average size of cells in the human body ranges from 10–100 microns, which is much smaller than the average size of the apical foramen of human teeth (0.2–0.3 mm) and the tip diameter of a hand stainless steel ISO #10 K-file (0.10). Therefore, cells from the periapical tissues should be able to migrate into the canal space through the apical foramen. However, enlargement of the apical foramen to a large size may facilitate the ingrowth of new tissue into the canal space from the periapical tissues after regenerative endodontic therapy of mature permanent teeth.

6. Regenerative Endodontics and Pulp Tissue Regeneration/Replacement

As previously mentioned, mesenchymal stem cells in the apical papilla of immature permanent teeth with necrotic pulps introduced into the canal space during regenerative endodontic procedures might be able to differentiate into odontoblasts and produce dentin [4,21], and Hertwig's epithelial root sheath, if intact after apical periodontitis, is capable of signaling mesenchymal stem cells in the dental follicle to differentiate into cementoblasts and regulate the root development [48,49]. Based on these presumptions, it was speculated that regenerative endodontic therapy of immature permanent teeth with necrotic pulps was able to regenerate the dentin-pulp complex and promote continued root development (Figure 1). However, histological studies of immature permanent teeth with necrotic pulps and apical periodontitis after regenerative endodontic therapy revealed that the tissues generated in the canal space were cementum-like, bone-like, or periodontal ligament–like tissue and not true pulp tissue in many animal models and humans [50–56] (Figure 2). Thickening of the canal walls and/or continued root maturation were due to deposition of cementum-like tissue or bone-like tissue on the canal walls and at the root apex, respectively. In one human study, nerve fibers were demonstrated in newly formed tissue in the canal space of a revascularized immature permanent tooth using immunohistochemical study [56]. Most vital tissues are supplied with blood vessels and nerve innervation because the biological function of blood vessels is largely controlled by the sympathetic and parasympathetic nervous system. Although the pulp replacement tissues are not true pulp tissue, they are vital tissues inherited with innate and adaptive immune defense mechanisms and innervated by sensory nerve fibers to detect and protect themselves from foreign invaders such as bacteria. If the primary goal of regenerative endodontic therapy of immature permanent teeth with necrotic pulps is to eliminate clinical symptoms/signs and resolve apical periodontitis, then repair by tissue different from pulp tissue, although not ideal in wound healing, is not a clinical treatment failure.

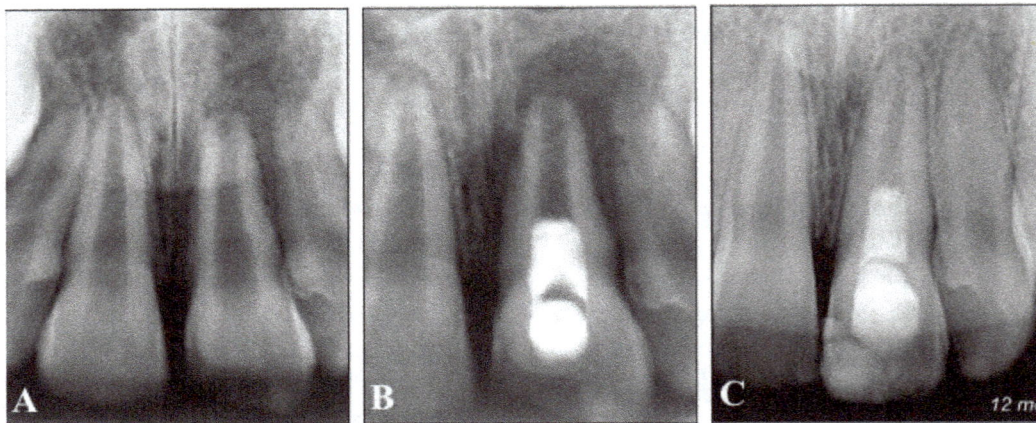

Figure 1. Radiographs of revascularized human immature permanent tooth #9. (**A**) Preoperative radiograph to show inflammatory periapical lesion; (**B**) Postoperative radiograph after regenerative endodontic procedures; (**C**) At 12-month follow-up, thickening of the canal walls and continued root maturation [54].

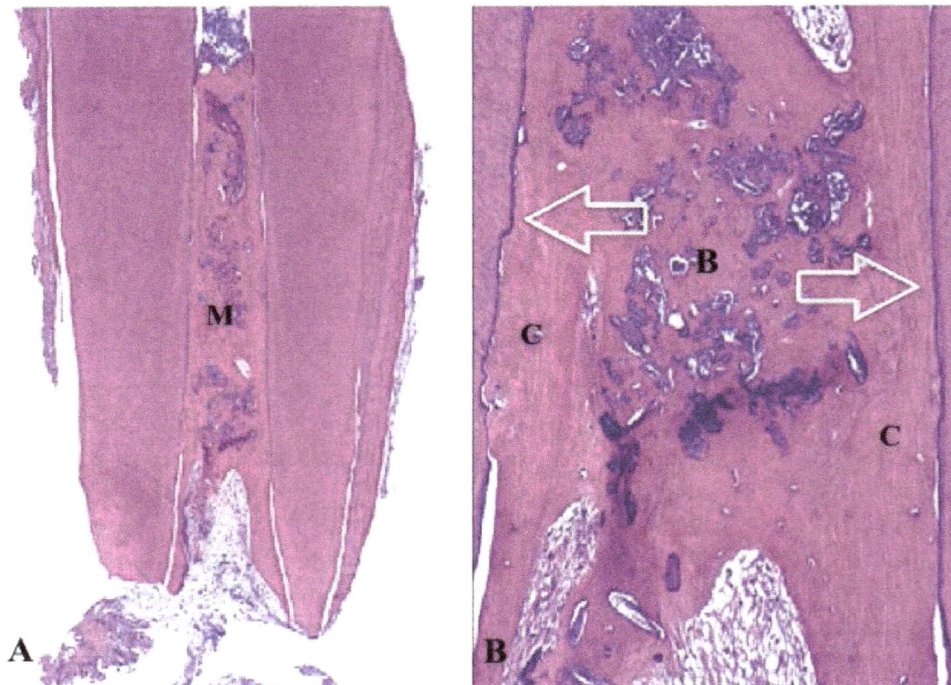

Figure 2. Histology of revascularized human immature permanent tooth (hematoxylin-eosin stain). (**A**) The canal space filled with mineralized tissue (M) (original magnification ×16); (**B**) High magnification of A. The mineralized tissue similar to bone (**B**) and cementum (**C**). The canal dentin walls covered by newly formed cellular cementum-like tissue (arrows) (original magnification ×100) [53].

7. Regenerative Endodontic ProceduresSuggested by AAE [15]

First appointment:

- Local anesthesia, dental dam isolation and access.
- Copious, gentle irrigation with 20 mL NaOCl using an irrigation system that minimizes the possibility of extrusion of irrigants into the periapical space (e.g., needle with closed end and side-vent, or EndoVac™). Lower concentrations of NaOCl are advised (1.5% NaOCl (20 mL/canal, 5 min) and then irrigated with saline (20 mL/canal, 5 min), with irrigation needle positioned about 1 mm from root end, to minimize cytotoxicity to stem cells in the apical tissues.
- Dry canals with paper points.
- Place calcium hydroxide or low concentration of triple antibiotic paste. If the triple antibiotic paste is used: (1) consider sealing pulp chamber with a dentin bonding agent (to minimize risk of staining) and (2) mix 1:1:1 ciprofloxacin:metronidazole:minocycline to a final concentration of 0.1 mg/mL.
- Deliver into canal system via syringe.
- If triple antibiotic is used, ensure that it remains below Cement-enamel junction (CEJ) (minimize crown staining).
- Seal with 3–4 mm of a temporary material such as Cavit™, IRM™, glass-ionomer or another temporary material. Dismiss patient for one to four weeks.

Second appointment (one to four weeks after first visit):

- Assess response to initial treatment. If there are signs/symptoms of persistent infection, consider additional treatment with antimicrobial or alternative antimicrobial.
- Anesthesia with 3% mepivacaine without vasoconstrictor, dental dam isolation.
- Copious, gentle irrigation with 20 mL of 17% EDTA.
- Dry with paper points.
- Create bleeding into canal system by over-instrumenting (endo file, endo explorer) (induce by rotating a pre-curved K-file at 2 mm past the apical foramen with the goal of having the entire canal filled with blood to the level of cement-enamel junction).
- Stop bleeding at a level that allows for 3–4 mm of restorative material.
- Place a resorbable matrix such as CollaPlug™, Collacote™, CollaTape™ or other material over the blood clot if necessary and white MTA/CaOH as capping material.
- A 3–4 mm layer of glass ionomer (e.g., Fuji IlLC™, GC America, Alsip, IL, USA) is flowed gently over the capping material and light-cured for 40 s. MTA has been associated with discoloration. Alternatives to MTA should be considered in teeth where there is an esthetic concern.

* Anterior and premolar teeth—Consider use of Collatape/Collaplug and restoration with 3 mm of Resin modified glass-ionomer (RMGI) followed by bonding a filled composite to the beveled enamel margin.
* Molar teeth or teeth with Porcelain fused to metal (PFM) crown—Consider use of Collatape/Collaplug and restoration with 3 mm of MTA, followed by RMGI or alloy.

Follow-up:

Clinical and radiographic examination

* No pain, soft tissue swelling or sinus tract (often observed between first and second appointments).
* Resolution of apical radiolucency (often observed six to 12 months after treatment).
* Increased width of root walls (this is generally observed before apparent increase in root length and often occurs 12–24 months after treatment).
* Increased root length.
* Pulp vitality test.

8. Treatment of Immature Permanent Teeth with Necrotic Pulps

Traditionally, immature permanent teeth with necrotic pulps are treated with calcium hydroxide apexification to induce an apical hard tissue barrier formation, or with a mineral trioxide aggregate (MTA) apical plug to create a barrier [57]. The disinfected root canal space is then filled with biocompatible materials, gutta-percha and sealer/cement to the apical barrier. The outcome of calcium hydroxide or MTA apexification treatment is predictable [57]. However, the possibility of the thickening of the canal walls and/or continued root development cannot occur after apexification, thus rendering the immature teeth with already thin canal walls more prone to cervical root fracture [58,59]. In addition, calcium hydroxide apexification usually takes several months to complete, which creates a problem for children and their parents to comply with treatment procedures.

Since the introduction of regenerative endodontic therapy for immature permanent teeth with apical periodontitis by Iwaya and associates [18], regenerative endodontic therapy has become a treatment option for immature permanent teeth with necrotic pulps [19]. The treatment could result in resolution of apical periodontitis and elimination of clinical symptoms, and in some cases radiographic thickening of the canal walls and/or continued root development [19]. Thickening of the canal walls and/or increased root length are considered to be the favorable outcomes of regenerative endodontic therapy of immature permanent teeth with necrotic pulps, because they may strengthen the root and increase the root/crown ratio. Although randomized, prospective studies of regenerative endodontic therapy of immature permanent teeth with necrotic pulps are still lacking, the best available evidence seems to indicate that regenerative endodontic therapy is a feasible treatment option for immature permanent teeth with necrotic pulps [60]. Importantly, the vitality, immunity, and sensibility of immature permanent teeth with necrotic pulps are restored after regenerative endodontic therapy.

9. Treatment of Mature Permanent Teeth with Necrotic Pulps

Mature permanent teeth with necrotic pulps are traditionally treated with pulpectomy and root canal filling. The outcome of primary root canal treatment varies considerably depending on the presence or absence of apical periodontitis [1]. The major contributing factor to the success of root canal treatment is effective control of root canal infection [39,40]. Endodontists have enjoyed the success of practicing non-surgical root canal therapy for teeth with infected, necrotic pulps and/or apical periodontitis for many decades, given that the treatment is properly performed [39,40]. Although the technology, devices, and materials used in root canal therapy have been greatly improved, the outcome of non-surgical root canal treatment for mature permanent teeth with apical periodontitis has not been improved significantly for the past two decades [1]. This further emphasizes the importance of infection control in root canal therapy.

Very recently, regenerative endodontic therapy has been employed to treat mature permanent teeth with necrotic pulps and apical periodontitis, based on the rationale of elimination of clinical symptoms/signs and resolution of apical periodontitis observed in immature permanent teeth with necrotic pulps after regenerative endodontic therapy [45–47,61]. Thickening of the canal walls and/or continued root development are not expected to occur in mature permanent teeth following regenerative endodontic therapy. However, apical closure can take place [47]. The major difference in regenerative endodontic procedures for mature teeth with infected, necrotic pulps is that complete mechanical debridement is required to help eliminate root canal infection and remove necrotic tissue. Similar to traditional non-surgical root canal therapy, regenerative endodontic therapy of mature permanent teeth with apical periodontitis is able to result in the elimination of clinical symptoms and resolution of apical periodontitis [45–47,61]. Therefore, regenerative endodontic therapy provides another treatment option for mature permanent teeth with necrotic pulps (Figure 3).

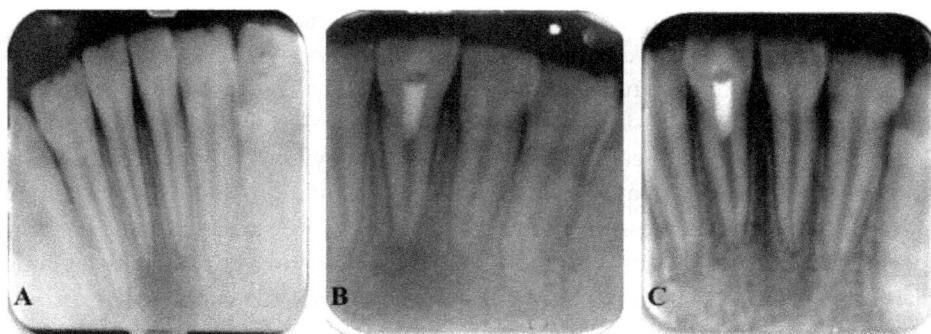

Figure 3. Radiographs of revascularized human mature teeth #25. (**A**) Preoperative radiograph to show inflammatory periapical lesion; (**B**) Postoperative radiograph after regenerative endodontic procedures; (**C**) At 12-month follow-up, resolution of apical periodontitis [61].

10. Treatment of Teeth with Persistent Apical Periodontitis after Root Canal Therapy

It is well established that persistent apical periodontitis after root canal therapy is caused by persistence of root canal infection or re-infection [62,63]. Traditionally, teeth with persistent apical periodontitis after root canal therapy are managed with non-surgical root canal therapy. Endodontic surgery is usually indicated if non-surgical treatment is not feasible. The outcome of secondary root canal treatment is less favorable than that of primary root canal treatment because of several possibly complicated factors, such as untreated extra canals, ledge formation, canal blockage, separated instrument, or irretrievable cement or post in the canals created by primary root canal therapy [1,64]. In principle, secondary and primary root canal treatments are similar, except that more complete root canal infection control procedures are required in secondary root canal therapy. Recently, regenerative endodontic therapy has also been used to manage teeth with persistent apical periodontitis after root canal therapy [65,66]. The treatment also achieved elimination of clinical symptoms and resolution of apical periodontitis. Interestingly, thickening of the canal walls and apical closure were demonstrated after regenerative endodontic therapy of teeth with persistent apical periodontitis after root canal treatment [65,66]. Therefore, regenerative endodontic therapy offers another potential for retreatment of teeth with persistent apical periodontitis after root canal treatment.

11. Treatment of Traumatized Teeth with External Inflammatory Root Resorption, Horizontal Root Fracture, and Avulsed Teeth

Traumatized teeth with external inflammatory root resorption, horizontal root fracture, and complete avulsion are traditionally managed with control of root canal infection using chemo-mechanical debridement and root canal filling [67]. Recently, regenerative endodontic procedures have been employed to manage traumatized teeth with horizontal root fracture, external inflammatory root resorption, and complete avulsion.

In order for external inflammatory root resorption to take place, the protective layer of precementum must be damaged, likely by trauma or inflammation, thus leading to exposure of the underlying dentin [68–70]. In addition, the canal space has to contain infected necrotic pulp tissue. The toxic products from bacteria and tissue breakdown in the canal space diffuse through the dentinal tubules, communicating with the root surface denuded of cementum, and initiate the inflammatory reaction [68–70]. Therefore, infected necrotic pulp is the primary cause of external inflammatory root resorption. Treatment of external inflammatory root resorption is usually carried out by complete chemomechanical debridement, long-term calcium hydroxide dressing, and root canal filling [71]. It was presumed that calcium hydroxide would penetrate through the dentinal tubules and change the acidic environment of the resorbed root surface to prevent osteoclast activity [72,73]. It has also been shown that long-term calcium hydroxide dressing in the canal space of immature permanent teeth weakens the fragile thin root structure, thus increasing the likelihood of root fractures [59].

External inflammatory root resorption of immature permanent teeth caused by trauma was successfully treated with regenerative endodontic procedures and resulted in the resolution of apical periodontitis and the arrest of external root resorption [74]. The traumatized tooth with horizontal root fracture resulting in pulp necrosis was also successfully treated with the concept of regenerative endodontic procedures, achieving healing of the root fracture by hard tissue formation [75].

Avulsed teeth are commonly treated with immediate replantation, followed by chemomechanical debridement, calcium hydroxide dressing and root canal filling if the pulps become necrotic. Recently, an avulsed permanent mature incisor with more than 8 h extra-oral dry time was replanted into the alveolar socket after complete chemomechanical debridement of the canal space and enlargement of the apical foramen to 1.5–2 mm. The tooth was then treated with regenerative endodontic therapy, using platelet-rich plasma instead of blood clot as a scaffold. At 12-month follow-up, the tooth showed resolution of apical periodontitis and arrest of internal and external inflammatory resorption [76]. Therefore, regenerative endodontic procedures have the potential to be used to manage external inflammatory root resorption, horizontal root fracture, and avulsed tooth and should be explored further.

12. Treatment Outcomes of Regenerative Endodontics

There are no randomized, prospective clinical trials of regenerative endodontics for immature and mature teeth with necrotic pulps available. The level of evidence of success rates and treatment outcomes of regenerative endodontics is very low because most studies are case reports and case series [60]. In addition, there was a lack of criteria of success used in various case reports and case series of regenerative endodontic therapy. One oft-cited cohort study investigated 20 cases of regenerative endodontic therapy for immature permanent teeth with necrotic pulps and showed that the success or survival rate of treated teeth was 100% in terms of regression of clinical symptoms/signs and resolution of apical periodontitis or retention of teeth [77]. The frequency of thickening of the canal walls and/or continued root development of immature permanent teeth with necrotic pulps after regenerative endodontic therapy is not always unpredictable [78,79] (Figure 4). For mature teeth with necrotic pulps, it was demonstrated that regenerative endodontic therapy could be an alternate treatment choice to non-surgical root canal therapy regarding elimination of clinical symptoms/signs and resolution of apical periodontitis [61]. Nevertheless, long-term follow-up studies of regenerative endodontic therapy of immature and mature teeth with necrotic pulps are necessary. In addition, randomized, prospective clinical trials have to be performed to obtain reliable success rates and treatment outcomes of regenerative endodontics.

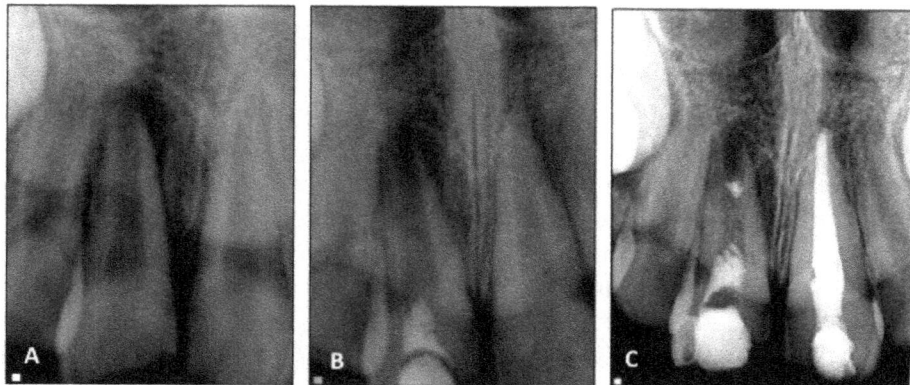

Figure 4. Radiographs of revascularized human immature permanent tooth #8. (**A**) Preoperative radiograph to show inflammatory periapical lesion; (**B**) Postoperative radiograph after regenerative endodontic procedures; (**C**) At 12-month follow-up, no thickening of the canal walls and no continued root maturation are seen.

13. Is Regenerative Endodontic Therapy for All Teeth with Necrotic Pulps?

If the primary goal of regenerative endodontics is to eliminate clinical symptoms/signs and achieve resolution of apical periodontitis [15], then regenerative endodontic procedures can be employed to manage most teeth with necrotic pulps. Similar to non-surgical root canal therapy, if root canal infection can be effectively controlled, regenerative endodontic therapy could also be successfully performed for the immature permanent tooth with apical periodontitis in one visit [80]. However, in some teeth, regenerative endodontics may not be suitable, for example in teeth requiring a post for adequate coronal restoration. Retreatment of failure of teeth treated with regenerative endodontic procedures can be a challenge. The teeth treated with root canal filling may have a poorer survival rate than the teeth treated with regenerative procedures because of lack of defense mechanisms such as immuno-inflammatory and sensory response.

14. Conclusions

The goal of treatment of a disease is to assist the host's natural wound healing processes by enhancing innate and adaptive immune defense mechanisms to eliminate irritants and create a favorable microenvironment conducive for tissue repair and/or regeneration to take place.

Infection is the main cause of primary and post-treatment apical periodontitis of immature and mature permanent teeth. Therefore, if infection is effectively under control, the tissue should be able to heal. Traditional root canal therapy of immature and mature permanent teeth with necrotic pulps is mechanically and materially based. The procedures involve removal of infected necrotic pulp, root canal disinfection, and filling of the canal space with biocompatible foreign material. Regenerative endodontic therapy is biologically based and intended to promote the host's natural wound healing process to restore vitality, immunity, and sensitivity of tissue in the canal space destroyed by infection or trauma. Similar to traditional root canal therapy, regenerative endodontic therapy of immature and mature teeth with necrotic pulps and apical periodontitis has been shown to be able to eliminate clinical symptoms and resolve apical periodontitis. Furthermore, teeth with persistent apical periodontitis after root canal therapy can also be treated with regenerative endodontic therapy. Biologically, it may be preferable to have the disinfected root canal space filled with the host's own vital tissues rather than with non-vital foreign materials. Like the revascularization of an immature tooth with an apical lesion reported in 2001 [18], regenerative endodontics for mature permanent teeth with necrotic pulps is still in the early stage of clinical trials. Nonetheless, regenerative procedures have become an important treatment choice for immature permanent teeth with necrotic pulps even though thickening of the canal walls and/or continued root maturation are not always predictable [78,79]. However, as previously mentioned, randomized, prospective clinical trials are required to compare the clinical outcomes of regenerative endodontic therapy and non-surgical root canal therapy for immature and mature teeth with necrotic pulps. The clinicians have to constantly follow the rapid advancement of regenerative endodontics to make appropriate treatment choices for the patients. Pulp biology and clinical endodontic therapy are slowly coming together [81]. Regenerative endodontics may bring about a new era in clinical endodontics as an alternative treatment option to non-surgical root canal treatment.

References

1. Ng, Y.-L.; Mann, V.; Gulabivala, K. Outcome of primary root canal treatment: A systematic review of the literature. *Int. Endod. J.* **2007**, *40*, 912–939.
2. Gronthos, S.; Mankani, M.; Brahim, J.; Gehron Robey, P.; Shi, S. Postnatal human dental pulp stem cells (DPCs) *in vitro* and *in vivo*. *Proc. Natl. Acad. Sci. USA* **2000**, *97*, 13625–13630. [CrossRef] [PubMed]
3. Miura, M.; Gronthos, S.; Zhao, M.; Lu, B.; Fisher, L.W.; Robey, P.G.; Shi, S. SHED: Stem cells from human exfoliated deciduous teeth. *Proc. Natl. Acad. Sci. USA* **2003**, *100*, 5807–5812. [CrossRef] [PubMed]

4.   Sonoyama, W.; Liu, Y.; Yamaza, T.; Wang, S.; Shi, S.; Huang, G.T.-J. Characterization of apical papilla and its residing stem cells from human immature permanent teeth—A pilot study. *J. Endod.* **2008**, *34*, 166–171. [CrossRef] [PubMed]

5.   Corderio, M.M.; Dong, Z.; Kaneko, T.; Zhang, Z.; Miyazawa, M.; Shi, S.; Smith, A.J.; Nör, J.E. Dental pulp engineering with stem cells from exfoliated deciduous teeth. *J. Endod.* **2008**, *34*, 962–969. [CrossRef] [PubMed]

6.   Huang, G.T.; Yamaza, T.; Shea, L.D.; Djouad, F.; Kuhn, N.Z.; Tuan, R.S.; Shi, S. Stem/progenitor cell-mediated *de novo* regeneration of dental pulp with newly deposited continuous layer of dentin in an *in vivo* model. *Tissue Eng. Part A* **2010**, *16*, 605–615. [CrossRef] [PubMed]

7.   Iohara, K.; Imabayashi, K.; Ishizaka, R.; Watanabe, A.; Nabekura, J.; Ito, M.; Matsushita, K.; Nakamura, H.; Nakashima, M. Complete pulp regeneration after pulpectomy by transplantation of CD105$^+$ stem cells with stromal cell-derived factor-1. *Tissue Eng. Part A* **2011**, *17*, 1911–1920. [CrossRef] [PubMed]

8.   Kim, J.Y.; Xin, X.; Moioli, E.K.; Chung, J.; Lee, C.H.; Chen, M.; Fu, S.Y.; Koch, P.D.; Mao, J.J. Regeneration of dentin-pulp-like tissue by chemotaxis-induced cell homing. *Tissue Eng. Part A* **2010**, *16*, 3023–3031. [CrossRef] [PubMed]

9.   Nygaard-Ostby, B. The role of the blood clot in endodontic therapy. *Acta Odontol. Scand.* **1961**, *19*, 324–353.

10. Nygaard-Ostby, B.; Hjordal, O. Tissue formation in the canal following pulp removal. *Scand. J. Dent. Res.* **1971**, *79*, 333–349. [CrossRef] [PubMed]

11. Nevins, A.; Finkelstein, F.; Borden, B.G.; Laporta, R. Revitalization of pulpless open apex teeth in rhesus monkeys using collagen-calcium phosphate gel. *J. Endod.* **1976**, *2*, 159–165. [CrossRef]

12. Nevins, A.; Wrobel, W.; Valachovic, R.; Borden, B.G. Hard tissue induction into pulpless open-apex teeth using collagen-calcium phosphate gel. *J. Endod.* **1977**, *3*, 431–433. [CrossRef]

13. Nevins, A.; Finkelstein, F.; Paports, R.; Borden, B.G. Induction of hard tissue into pulpless open-apex teeth using collagen-calcium phosphate gel. *J. Endod.* **1978**, *4*, 76–81. [CrossRef]

14. American Association of Endodontists. *Glossary of Endodontic Terms*, 8th ed.; American Association of Endodontists: Chicago, IL, USA, 2012.

15. American Association of Endodontists. AAE Clinical Considerations for a Regenerative Procedure. Available online: https://www.aae.org/uploadedfiles/publications_and_research/research/currentregenerativeendo donticconsiderations.pdf (accessed on 25 February 2016).

16. Kling, M.; Cvek, M.; Mejare, I. Rate and predictability of pulp revascularization in therapeutically reimplanted permanent incisors. *Endod. Dent. Traumatol.* **1986**, *2*, 83–89. [CrossRef] [PubMed]

17. Andreasen, J.O.; Borum, M.; Jacobsen, H.L.; Andreasen, F.M. Replantation of 400 avulsed permanent incisors. II. Factors related to pulp healing. *Endod. Dent. Traumatol.* **1995**, *11*, 59–68. [CrossRef] [PubMed]

18. Iwaya, S.I.; Ikawa, M.; Kubota, M. Revascularization of an immature permanent tooth with apical periodontitis and sinus tract. *Dent. Traumatol.* **2001**, *17*, 185–187. [CrossRef] [PubMed]

19. Diogenes, A.; Henry, M.A.; Teizeira, F.B.; Hargreaves, K.M. An update on clinical regenerative endodontics. *Endod. Top.* **2013**, *28*, 2–23. [CrossRef]

20. Thibodeau, B.; Teixeira, F.; Yamauchi, M.; Caplan, D.J.; Trope, M. Pulp revascularization of immature dog teeth with apical periodontitis. *J. Endod.* **2007**, *33*, 680–689. [CrossRef] [PubMed]

21. Lovelace, T.W.; Henry, M.A.; Hargreaves, K.M.; Diogenes, A. Evaluation of the delivery of mesnechymal stem cells into the canal space of necrotic immature teeth after clinical regenerative endodontic procedure. *J. Endod.* **2011**, *17*, 133–138. [CrossRef] [PubMed]

22. Civinini, R.; Mecera, A.; Redi, B.; Innocenti, M. Blood-derived growth factors. *Clin. Cases Miner Bone Metab.* **2010**, *7*, 194.

23. Lubkowska, A.; Dolegowska, B.; Banfi, G. Growth factor content in PRP and their applicability in medicine. *J. Biol. Regul. Homeost. Agents* **2012**, *26*, 3S–22S. [PubMed]

24. Galler, K.M.; Buchalla, W.; Hiller, K.-A.; Federlin, M.; Eidt, A.; Schiefersteiner, M.; Schmalz, G. Influence of root canal disinfections on growth factor release from dentin. *J. Endod.* **2015**, *41*, 363–368. [CrossRef] [PubMed]

25. Abbas, A.K.; Lichman, A.H.; Pillai, S. *Cellular and Molecular Immunology*, 6th ed.; Saunders: Philadelphia, PA, USA, 2007.

26. Krasnodembskaya, A.; Song, Y.; Fang, X.; Gupta, N.; Serikov, V.; Lee, J.W.; Matthay, M.A. Antibacterial effect of human mesenchymal stem cells is mediated in part from secretion of the antimicrobial peptide LL-37. *Stem Cells* **2010**, *28*, 2229–2238. [CrossRef] [PubMed]

27. Mei, S.H.J.; Haitsma, J.J.; Dos Santos, C.C.; Deng, Y.; Lai, P.F.; Slutsky, A.S.; Liles, W.C.; Stewart, D.J. Mesenchymal stem cells reduce inflammation while enhancing bacterial clearance and improving survival in sepsis. *Am. J. Repir. Crit. Care Med.* **2010**, *182*, 1047–1057. [CrossRef] [PubMed]

28. Brandau, S.; Jakob, M.; Bruderek, K.; Bootz, F.; Giebel, B.; Radtke, S.; Mauel, K.; Jäger, M.; Flohé, S.B.; Lang, S. Mesenchymal stem cells augment the antibacterial activity of neutrophil granulocytes. *PLoS ONE* **2014**, *9*, e14201. [CrossRef] [PubMed]

29. Kajiya, M.; Shiba, H.; Komatsuzawa, H.; Ouhara, K.; Fujita, T.; Takeda, K.; Uchida, Y.; Mizuno, N.; Kawaguchi, H.; Kurihara, H. The antimicrobial peptide LL-37 induces the migration of human pulp cells: A possible adjunct for regenerative endodontics. *J. Endod.* **2010**, *36*, 1009–1013. [CrossRef] [PubMed]

30. Wu, M.K.; Dummer, P.M.; Wesselink, P.R. Consequence and strategies to deal with residual post-treatment root canal infection. *Int. Endod. J.* **2006**, *39*, 343–356. [CrossRef] [PubMed]

31. Siqueira, J.F.; Rocas, I.N. Clinical implications and microbiology of bacterial persistence after treatment procedures. *J. Endod.* **2008**, *34*, 1291–1301.e3. [CrossRef] [PubMed]

32. Portenier, I.; Haapasalo, H.; Rye, A.; Waltimo, T.; Ørstavik, D.; Haapasalo, M. Inactivation of root canal medicaments by dentin, hydroxylapatite, and bovine serum albumin. *Int. Endod. J.* **2001**, *34*, 184–188. [CrossRef] [PubMed]

33. Haapasalo, M.; Qian, W.; Portenier, I.; Waltimo, T. Effects of dentin on the antimicrobial properties of endodontic medicaments. *J. Endod.* **2007**, *33*, 917–925. [CrossRef] [PubMed]

34. Sato, I.; Ando-Kurihara, N.; Kota, K.; Iwaku, M.; Hoshino, E. Sterilization of infected root-canal dentin by topical application of mixture of ciprofloxacin, metronidazole and minocycline *in situ*. *Int. Endod. J.* **1996**, *29*, 118–124. [CrossRef] [PubMed]

35. Hoshino, E.; Kurihara-Ando, N.; Sato, I.; Uematsu, H.; Sato, M.; Kota, K.; Iwaku, M. *In-vitro* antibacterial susceptibility of bacteria taken from infected root dentin to a mixture of ciprofloxacin, metronidazole and minocycline. *Int. Endod. J.* **1996**, *29*, 125–130. [CrossRef] [PubMed]

36. Windley, W.; Teixeira, F.; Levine, L.; Sigurdsson, A.; Trope, M. Disinfection of immature teeth with a triple antibiotic paste. *J. Endod.* **2005**, *31*, 439–443. [CrossRef] [PubMed]

37. Mims, C.; Dockrell, H.; Goering, R. *Medical Microbiology*; Mosby: St Louis, MO, USA, 2004.

38. Lin, L.M.; Shimizu, E.; Gibbs, J.L.; Loghin, S.; Ricucci, D. Histologic and histobacteriologic observations of failed revascularization/revitalization therapy: A case report. *J. Endod.* **2014**, *40*, 291–295. [CrossRef] [PubMed]

39. Sjogren, U.; Figdor, D.; Persson, S.; Sundqvist, G. Influence of infection at the time of root filling on the outcome of endodontic treatment of teeth with apical periodontitis. *Int. Endod. J.* **1997**, *30*, 297–306. [CrossRef] [PubMed]

40. Fabricius, L.; Dahlin, G.; Sundqvist, G.; Happonen, R.P.; Möller, A.J. Influence of residual bacteria on periapical tissue healing after chemomechanical treatment and root filling of experimentally infected monkey teeth. *Eur. J. Oral Sci.* **2006**, *114*, 278–285. [CrossRef] [PubMed]

41. Klevant, F.J.; Eggink, C.O. The effect of canal preparation on periapical disease. *Int. Endod. J.* **1983**, *16*, 68–75. [CrossRef] [PubMed]

42. Sabeti, M.A.; Nekofar, M.; Motahhary, P.; Ghandi, M.; Simon, J.H. Healing of apical periodontitis after endodontic treatment with and without obturation in dogs. *J. Endod.* **2006**, *32*, 6128–6133. [CrossRef] [PubMed]

43. Laureys, W.G.; Guvelier, G.A.; Dermaut, I.R.; De Pauw, G.A. The critical apical diameter to obtain regeneration of the pulp tissue after tooth transplantation, replantation, or regenerative endodontic therapy. *J. Endod.* **2013**, *39*, 759–763. [CrossRef] [PubMed]

44. Gomes-Filho, J.E.; Tobias Duarte, P.G.; Ervolino, E.; Mogami Bomfim, S.R.; Xavier Abimussi, C.J.; Mota da Silva Santos, L.; Lodi, C.S.; Penha De Oliveira, S.H.; Dezan, E., Jr.; Cintra, L.T. Histological characterization of engineering tissues in the canal space of close-apex teeth with apical periodontitis. *J. Endod.* **2013**, *39*, 1549–1556. [CrossRef] [PubMed]

45. Shah, N.; Logani, A. SealBio: A novel, non-obturation endodontic treatment based on concept of regeneration. *J. Conserv. Dent.* **2012**, *15*, 328–332. [CrossRef] [PubMed]

46. Paryani, K.; Kim, S.G. Regenerative endodontic treatment of permanent teeth after completion of root development: A report of 2 cases. *J. Endod.* **2013**, *39*, 929–934. [CrossRef] [PubMed]

47. Saoud, T.M.; Sigurdsson, A.; Rosenberg, P.A.; Lin, L.M.; Ricucci, D. Treatment of a large cystlike inflammatory periapical lesion associated with mature necrotic teeth using regenerative endodontic therapy. *J. Endod.* **2014**, *40*, 2081–2086. [CrossRef] [PubMed]

48. Zeichner-David, M. Regeneration of periodontal tissues: Cementogenesis revisited. *Periodontology 2000* **2006**, *41*, 196–217. [CrossRef] [PubMed]

49. Sonoyama, W.; Seo, B.-M.; Yamaza, T.; Shi, S. Human Hertwig's epithelial root sheath cells ply crucial roles in cementum formation. *J. Dent. Res.* **2007**, *86*, 594–599. [CrossRef] [PubMed]

50. Wang, X.; Thibodeau, B.; Trope, M.; Lin, L.M.; Huang, G.T.-J. Histological characterization of regenerated tissues in canal space after revitalization/revascularization procedure of immature dog teeth with apical periodontitis. *J. Endod.* **2010**, *36*, 56–63. [CrossRef] [PubMed]

51. Bezerra da Silva, L.A.; Nelson-Filho, P.; Bezerra da Silva, R.A.; Flores, D.S.; Heilborn, C.; Johnson, J.D.; Cohenca, N. Revascularization and periapical repair after endodontic treatment using apical negative pressure irrigation versus conventional irrigation plus triantibiotic intracanal dressing in dog's teeth with apical periodontitis. *Oral Surg. Oral Med. Oral Pathol. Oral Radiol. Endod.* **2010**, *109*, 779–787. [CrossRef] [PubMed]

52. Yamauchi, N.; Yamauchi, S.; Nakaoka, H.; Duggan, D.; Zhong, S.; Lee, S.M.; Teixeira, F.B.; Yamauchi, M. Tissue engineering strategies for immature teeth with apical periodontitis. *J. Endod.* **2011**, *37*, 390–397. [CrossRef] [PubMed]

53. Martin, G.; Ricucci, D.; Gibbs, J.L.; Lin, L.M. Histological findings of revascularized/revitalized immature permanent molar with apical periodontitis using platelet-rich plasma. *J. Endod.* **2013**, *39*, 138–144. [CrossRef] [PubMed]

54. Shimizu, E.; Ricucci, D.; Albert, J.; Alobaid, A.S.; Gibbs, J.L.; Huang, G.T.; Lin, L.M. Clinical, radiographic, and histological observation of a human immature permanent tooth with chronic apical abscess after revitalization treatment. *J. Endod.* **2013**, *39*, 1078–1083. [CrossRef] [PubMed]

55. Becerra, P.; Ricucci, D.; Loghin, S.; Gibbs, J.L.; Lin, L.M. Histological study of a human immature permanent premolar with chronic apical abscess after revascularization/revitalization. *J. Endod.* **2014**, *40*, 133–139. [CrossRef] [PubMed]

56. Lei, L.; Chen, Y.; Zhou, R.; Huang, X.; Cai, Z. Histologic and immunohistochemical findings of a human immature permanent tooth with apical periodontitis after regenerative endodontic therapy. *J. Endod.* **2015**, *41*, 1172–1179. [CrossRef] [PubMed]

57. Rafter, M. Apexification: A review. *Dent. Traumatol.* **2005**, *21*, 1–8. [CrossRef] [PubMed]

58. Cvek, M. Prognosis of luxated non-vital maxillary incisors treated with calcium hydroxide and filled with gutta-percha. A retrospective clinical study. *Endod. Dent. Traumatol.* **1992**, *8*, 45–55. [CrossRef] [PubMed]

59. Andreasen, J.O.; Farik, B.; Munksgaard, E.C. Long-term calcium hydroxide as a root canal dressing may increase risk of root fracture. *Dent. Traumatol.* **2002**, *18*, 134–137. [CrossRef] [PubMed]

60. Kontakiotis, E.G.; Filippatos, C.G.; Agrafioti, A. Levels of evidence for the outcome of regenerative endodontic therapy. *J. Endod.* **2014**, *40*, 1045–1053. [CrossRef] [PubMed]

61. Saoud, T.M.; Martin, G.; Chen, Y.-H.M.; Chen, K.L.; Chen, C.A.; Songtrakul, K.; Malek, M.; Sigurdsson, A.; Lin, L.M. Treatment of mature permanent teeth with necrotic pulps and apical periodontitis using regenerative endodontic procedures: A case series. *J. Endod.* **2016**, *42*, 57–65. [CrossRef] [PubMed]

62. Siqueira, J.F., Jr. Aetiology of root canal treatment failures: Why well-treated teeth can fail. *Int. Endod. J.* **2001**, *34*, 1–10. [CrossRef] [PubMed]

63. Nair, P.N. Pathogenesis of apical periodontitis and the causes of endodontic failures. *Crit. Rev. Oral Biol. Med.* **2004**, *15*, 348–381. [CrossRef] [PubMed]

64. Ng, Y.-L.; Mann, V.; Gulabivala, K. Outcome of secondary root canal treatment: A systematic review of the literature. *Int. Endod. J.* **2008**, *41*, 1026–1046. [CrossRef] [PubMed]

65. Nevins, A.J.; Cymerman, J.J. Revitalization of open apex teeth with apical periodontitis using a collagen-hydroxyapatite scaffold. *J. Endod.* **2015**, *41*, 966–973. [CrossRef] [PubMed]

66. Saoud, T.M.A.; Huang, G.T.-J.; Gibbs, J.L.; Sigurdsson, A.; Lin, L.M. Management of teeth with persistent apical periodontitis after root canal treatment using regenerative endodontic therapy. *J. Endod.* **2015**, *41*, 1743–1748. [CrossRef] [PubMed]

67. Andreasen, J.O.; Andreasen, F.M.; Anderson, J. *Textbook and Color Atlas of Traumatic Injuries to The teeth*, 4th ed.; Wiley-Blackwell: Chichester, UK, 2007.

68. Andreasen, J.O. External root resorption: Its implication in dental traumatology, paedodontics, periodontics, orthodontics and endodontics. *Int. Endod. J.* **1985**, *18*, 109–118. [CrossRef] [PubMed]

69. Tronstad, L. Root resorption—Etiology, terminology, and clinical manifestations. *Endod. Dent. Traumatol.* **1988**, *4*, 241–252. [CrossRef] [PubMed]

70. Trope, M. Root resorption due to dental trauma. *Endod. Top.* **2002**, *1*, 79–100. [CrossRef]

71. Cvek, M. Treatment of non-vital permanent incisors with calcium hydroxide. II. Effect on external root resorption in luxated teeth compared with effect of root filling with gutta-percha. A follow-up. *Odontol. Revy* **1973**, *24*, 343–354. [PubMed]

72. Tronstad, L.; Andreasen, J.O.; Hasselgren, G.; Kristenson, L. pH changes in dental tissues after root canal filling with calcium hydroxide. *J. Endod.* **1981**, *7*, 17–21. [CrossRef]

73. Hammarstrom, L.; Blomlof, L.; Feiglin, B.; Lindskog, S. Effect of calcium hydroxide treatment on periodontal repair and root resorption. *Dent. Traumatol.* **1986**, *2*, 184–189. [CrossRef]

74. Santiago, C.N.; Pinto, S.S.; Sassone, L.M.; Hirata, R., Jr.; Fidel, S.R. Revascularization technique for the treatment of external inflammatory root resorption: A report of 3 cases. *J. Endod.* **2015**, *41*, 1560–1564. [CrossRef] [PubMed]

75. Chaniotis, A. The use of MTA/blood mixture to induce hard tissue healing in a root fractured maxillary central incisor. Case report and treatment considerations. *Int. Endod. J.* **2014**, *47*, 989–999. [CrossRef] [PubMed]

76. Priya, H.; Tambakad, P.B.; Naidu, J. Pulp and periodontal regeneration of an avulsed permanent mature incisor using platelet-rich plasma after delayed replantation: A 12-month clinical case study. *J. Endod.* **2016**, *42*, 66–71. [CrossRef] [PubMed]

77. Jeeruphan, T.; Jantarat, J.; Yanpiset, K.; Suwannapan, L.; Khewsawai, P.; Hargreaves, K.M. Mahilod study 1: Comparison of radiographic and survival outcomes of immature teeth treated with either regenerative endodontics or apexification methods—A retrospective study. *J. Endod.* **2012**, *38*, 1330–1336. [CrossRef] [PubMed]

78. Chen, M.Y.; Chen, K.L.; Chen, C.A.; Tayebaty, F.; Rosenberg, P.A.; Lin, L.M. Response of immature permanent teeth with infected necrotic pulp tissue and apical periodontitis/abscess to revascularization procedures. *Int. Endod. J.* **2012**, *45*, 294–305. [CrossRef] [PubMed]

79. Saoud, T.M.A.; Zaazou, A.; Nabil, A.; Moussa, S.; Lin, L.M.; Gibbs, J.L. Clinical and radiographic outcomes of traumatized immature permanent necrotic teeth after revascularization therapy. *J. Endod.* **2014**, *40*, 1946–1952. [CrossRef] [PubMed]

80. Shin, S.Y.; Albert, J.S.; Mortman, R.E. One step pulp revascularization treatment of an immature permanent tooth with chronic apical abscess: A case report. *Int. Endod. J.* **2009**, *42*, 1118–1126. [CrossRef] [PubMed]

81. Hargreaves, K.M.; Diogenes, A.R.; Teixeira, F.B. Treatment options: Biological basis of regenerative endodontic procedures. *J. Endod.* **2013**, *39*, 30–43. [CrossRef] [PubMed]

2

Oral and Dental Health Status among Adolescents with Limited Access to Dental Care Services in Jeddah

Salma A. Bahannan [1,*], Somaya M. Eltelety [2], Mona H. Hassan [3], Suzan S. Ibrahim [4],
Hala A. Amer [5], Omar A. El Meligy [6] , Khalid A. Al-Johani [7], Rayyan A. Kayal [8] ,
Abeer A. Mokeem [9], Akram F. Qutob [10] and Abdulghani I. Mira [11]

[1] Oral and Maxillofacial Prosthodontics Department, Faculty of Dentistry, King Abdulaziz University, Jeddah 21589, Saudi Arabia
[2] Dental Public Health Department, Faculty of Dentistry, Al Mansoura and King Abdulaziz Universities, Jeddah 21589, Saudi Arabia; saltalety@kau.edu.sa
[3] Biostatistics Department, High Institute of Public Health, Alexandria University and Dental Public Health Department, Faculty of Dentistry, King Abdulaziz University, Jeddah 21589, Saudi Arabia; monaha59@hotmail.com
[4] Oral Diagnostic Sciences Department, Faculty of Dentistry, Ain Shams and King Abdulaziz Universities, Jeddah 21589, Saudi Arabia; suzan_ibrahim2000@yahoo.com
[5] Dental Public Health Department, Faculty of Dentistry, Alexandria and King Abdulaziz Universities, Jeddah 21589, Saudi Arabia; halaamerdr@gmail.com
[6] Pediatric Dentistry Department, Faculty of Dentistry, King Abdulaziz and Alexandria Universities, Jeddah 21589, Saudi Arabia; omeligy@kau.edu.sa
[7] Oral Diagnostic Sciences Department, Faculty of Dentistry, King Abdulaziz University, Jeddah 21589, Saudi Arabia; kauoralmed@gmail.com
[8] Periodontics Department, Faculty of Dentistry, King Abdulaziz University, Jeddah 21589, Saudi Arabia; rkayal@kau.edu.sa
[9] Endodontics Department, Faculty of Dentistry, King Abdulaziz University, Jeddah 21589, Saudi Arabia; aasaleh@kau.edu.sa
[10] Dental Public Health Department, Faculty of Dentistry, King Abdulaziz University, Jeddah 21589, Saudi Arabia; aqutob@kau.edu.sa
[11] Conservative Dentistry Department, Faculty of Dentistry, King Abdulaziz University, Jeddah 21589, Saudi Arabia; amira@kau.edu.sa
* Correspondence: sbahannan@kau.edu.sa or sbahannan@gmail.com;

Abstract: The purpose of this study was to assess the prevalence and associated factors of dental caries and periodontal diseases among 14–19-year-old schoolchildren with limited access to dental care services. A cross sectional study design was conducted during field visits to seven governmental schools in Al-Khomrah district, South Jeddah, over the period from September 2015 to May 2016. Clinical examinations and administered questionnaires were carried out in mobile dental clinics. The dentists carried out oral examinations using the dental caries index (DMFT), the simplified oral hygiene index (OHI-S), and the community periodontal index for treatment needs (CPITN). Statistical analyses were performed using SPSS 20. A total of 734 schoolchildren were examined. The prevalence of decayed teeth was 79.7% and was significantly higher among boys (88.9%) than girls (69.0%). About 11% of students had missing teeth, with a significantly higher figure among females than males (15.9% versus 7.3%); 19.8% of students had filled teeth. Moreover, a DMFT of seven or more was significantly more prevalent among males (43.3%) than females (26.8%), while the percentage of females with sound teeth was significantly higher than for males (20.4% and 9.6% respectively). The CPITN revealed 0, 1 and 2 scores among 14.6%, 78.2%, and 41.6% respectively. Males had a significantly higher percentage of healthy periodontal condition (23.8%) than females (3.8%). Dental caries prevalence was moderate to high, calculus and gingival bleeding were widespread among schoolchildren, and were more prevalent among students with low socioeconomic status.

Keywords: oral health; caries; student; habits; risk factors; limited access; oral health survey

1. Introduction

Oral hygiene is essential to general health and quality of life. The common oral diseases are caries, periodontal disease, erosion, abfraction lesions and oral cancer [1]. Oral health is a state of being in which an individual is free from mouth and facial pain, oral and throat cancer, oral infection and sores, periodontal disease, tooth decay, tooth loss, and other diseases and disorders that limit an individual's capacity to bite, chew, smile, speak, as well as his or her psychosocial wellbeing. Risk factors for oral diseases include an unhealthy diet, tobacco use, harmful alcohol use, poor oral hygiene, and social determinants [1]. The United States Department of Health and Human Services (HHS) reported in 2014 that dental caries is the most common chronic disease. It is five times more common than asthma, and seven times more common than seasonal allergies [2]. In a recent review, it was documented that the prevalence of caries is high across Saudi Arabia: about 70% in children's permanent teeth, with a mean DMFT score of 3.5 [3]. Al Dosari et al., reported that the prevalence of caries in the dentition of Saudi children aged 15–18-year old ranged from 59–80%, depending on the fluoride level of the area, and the mean DMFT scores was 2.24–4.08 [4].

It is clearly known that the prevalence of oral disease varies according to geographical region and accessibility of oral health services. With contemporary understanding of social sciences, it has been acknowledged that oral health is influenced by many social and environmental factors. One such factor is accessibility to oral health care services. Limited access to oral health care can be accounted for on the level of the patient, community, inadequate insurance coverage, and a limited supply of oral health care providers. While the delivery of quality care is important, access to oral health is an important factor in maintaining oral health. Individual knowledge, the perceptions of one's need for oral health care, financial concerns, and cultural preferences can influence patients' pursuit for oral health care [5]. While the delivery of quality care is important, access to oral health is an equally important determinant of oral health [1].

Many studies have reported that oral diseases are significantly more prevalent among poor and disadvantaged population groups [1,6–9]. It has been reported that oral diseases have a negative impact on the quality of life, in both developing and developed countries [10,11]. In addition, they restrict activities in school and home, and present challenges for maintaining self-esteem and attentiveness to learning [12].

Although Saudi Arabia has a considerable number of dental colleges, there is glaring disparity in the distribution of these institutions. A geographic imbalance in the availability of oral health care services affect the dentist–population ratio. Most of the Saudi population who reside in rural areas have limited access to oral health care facilities [3].

The objective of the current study was to assess the prevalence and associated factors of caries and periodontal diseases among school students with limited access to dental care services in the Al-Khomrah district in South Jeddah, Saudi Arabia.

2. Methods

This was a cross sectional study design that took place in Al-Khomrah district in South Jeddah, Saudi Arabia, during the period from September 2015 to May 2016. The target population was chosen based on its low socioeconomic classification among the Districts of South Jeddah. This classification was obtained from the Ministry of Social Affairs.

Initial site visits then took place to check the logistics of the field visits, and to obtain verbal consent from the principals of Al-Khomrah intermediate and secondary schools. Ethical approval was then obtained from the Ethics Committee of the Faculty of Dentistry at King Abdulaziz University (KAU), Jeddah (REC-FD # 006-15). This was followed by contacting all concerned authorities (the Ministry of Education, the local municipality, and the District's Governor's Office), in order to obtain official approval and to facilitate the field visits.

Clinical examination forms and administered questionnaires were developed and tested during the period of examiner calibration at the Faculty of Dentistry, KAU. Questionnaire items were developed after taking input from different clinical expert focus groups, in order to establish validity. These items reflected factors related to oral health status, such as social history, and barriers to care. Designated examiners went through calibration sessions to standardize inter- and intra-examiner reliability. Each examiner conducted five patient examinations to assess dental caries, oral hygiene status, and the gingival condition using the DMFT [13], OHI-S [14] and CPITN [13] indices respectively. Calibration sessions were repeated until the level of consistency reached 85% or higher.

Prior to the start of the field visits, parental informed consent forms were distributed by the participating school. The latter collected signed forms and prepared a list of consensual students in preparation for the field visits. These consents included permission to perform the administered questionnaire, a clinical examination, and provision of basic dental treatments (preventive, restorative, and surgical). Participants requiring advanced dental treatments were given referral slips to continue their treatment at the KAU Faculty of Dentistry clinics, or at the nearest local Ministry of Health primary health care center. At the end of each visit, students were given a summary report of the treatment provided, to inform their parents or care givers. The field visits were undertaken at seven schools: four intermediate schools, and three secondary schools.

The dental team consisted of six general dentists and four dental assistants. The mobile dental clinic car was parked at each school until all participating schoolchildren have been examined. The examiners conducted clinical examinations and provided basic dental treatment in the two mobile clinics (which were stationed in the carpark), and in the first aid rooms of the schools using two portable dental units (ProCart II, South Pointe Surgical Supply, Inc., Coral Springs, FL, USA). Infection control and sterilization standards were employed at all examination sites to ensure the safety of participants.

Data was entered after removing all participants' identifiers to protect confidentiality, and group analyses were performed using IBM SPSS 20, (IBM, Armonk, NY, USA). Descriptive statistics and odds ratios were calculated and presented, as seen in the results section. All tests were two-sided, and the 0.05 level was used to indicate statistical significance.

3. Results

Demographic characteristics of students by gender is shown in Table 1. The current study included 734 students (53.8% males and 46.2% females), with a mean age of 16.02 ± 1.61 years, with a similar mean age of males and females. The distribution of students according to the education level of their fathers and mothers showed a similar distribution for both boys and girls. A considerable percentage of students' parents had less than a secondary level of education (in males and females 79.1% and 69.1% respectively). Regarding parents working status, 73.4% of fathers were working, whereas only 11.3% of mothers were working. Considering citizenship, 37 (5%) were non-Saudi, while 697 (95%) were Saudi. Regarding residence, 89 (12.2%) reported rented residence, while 640 (87.8%) reported owned residence. Non-Saudi females reported a significantly higher rate of residence in rented houses than that of males.

As shown in Table 2, males and females are significantly different in both oral hygiene status and habits. The percentage of females who brush their teeth twice daily was significantly higher than that of males (57.8% and 14.9% respectively), while the rate of males who did not brush their teeth, or who brush irregularly, was significantly higher compared to that of females (59.7% versus 19.2% respectively). On the other hand, males use Miswak significantly more than females (32.7% compared to 19.5% respectively). Miswak is a stem or root of the plant Salvadora persica; it becomes brushlike after treatment and is suitable for oral hygiene. The basic technique employed for removing plaque mechanically is similar to that of the toothbrush, i.e., vertical and horizontal brushing [10]. About 9%

of students were smokers, without significant difference between males and females. Considering the oral hygiene index (soft deposit), significantly more males had good oral hygiene than females (33.7% and 13.6% respectively), while the percentage of fair oral hygiene was higher among females (71.4%) compared to males (47.3%).

Table 1. Demographic characteristics of students by gender.

Characteristics		No. Examined 734		Males 395 (53.8%)		Females 339 (46.2%)		χ^2	p
Age (Years)	14–	326	44.4	176	44.6	150	44.2		0.774
	16–	239	32.6	132	33.4	107	31.6	0.57	
	18–19	169	23.0	87	22.0	82	24.2		
	Mean (SD)	16.02	(1.61)	16.02	(1.59)	16.02	(1.64)	t = 0.02	0.983
Father's Education ◊	No education	105	15.2	61	16.1	44	14.1		0.563
	Primary school	158	22.8	93	24.5	65	20.8		
	Intermediate school	146	21.1	73	19.2	73	23.3	2.97	
	Secondary school	186	26.8	100	26.3	86	27.5		
	University or higher	98	14.1	53	13.9	45	14.4		
Mother's education ⸪	No education	179	25.3	111	29.3	68	20.7		0.052
	Primary school	163	23.1	78	20.6	85	25.9		
	Intermediate school	146	20.7	70	18.5	76	23.2	9.42	
	Secondary school	149	21.1	83	21.9	66	20.1		
	University or higher	70	9.9	37	9.8	33	10.1		
Fathers' work	Yes	519	73.4	278	72.8	241	74.2	0.17	0.679
	No	188	26.6	104	27.2	84	25.8		
Mothers' work	Yes	81	11.3	45	11.7	36	10.9	0.12	0.732
	No	635	88.7	340	88.3	295	89.1		
Citizenship	Saudi	697	95.0	381	96.5	316	93.2	4.00 *	0.045
	Non-Saudi	37	5.0	14	3.5	23	6.8		
Residence	Owned	640	87.8	352	90.0	288	85.2		
	Rented	89	12.2	39	10.0	50	14.8	3.93 *	0.048

◊ 16 males and 11 females with missing mothers' education; ⸪ 15 males and 26 females with missing fathers' education; * $p < 0.05$ (Significant).

The prevalence of decayed permanent teeth (Table 3) was 79.7% and was significantly higher among boys (88.9%) than girls (69.0%). About 11% of students had missing teeth; this rate was significantly higher among females (15.9% versus 7.3%); 19.8% of students had filled teeth, with a significantly higher rate among females (13.9% and 26.5% respectively).

The prevalence of decayed teeth revealed a decreasing significant trend by age, from 83.7% among children aged 14 ≤ 16 years, down to 69.8% for 18–19 years. A reverse pattern could be observed for missing teeth, where the percentage increased from 7.4% at age 14 ≤ 16 years, up to 16% at the age of 18–19 years. The percentage of filled teeth did not show a statistically significant trend by age.

DMFTs of 7 or more (Table 4) were significantly higher among males (43.3%) than females (26.8%). Moreover, the percentage of females with sound teeth was significantly higher than that of males (20.4% and 9.6% respectively). Non-Saudi students showed a significantly higher prevalence of a DMFT index of 7 or more (59.5%) than Saudi students (34.4%). Students who brush their teeth twice daily showed the lowest prevalence of severe dental caries (29.8%), compared to those who never brush their teeth (44.4%). The percentage of students who have severe dental caries was higher among those who visit dentists regularly every six months (43.6%) or every 12 months (72.7%) than those who did not visit dentists (29.1%).

Students with good oral hygiene (soft deposits) had a significantly higher percentage of sound teeth (14%) and a lower percentage of DMFT of 7 or more (35.8%) than those with poor oral hygiene (8.7% and 49.2% respectively). No significant relationship could be detected between DMFT categories and other socio-demographic variables.

The CPITN is presented in Table 5. Males have a significantly higher percentage of healthy periodontal conditions (23.8%) than females (3.8%). While the percentage with bleeding was higher among females (92% versus 66.3% respectively), and 53.1 versus 31.6% respectively with calculus. The youngest age category was more likely to have healthy gingiva in contrast to the 18–19 age category (OR 2.0, 95% CI 1.2 to 3.4), while the latter age category are 1.5 times more prone to calculus deposits, in contrast to the $14 \leq 16$ years age category.

Table 2. Oral hygiene status and habits of students by gender.

Characteristics		No. Examined 734		Males 395 53.8%		Females 339 46.2%		X^2	p
Daily tooth brushing	Twice	255	34.7	59	14.9 A	196	57.8 A	191.07 *	<0.001
	Once	178	24.3	100	25.3	78	23.0		
	Not frequently	184	25.1	125	31.6 B	59	17.4 B		
	Never	117	15.9	111	28.1 C	6	1.8 C		
Miswak	Yes	195	26.6	129	32.7	66	19.5	16.27 *	<0.001
	No	539	73.4	266	67.3	273	80.5		
Tooth flossing	Yes	43	5.9	19	4.8	24	7.1	1.70	0.192
	No	691	94.1	376	95.2	315	92.9		
Dental visits	Every 6 months	39	5.3	27	6.8 A	12	3.5 A	32.12 *	<0.001
	Every 12 months	11	1.5	8	2.0	3	0.9		
	Irregular	21	2.9	7	1.8	14	4.1		
	When needed	336	45.8	148	37.5 B	188	55.5 B		
	Never	327	44.6	205	51.9 C	122	36.0 C		
Smoking	No	669	91.1	354	89.6	315	92.9	2.46	0.117
	Yes	65	8.9	41	10.4	24	7.1		
OHI-S (Soft deposit)	<1 (Good)	179	24.4	133	33.7 A	46	13.6 A	49.93	<0.001
	1– (Fair)	429	58.4	187	47.3 B	242	71.4 B		
	2+ (Poor)	126	17.2	75	19.0	51	15.0		

Percent with common superscripts for the same variable are significantly different; * $p < 0.05$ (Significant).

Table 3. Dental caries by age and gender.

		No. Examined	Caries prevalence						Median DMFT	95% CI	
			D		M		F				
			No.	%	No.	%	No.	%			
Overall		734	585	79.7	83	11.3	145	19.8	4.0	4.0	5.0
Gender	Males	395	351	88.9	29	7.3	55	13.9	6.0	5.0	6.0
	Females	339	234	69.0	54	15.9	90	26.5	3.0	3.0	4.0
	Test (p)		$X^2 = 44.36$ * (<0.001)		$X^2 = 13.41$ * (<0.001)		$X^2 = 18.34$ * (<0.001)		Mann-Whitney Z = 50.75 * (<0.001)		
Age (Years)	14–	326	273	83.7 A	24	7.4 A	58	17.8	4.0	4.0	5.0
	16–	239	194	81.2 A	32	13.4 AB	55	23.0	5.0	4.0	6.0
	18–19	169	118	69.8 B	27	16.0 B	32	18.9	4.0	3.0	5.0
	Test (p)		$X^2 = 13.8$ * (0.001)		$X^2 = 9.77$ * (0.008)		$X^2 = 2.47$ (0.292)		Kruskal-Wallis X^2 = 3.32 (0.190)		

Groups with different subscripts in the same column are significantly different; * $p < 0.05$ (Significant).

Table 4. Caries prevalence by students' characteristics.

		Examined	DMFT (%)				χ^2	p
			0	1–3	4–6	7+		
Overall		734	14.6	26.4	23.3	35.7		
Gender	Males	395	9.6	20.8	26.3	43.3	42.03 *	<0.001
	Females	339	20.4	33.0	19.8	26.8		
Age (Years)	14–	326	12.0	26.4	23.6	38.0	11.41	0.076
	16–	239	13.8	25.5	27.2	33.5		
	18–19	169	20.7	27.8	17.2	34.3		
Father's Education ◊	No education	105	16.2	25.7	23.8	34.3	10.50	0.572
	Primary school	158	13.3	20.9	23.4	42.4		
	Intermediate school	146	10.3	30.1	24.0	35.6		
	Secondary school	186	16.7	25.3	27.4	30.6		
	University or higher	98	16.3	28.6	21.4	33.7		
Mother's Education ⁑	No education	179	14.5	25.1	23.5	36.9	9.57	0.654
	Primary school	163	14.1	26.4	23.3	36.2		
	Intermediate school	146	16.4	23.3	26.7	33.6		
	Secondary school	149	16.8	31.5	18.1	33.6		
	University or higher	70	10.0	25.7	32.9	31.4		
Fathers' work	Yes	519	13.9	25.0	23.9	37.2	1.82	0.611
	No	188	16.0	28.2	23.4	32.4		
Mothers' work	Yes	81	8.6	30.9	24.7	35.8	2.92	0.405
	No	635	15.3	25.8	23.5	35.4		
Citizenship	Saudi	697	15.1	27.0	23.5	34.4	10.27 *	0.016
	Non-Saudi	37	5.4	16.2	18.9	59.5		
Residence	Owned	640	15.2	27.2	23.1	34.5	3.38	0.337
	Rented	89	11.2	22.5	22.5	43.8		
Daily tooth brushing	Twice	178	18.0	33.3	18.8	29.8	34.64 *	<0.001
	Once	255	16.9	25.3	17.4	40.4		
	Not frequently	184	12.5	21.2	32.6	33.7		
	Never	117	6.8	21.4	27.4	44.4		
Miswak	Yes	195	14.9	22.1	27.7	35.4	4.15	0.246
	No	539	14.5	28.0	21.7	35.8		
Tooth flossing	Yes	43	11.6	23.3	30.2	34.9	1.40	0.706
	No	691	14.8	26.6	22.9	35.7		
Dental visits	Every 6 months	39	5.1	23.1	28.2	43.6	*	MCP = 0.002
	Every 12 months	11	0.0	9.1	18.2	72.7		
	Irregular	21	14.3	14.3	19.0	52.4		
	When needed	336	10.4	28.3	22.3	39.0		
	Never	327	20.5	26.3	24.2	29.1		
Smoking	No	669	14.6	25.6	23.9	35.9	3.50	0.321
	Yes	65	13.8	35.4	16.9	33.8		
OHI-S (Soft deposit)	<1 (Good)	179	14.0	21.2	29.1	35.8	21.09 *	0.002
	1– (Fair)	429	16.6	30.1	21.7	31.7		
	2+ (Poor)	126	8.7	21.4	20.6	49.2		

◊ 16 males and 11 females with missing mothers' education; ⁑ 15 males and 26 females with missing fathers' education; MCP = Monte Carlo exact P; * $p < 0.05$ (Significant).

Table 5. Community periodontal index for treatment needs by students' characteristics.

		Examined	% Healthy	OR (95% CI)	% with Bleeding	OR (95% CI)	% with Calculus	OR (95% CI)
Overall		734	14.6		78.2		41.6	
Gender	Males	395	23.8	7.8 * (4.3–14.3)	66.3	1.0	31.6	1.0
	Females	339	3.8	1.0	92.0	5.9 * (3.8–9.2)	53.1	2.4 * (1.8–3.3)
Age (Years)	14–	326	11.0	2.0 * (1.2–3.4)	81.0	1.0	39.3	1.0
	16–	239	15.5	1.4 (0.8–2.3)	81.2	1.0 (0.7–1.6)	39.3	1.0 (0.7–1.4)
	18–19	169	20.1	1.0	68.6	0.5 (0.3–0.8)	49.1	1.5 * (1.0–2.2)
Father's Education ◈	No education	105	14.3	1.0	83.8	1.9 (0.9–3.7)	37.1	0.8 (0.4–1.4)
	Primary school	158	15.2	0.9 (0.5–1.9)	70.9	0.9 (0.5–1.5)	44.3	1.1 (0.6–1.8)
	Intermediate school	146	11.0	1.4 (0.6–2.9)	82.9	1.7 (0.9–3.3)	43.8	1.0 (0.6–1.7)
	Secondary school	186	14.5	1.0 (0.5–1.9)	79.6	1.4 (0.8–2.5)	39.2	0.9 (0.5–1.4)
	University or higher	98	20.4	0.7 (0.3–1.4)	73.5	1.0	42.9	1.0
Mother's Education ⁑	No education	179	18.4	1.0	72.1	0.9 (0.5–1.7)	38.5	0.9 (0.5–1.7)
	Primary school	163	13.5	1.0 (0.5–2.1)	81.0	1.5 (0.8–2.9)	41.7	1.1 (0.6–1.9)
	Intermediate school	146	8.9	1.5 (0.7–3.1)	86.3	2.2 * (1.1–4.5)	42.5	1.1 (0.6–2.0)
	Secondary school	149	15.4	2.3 * (1.0–5.3)	75.8	1.1 (0.6–2.1)	43.0	1.1 (0.6–2.0)
	University or higher	70	18.6	1.2 (0.6–2.6)	74.3	1.0	40.0	1.0
Fathers' work	Yes	519	14.5	1.0 (0.6–1.5)	78.0	1.0	41.8	1.0
	No	188	14.9	1.0	78.7	1.0 (0.7–1.6)	40.4	0.9 (0.7–1.3)
Mothers' work	Yes	81	17.3	1.3 (0.7–2.3)	72.8	1.0	46.9	1.0
	No	635	14.2	1.0	79.1	1.4 (0.5–1.2)	40.5	0.8 (0.5–1.2)
Citizen-ship	Saudi	697	14.5	0.9 (0.4–2.2)	78.8	1.0	40.9	1.0
	Non-Saudi	37	16.2	1.0	67.6	0.6 (0.3–1.1)	54.1	1.7 (0.9–3.3)
Residence	Owned	640	14.1	0.7 (0.4–1.2)	80.2	1.0	39.5	1.0
	Rented	89	19.1	1.0	66.3	0.5 * (0.3–0.8)	52.8	1.7 * (1.1–2.7)

Table 5. Cont.

		Examined	% Healthy	OR (95% CI)	% with Bleeding	OR (95% CI)	% with Calculus	OR (95% CI)
Daily tooth brushing	Twice	255	11.4	0.7 (0.4-1.2)	83.5	1.0	42.7	1.0
	Once	178	12.9	0.8 (0.4-1.5)	79.8	0.8 (0.5-1.3)	42.7	1.0 (0.7-1.5)
	Not frequently	184	19.6	1.3 (0.7-2.3)	73.9	0.6 * (0.4-0.9)	39.1	0.9 (0.6-1.3)
	Never	117	16.2	1.0	70.9	0.5 * (0.3-0.8)	41.0	0.9 (0.6-1.5)
Miswak	Yes	195	16.4	1.2 (0.8-1.9)	76.4	1.0	36.4	1.0
	No	539	13.9	1.0	78.8	1.2 (0.8-1.7)	43.4	1.3 * (1.0-1.9)
Tooth flossing	Yes	43	9.3	0.6 (0.2-1.7)	79.1	1.0	44.2	1.0
	No	691	14.9	1.0	78.1	0.9 (0.4-2.0)	41.4	0.9 (0.5-1.7)
Dental visits	Every 6 months	39	15.4	1.1 (0.4-2.8)	71.8	1.0	43.6	1.0
	Every 12 months	11	9.1	2.0 (0.3-16.1)	90.9	3.9 (0.4-34.4)	18.2	0.3 (0.1-1.5)
	Irregular	21	9.5	1.9 (0.4-8.5)	81.0	1.7 (0.5-6.1)	42.9	1.0 (0.3-2.8)
	When needed	336	12.8	1.4 (0.9-2.1)	81.0	1.7 (0.8-3.5)	42.9	1.0 0.5-1.9)
	Never	327	16.8	1.0	75.5	1.2 (0.6-2.5)	40.7	0.9 (0.5-1.7)
Smoking	No	669	14.2	0.7 (0.4-1.4)	79.2	1.0	41.3	1.0
	Yes	65	18.5	1.0	67.7	0.6 (0.3-1.0)	44.6	1.1 (0.7-1.9)
OHI-S (Soft deposit)	<1 (Good)	179	50.3	126.4 * (17.3-924.2)	45.3	1.0	18.4	1.0
	1- (Fair)	429	3.7	4.8 (0.6-36.9)	91.8	13.6 * (8.7-21.4)	45.2	3.7 * (2.4-5.6)
	2+ (Poor)	126	0.8	1.0	78.6	4.4 * (2.6-7.4)	61.9	7.2 * (4.3-12.1)

◈ 16 males and 11 females with missing mothers' education; ‡ 15 males and 26 females with missing fathers' education.

Non- and infrequent-users of tooth brushes were less likely to have bleeding, while non-users of Miswak were more likely to have calculus. Students with good oral hygiene were more likely to have sound teeth regarding CPITN, while those with fair or poor oral hygiene were more likely to have bleeding or calculus.

Regarding standardization and measurement processes for oral and dental health, a comparison among the results of the examiners and the analysis was done to determine the level of consistency between them. An acceptable level of consistency was 85% or more [13]. Inter- and intra-examiner agreement ranged from 0.75 to 0.866, and 0.933 to 0.989 respectively.

4. Discussion

Our data shows a high prevalence of dental caries, calculus, and gingival bleeding among 14–19-year-old schoolchildren from low socioeconomic status background in the Al-Khomrah district, South Jeddah, Saudi Arabia. This data may be of importance in the evaluation of past and future planning of oral health prevention and treatment programs targeting schoolchildren. This calls for early preventive strategies and treatment services. We recommend the incorporation of oral health education in school curricula to help in improving the oral health status of schoolchildren with limited access to oral health care services.

With a contemporary understanding of social sciences, it has been acknowledged that oral health is influenced by many social and environmental factors. One such factor is accessibility to oral health care services. Individual knowledge, the perceptions of one's need for oral health care, financial concerns, and cultural preferences can influence the priority that patients place upon oral health care [5].

The impact of such limited access to health care services is of even greater consequence on strata of the population, such as children. They depend entirely on their parents to utilize health care services [5]. Hence, this study aimed to assess the oral health status of intermediate and secondary schoolchildren with limited access to oral health care services in the districts of Al-Khomrah in South Jeddah, in order to raise the level of health awareness and to promote good habits for oral health. In addition, early treatment and following preventive methods can decrease dental caries and tooth loss [11].

As for behavior, tooth brushing was the most common method used for cleaning teeth, followed by Miswak. The least common method was the dental floss. This agrees with previous studies [15–17]. This might suggest a lack of awareness and understanding of the procedure, and its value in preventing oral disease among the subjects.

Because of the scientific merit of using Miswak and the special importance of the cultural and religious beliefs deeply rooted in, and affecting the behaviors of, the Saudi population, the right method of using a Miswak as a cleaning technique to achieve maximum benefits should be stressed through various interventions [16]. Regarding the frequency of brushing, flossing, and use of Miswak in relation to gender, it was found that females used brushing and flossing more than males. The significant difference ($p < 0.001$) was attributed to a higher concern regarding personal hygiene and health care among females [15,18]. However, males used Miswak more than females; the difference was statistically significant ($p < 0.001$). This result could be justified by cultural beliefs among Saudi communities [16]. The result indicates that improvements in knowledge of the role of dental floss are needed; this agrees with other studies [15–18].

In relation to dental visits, the majority (45.8%) of students only visited their dentist when needed, followed by those who never visited a dentist (44.6%); a minority visited a dentist every 6 to 12 months (6.8%). This agrees with previous studies [19,20]. This may be due to the lack of oral health knowledge among these students. Delay in seeking dental care could be also attributed to other factors, like parental beliefs and practices, lack of economic resources, and the accessibility of dental services [21]. Such a negative attitude towards visiting a dentist leads to an inability to avail sound advice on preventive oral health practices and counseling, a high prevalence of dental caries, and delayed recognition and management of carious teeth [20]. In the current study, there was a significant difference in the frequency of dental visits by gender ($p < 0.001$). Females showed more frequent visits than males.

Four hundred and twenty-nine students (58.4%) had fair oral hygiene (soft deposits), which is less than reported in Kuwait (67%) [22] and in Nigeria (72%) [23]. There were significant sex differences in oral hygiene status, where fair status was observed to be higher in females than males. It was reported that females pay more attention to their personal hygiene, and tend to practice better oral hygiene than males, because of their greater social awareness and grooming habits [24].

Despite incredible scientific advances and the fact that caries are preventable, the disease continues to be a major public health problem. The World Health Organization (WHO) has ranked it as number three among all chronic non-communicable diseases that require worldwide attention for prevention and treatment [1]. Moreover, decayed teeth are particularly harmful to children's growth and development and can severely jeopardize their health [25]. Therefore, reliable estimations of its prevalence will play an important role in improving oral health.

This study showed that only 14.6% were free from caries, which indicates a high prevalence of caries (85.6%) and DMFT (>7). This is in accordance with findings of previous studies in Saudi Arabia [20,26,27]. This rate was higher than Riyadh (70%) [4], or Iran, where the prevalence of dental caries was 75.5% [28]; in Istanbul, the rate is 80% [29].

In a previous study by Al-Ansari, [30] it was found that the increased prevalence of caries in Saudi communities was related to tremendous growth in population coupled with social changes, unhealthy oral health behaviors and practices, inadequate access to oral health care, particularly in remote areas, non-availability of fluoridated water, and paucity of clinical and population-based research.

Dental decay was the major component of the DMFT scores in this study, as evidenced by the high prevalence of decayed teeth (79.7%), which agrees with studies in the Riyadh and Qasim regions. Several studies of younger children in Riyadh have also reported decay as the major component of DMFT [26,31,32]. Such a large proportion of untreated caries indicates the extent of restorative needs among the studied population; consequently, a considerable effort will be required to provide restorative services to them.

Regarding gender, it has been found that boys showed a significantly higher prevalence of caries and missing teeth than girls. This may be because Saudi girls are more concerned about their oral health than Saudi boys. This agrees with other studies in Riyadh [33], while the prevalence of filled teeth was higher in females, suggesting that girls showed a preference for receiving dental treatment compared to boys.

The result of this study showed a significant relationship between DMFT and the frequency of oral hygiene practices: students who brushed regularly (twice/day) had the lowest prevalence of severe dental caries (29.8%), in comparison to those who never brush their teeth (44.4%); this is consistent with the findings of Dummer et al. [24].

Moreover, severe dental caries were more common among those who visited a dentist regularly (every 6 or every 12 months) than those who did not. This agrees with a study in China [34]. The higher DMFT score can be attributed to the dental visit patterns of the studied group. Most of those in this group visited dentists only when they had a problem that required treatment. Studies have also shown that there is a relationship between dental caries and socioeconomic status. In addition, parental income level, educational level, employment status, and other socioeconomic factors have a considerable impact on the prevalence of dental caries [35].

The results of the current study showed that children with the highest prevalence of sound teeth (16.7%) were those having parents with higher levels education, and those who owned a house (15.2%), factors which could reflect a high socioeconomic status. The high prevalence of caries among individuals from lower social class may be linked to the increasing availability of cheap sugar-rich products, coupled with low income and poor access to health services and health education. The low prevalence of caries in members of high social classes may be attributed to increased oral health care awareness among and access to dental care at an earlier age [36].

Regarding the periodontal status, the current study revealed that healthy gingiva was found only in 14.6% of the studied group. Calculus was the most frequently observed condition (78%), while gingivitis was less common (41.6%). This finding agrees with a study by Hessari et al. [37].

Regarding gender, the rates of individuals with bleeding and calculus were higher among females than males. This agrees with the findings of other studies that recorded better gingival health among girls than boys, because the females give more importance to aesthetics and are more inclined to brush and seek dental care regularly [37,38].

This study showed that both socioeconomic background and the utilization of dental services had no effect on periodontal health status, which indicated that some other factors may be at play. This result agrees with that of a comparable study undertaken in Hong Kong [39]. It was also found that students who had good oral hygiene had more favorable periodontal condition, since dental plaque plays an important role in the development of gingival inflammation [40]. More promotion of oral health, and community-based activities, are needed among adolescents.

There are some limitations to this study that should be considered. First, as a cross sectional study, it cannot provide proof for causality, especially in the absence of a control group with better access to dental care services. Second, the sample size was small, and it was conducted in a single, low socioeconomic district. Therefore, further studies are recommended which would include more districts in different areas in Saudi Arabia.

5. Conclusions

Dental caries prevalence was moderate to high, and calculus and gingival bleeding were widespread among Al-Khomrah schoolchildren and were more prevalent among students of low socioeconomic status. Furthermore, males had a significantly higher prevalence of caries and missing teeth than females. More oral health promotion, and community-based activities are needed among the surveyed adolescents.

Author Contributions: S.A.B. developed study idea, field trips' supervising and participated in editing; S.M.E. developed study methods and participated in editing; M.H.H. performed statistical analysis and participated in editing; S.S.I. collected data and participated in editing; H.A.A. developed study methods and drafted the manuscript; O.A.E.M. performed field trips' supervising and participated in editing; K.A.A.-J. drafted the manuscript; R.A.K. drafted the manuscript; A.A.M. performed field trips' supervising and approved final manuscript; A.F.Q. performed writing review; A.I.M. approved final manuscript.

Acknowledgments: The authors would like to thank the Saudi Arabian Ministry of Education for their generous contribution to fund this project (grant number MB/74/435). The authors also thank Ebtehal Ghazal and Shuroog Aldosari for their valuable help in collecting and entering the data.

References

1. World Health Organization (WHO). *Oral Health. FACT Sheet No 318*; WHO: Geneva, Switzerland, 2012.
2. U.S. Department of Health and Human Services. Oral Health in America: A Report of the Surgeon General-Executive Summary. Rockville, MD, National Institute of Health and Craniofacial Research. Available online: https://www.nidcr.nih.gov/research/data-statistics/surgeon-general (accessed on 21 February 2014).
3. Al Agili, D.E. A systematic review of population-based dental caries studies among children in Saudi Arabia. *Saudi Dent. J.* **2013**, *25*, 3–11. [CrossRef] [PubMed]
4. Al Dosari, A.M.; Akpata, E.S.; Khan, N. Associations among dental caries experience, fluorosis, and fluoride exposure from drinking water sources in Saudi Arabia. *J. Public Health Dent.* **2010**, *70*, 220–226. [CrossRef] [PubMed]
5. Kumar, S.A.; Kumar, P.D.; Sivasamy, S.; Balan, I.N. Oral health status of 5 and 12-year-old rural school going children with limited access to oral health care-A cross sectional survey. *Carib. J. Sci. Tech.* **2014**, *2*, 336–339.
6. Al Darwish, M.A.; El Ansari, W.B.; Bener, A. Prevalence of dental caries among 12–14-year-old children in Qatar. *Saudi Dent. J.* **2014**, *26*, 115–125. [CrossRef] [PubMed]

7. Hooley, M.; Skouteris, H.; Boganin, C.; Satur, J.; Kilpatrick, N. Parental influence and the development of dental caries in children aged 0–6 years: A systematic review of the literature. *J. Dent.* **2012**, *40*, 873–885. [CrossRef] [PubMed]

8. Al-Jewair, T.S.; Leake, J.L. The prevalence and risks of early childhood caries (ECC) in Toronto, Canada. *J. Contemp. Dent. Pract.* **2010**, *11*, 1–8.

9. Fontana, M.; Jackson, R.; Eckert, G.; Swigonski, N.; Chin, J.; Zandona, A.F.; Ando, M.; Stookey, G.K.; Downs, S.; Zero, D.T. Identification of caries risk factors in toddlers. *J. Dent. Res.* **2011**, *90*, 209–214. [CrossRef] [PubMed]

10. Alsubait, A.; Alousaimi, M.; Geeverghese, A.; Ali, A.; El Metwally, A. Oral health knowledge, attitude and behavior among students of age 10–18 years old attending Jenadriyah festival Riyadh; a cross-sectional study. *Saudi J. Dent. Res.* **2016**, *7*, 45–50. [CrossRef]

11. Petersen, P.E. The World Oral Health Report 2003: Continuous improvement of oral health in the 21st century-the approach of the WHO Global Oral Health Program. *Commun. Dent. Oral Epidemiol.* **2008**, *31*, 3–24. [CrossRef]

12. Petersen, P.E.; Bourgeois, D.; Ogawa, H.; Estupinan-Day, S.; Ndiaye, C. The global burden of oral diseases and risks to oral health. *Bull World Health Organ* **2005**, *83*, 661–669. [PubMed]

13. World Health Organization (WHO). *Oral Health Surveys: Basic Methods*, 6th ed.; WHO: Geneva, Switzerland, 2013.

14. Green, J.C.; Vermillion, J.R. Simplified Oral Hygiene Index. *J. Am. Dent. Assoc.* **1964**, *68*, 7–13. [CrossRef]

15. Al-Sadhan, A.S. Oral health practices and dietary habits of intermediate school children in Riyadh Saudi Arabia. *Saudi Dent. J.* **2003**, *15*, 81–87.

16. Farsi, J.M.A.; Farghaly, M.M.; Farsi, N. Oral health knowledge, attitude and behavior among Saudi school students in Jeddah city. *J. Dent.* **2004**, *32*, 47–53. [CrossRef] [PubMed]

17. Al-Omiri, M.K.; Al-Wahadni, A.M.; Saeed, K.N. Oral health attitudes, knowledge, and behavior among school children in North Jordan. *J. Dent. Educ.* **2006**, *70*, 179–187. [PubMed]

18. Al-Ansari, J.; Honkala, E.; Honkala, S. Oral health knowledge and behavior among male health sciences college students in Kuwait. *BMC Oral Health* **2003**, *3*, 2. [CrossRef]

19. Al-Kheraif, A.A.; Al-Bejadi, A.S. Oral hygiene awareness among female Saudi school children. *Saudi Med. J.* **2008**, *29*, 1332–1336. [PubMed]

20. Al-Majed, M.I. Dental caries and its association with diet among female primary school children in Riyadh City. *Pakistan Oral Dent. J.* **2011**, *31*, 314–320.

21. Sa'adu, L.; Musa, O.I.; Abu-Saeed, K.; Abu-Saeed, M.B. Knowledge and practices on oral health among junior secondary school students in ILORIN West Local Government Area Of NIGERIA. *J. Dent.* **2012**, *2*, 170–175.

22. Al-Mutawa, S.A.; Shyama, M.; Al-Duwairi, Y.; Soparkar, P. Oral hygiene status of Kuwaiti school children. *East. Mediterr. Health J.* **2011**, *17*, 387–391. [CrossRef] [PubMed]

23. Lateefat, S.; Musa, O.I.; Muhammed As Saka, O.I. Determinants of oral hygiene status among junior secondary school students in Ilorin west local area of Nigeria. *Int. J. Pharm. Bio. Sci.* **2012**, *1*, 44–48. [CrossRef]

24. Dummer, P.M.; Addy, M.; Hicks, R.; Kingdon, A.; Shaw, W.C. The effect of social class on the prevalence of caries, plaque, gingivitis and pocketing in 11–12-year-old children in South Wales. *J. Dent.* **1987**, *15*, 185–190. [CrossRef]

25. Marrs, J.A.; Trumbley, S.; Malik, G. Early childhood caries: Determining the risk factors and assessing the prevention strategies for nursing intervention. *Pediatr. Nurs.* **2011**, *37*, 9–15. [PubMed]

26. AlDosari, A.M.; Wyne, A.H.; Akpata, E.S.; Khan, N.B. Caries prevalence among secondary school children in Riyadh and Qaseem. *Saudi Dent. J.* **2003**, *15*, 96–99.

27. Al-Sadhan, S.A. Dental caries prevalence among 12–14-year-old schoolchildren in Riyadh: A follow-up study of the Oral Health Survey of Saudi Arabia Phase I. *Saudi Dent. J.* **2006**, *18*, 2–7.

28. Hamissi, J.; Ramezani, G.H.; Ghodousi, A. Prevalence of dental caries among high school attendees in Qazvin, Iran. *J. Indian Soc. Pedod. Prev. Dent.* **2008**, *26*, 53–55.

29. Namal, N.L.; Can, G.; Vehid, S.; Koksal, S.; Kaypmaz, A. Dental health status and risk factors for dental caries in adults in Istanbul, Turkey. *East. Mediterr. Health J.* **2008**, *14*, 110–118. [PubMed]

30. Al-Ansari, A.A. Prevalence, severity, and secular trends of dental caries among various Saudi populations: A literature review. *Saudi J. Med. Sci.* **2014**, *2*, 142–150. [CrossRef]

31. Wyne, A.; Darwish, S.; Adenubi, J.; Battata, S.; Khan, N. The prevalence and pattern of nursing caries in Saudi preschool children. *Int. J. Paediatr. Dent.* **2000**, *11*, 361–364. [CrossRef]

32. Wyne, A.H.; Al-Ghoraibi, B.M.; Al-Asiri, Y.; Khan, N.B. Caries prevalence in Saudi primary school children of Riyadh and their teachers' oral health knowledge, attitude and practices. *Saudi Med. J.* **2002**, *23*, 77–81. [PubMed]

33. Al-Wazzan, K.A. Dental caries prevalence in 6–7-year-old school children in Riyadh region: A comparative study with the 1987 Oral Health Survey of Saudi Arabia Phase I. *Saudi Dent. J.* **2004**, *16*, 54–60.

34. Xu, W.; Lau, H.X.; Li, C.R.; Zeng, L.X. Dental caries status and risk indicators of dental caries among middle-aged adults in Shanghai, China. *J. Dent. Sci.* **2014**, *9*, 151–157. [CrossRef]

35. Amstutz, R.D.; Rozier, R.G. Community risk indicators for dental caries in school children: An ecologic study. *Commun. Dent. Oral Epidemiol.* **1995**, *23*, 129–137. [CrossRef]

36. Popoola, B.O.; Denloy, O.O.; Iyun, O.I. Influence of parental socioeconomic status on caries prevalence among children seen at the University Hospital, IBADAN. *Ann. Ib. Postgrad. Med.* **2013**, *11*, 81–86. [PubMed]

37. Hessari, H.; Vehkalahti, M.M.; Samadzan, H.; Eghbal, M.J. Oral health and treatment needs among 18-year-old Iranians. *Med. Princ. Pract.* **2008**, *17*, 302–307. [CrossRef] [PubMed]

38. Jacob, S.P. Global prevalence of periodontitis: A literature review. *Int. Arab J. Dent.* **2012**, *3*, 26–30.

39. Lu, X.H.; Wong, M.M.; Manlo, C.E.; Mcgrath, C. Risk indicators of oral health status among 18 years analyzed by negative binomial regression. *BMC Oral Health.* **2013**, *13*, 13–40. [CrossRef] [PubMed]

40. Albandar, J.M.; Rams, T.E. Risk factors for periodontal disease in children and young persons. *Periodontol. 2000* **2002**, *29*, 207–222. [CrossRef] [PubMed]

3

Paediatric Over-the-Counter (OTC) Oral Liquids Can Soften and Erode Enamel

Dan Zhao [1,2], James Kit-Hon Tsoi [1,*], Hai Ming Wong [3], Chun Hung Chu [4] and Jukka P. Matinlinna [1]

[1] Dental Materials Science, Applied Oral Sciences, Faculty of Dentistry, the University of Hong Kong, Hong Kong SAR, China; hannahziu@163.com (D.Z.); jpmat@hku.hk (J.P.M.)

[2] School of Stomatology, Zhejiang Chinese Medical University, Hangzhou 310053, Zhejiang, China

[3] Paediatric Dentistry, Faculty of Dentistry, the University of Hong Kong, Hong Kong SAR, China; wonghmg@hku.hk

[4] Operative Dentistry, Faculty of Dentistry, the University of Hong Kong, Hong Kong SAR, China; chchu@hku.hk

* Correspondence: jkhtsoi@hku.hk;

Academic Editor: Jeffrey A. Banas

Abstract: This study investigated the softening and erosive effects of various paediatric over-the-counter (OTC) oral liquids on deciduous teeth. Twenty sectioned and polished deciduous enamel blocks were ground on the buccal surface (2×2 mm^2) and randomly divided into five groups, immersed into four commercially-available paediatric OTC oral liquids (two for paracetamol, both sugared; and two for chlorpheniramine, one sugared and one sugar-free), with deionized water as control. The pH of the oral liquids ranged from 2.50 to 5.77. Each block was immersed into the test or control groups for 15 s, rinsed with deionized water, and Vickers micro-hardness ($n = 5$) was measured. After twenty cycles of immersion and hardness measurements, Scanning Electron Microscope (SEM) and Energy Dispersive X-ray Spectrometry (EDS) were used to evaluate the surface morphology and chemistry of the tooth blocks, respectively. The pH values of the liquids were also recorded. Rapidly descending trends in the micro-hardness ratios of the four test groups were observed that were statistically different from the control group ($p < 0.001$). EDS showed an increase of Ca/C ratio after drug immersion, whereas SEM showed an enamel loss in all the test groups. Paediatric OTC oral liquids could significantly soften the enamel and render them more susceptible to caries, such that the formulation of the oral liquids is the major factor.

Keywords: OTC drugs; paediatrics; enamel; hardness; pH; oral liquids

1. Introduction

Dental erosion is defined as the "irreversible loss of tooth structure due to chemical dissolution by acids without the involvement of bacteria" [1], and may combine with mechanical activities such as abrasion and attrition [2]. The sources could be intrinsic or extrinsic. Intrinsic sources include acid reflux, emesis or regurgitation due to some gastrointestinal diseases; on the other hand, extrinsic sources of acids are derived from acidic foods, beverages such as sport drinks and wines, and acidic medications [3].

Erosion begins on the enamel surfaces and then proceeds to the underlying dentine if no timely intervention is instituted. In brief, the initial stage is softening of enamel surface and the degree varies with the immersion time and the type of acids involved. Subsequently, if the erosive attack continues, dissolution of enamel crystals takes place, which is a permanent loss with a rough layer on top of the remaining tissue [4]. Indeed, in a chemical sense, there is a "critical pH of enamel", which is defined as the pH at which a solution is just saturated with respect to mineral of enamel, and the enamel on tooth surface will be in equilibrium with no dissolution or mineral precipitation occurring [5]. That means below the critical pH, the solution is going to be under-saturated and the potential for enamel dissolution exists.

Epidemiological surveys about dental erosion in preschool children have been conducted worldwide. The occurrence of dental erosion indeed varies from 25% to 75% due to the different factors including but not limited to countries, dietary habits and the lack of a standardised diagnosis guideline. For example, one survey [6] in Hong Kong was conducted to assess the prevalence of erosion among 12-year-old children in seven primary schools, and it was found that most children (75%) had at least some sign of erosion. It may thus be inferred that the occurrence of dental erosion in children is quite high, which should raise a concern among paedodontists.

With a considerably increasing intake of beverages such as soft drinks, energy drinks and soda, which contain a high concentration of fermentable carbohydrates [7], dental erosion among children becomes a public health concern due to its high prevalence [6,8,9]. Clinically, the early stages of erosion are often overlooked by the children themselves and doctors, possibly due to a lack of perceivable clinical signs and symptoms [10]. Thus, if there is no timely intervention, children may suffer from severe enamel surface loss, tooth sensitivity, poor aesthetics or even dental pulpitis, which will necessitate complicated treatment and lead to a compromised dentition for the entire life [10]. While in some cases dental erosion can be controlled through modification of the children's dietary habits, other children may be on long term medication which predisposes them to dental erosion, in particular those who are suffering from chronic diseases like respiratory allergies, asthma, cardiopathy and epilepsy, and it is in these cases where the possible incidence of dental erosion cannot be neglected [11].

As a matter of fact, some drugs, e.g., respiratory drugs, are commonly prescribed to children before two years of age [9]. Although many solid forms of oral medication such as pills or capsules have a coating to mask their bitter tastes, such methods are impractical for many children since the children are too young to swallow the pills and capsules. The situation varies greatly among older children [12]. Consequently, the most common choice of formulations for children are in liquid form. One of the biggest challenges of administering medicine in children is a "matter of taste", as drugs often taste bitter due to their chemical nature. In order to minimise the unpleasant taste of bitterness, paediatric medications are usually coloured, flavoured and sweetened with various excipients besides containing the main active ingredients. These additives include bulk materials (such as for thickening), flavourings, sweeteners, buffers, acids, preservatives and colouring agents, which are prevalent among formulations for children [12]. The frequent use of acids in paediatric medicine is associated with an improvement in flavour [13,14]. Meanwhile, proper liquid formulations have high requirements regarding the maintenance of solubility, chemical stability, taste masking and preservation. For liquid drugs, a suitable pH is needed at which the drug is both sufficiently soluble and chemically stable. Acidic contents are added into formulations as buffering agents, and are responsible for controlling tonicity and ensuring the drugs' physiological compatibility [13].

However, frequent use of syrups sweetened with sucrose or fructose or with a combination of both has been linked to dental caries and a drop of plaque pH in the long term [15–20], and the cariogenic potential of paediatric liquid medicines is probably the result of a high concentration of fermentable carbohydrates and their acidogenicity [21]. It has been reported in one study that about half of 97 regularly-used paediatric medication formulations have an endogenous pH below 5.5 and thus are capable of damaging tooth enamel [13]. In addition, consumption of such drugs at night could aggravate the dental caries and dental erosion, because during this period the salivary flow rate is reduced and the time of elimination from the oral cavity increases [22].

Nowadays, pharmaceutical companies recommend using sugar-free medicines that are oral liquid formulations without fructose, glucose, or sucrose. It seems to be a plausible option to replace the sugar-containing medications, but there is still no consensus as to whether they have true benefits or not. According to one report, it was found that the replacement sugar-free medicines might themselves damage teeth, which was not desirable. In fact, a reduction of the sugary ingredients in the medicines might entail the addition of weak acids to make up for their palatability concerns and optimise formulation properties, which would bring up dental erosion [20]. A comprehensive review [23] by Strickley et al. has illustrated various functions of the excipients in paediatric drug formulation, whilst a recent report [24] has expressed a very great concern about the potential risk of drug-induced caries from sugar or its carbohydrates and their negative effects on the oral health (and the future growth of adult dentition) of children. However, data about erosive potential and enamel softening of commonly-used over-the-counter (OTC) paediatric oral liquids is lacking.

The aim of this study was to evaluate the erosive effect of the paediatric oral liquid medicines on deciduous teeth. The null hypothesis for the study was that there was no difference of enamel between the test and control groups after immersion challenge, which means the liquids would not cause erosive damage.

2. Results

2.1. pH Values

Table 1 shows the pH value of the test groups. The pH values ranged from 2.50 (group GC) to 7.17 (group GE) with similar endogenous pH among paracetamol groups and only one medication that was slightly higher than 5.5 (group GD). These measurements indicate that all the tested paediatric OTC medications exhibited an acidic pH.

Table 1. The information of test medicines and their pH in this study.

Test Group	Main Component and Concentration	Brand	Manufacturer of Drugs	pH ($\pm$ SD); ($n = 3$)
GA	Paracetamol (120 mg per 5 mL)	Jean-Marie Paracetamol syrup	Jean-Marie Pharmcal, Hong Kong	4.97 ± 0.01
GB		Uni-Febrin syrup	Universal Pharm, Hong Kong	4.74 ± 0.01
GC	Chlorpheniramine (2 mg per 5 mL)	Jean-Marie Chlorpheniramine syrup	Jean-Marie Pharmcal, Hong Kong	2.50 ± 0.01
GD		Allerief syrup	Percuro Medica Ltd, UK	5.77 ± 0.01
GE	Control group	Deionised water		7.17 ± 0.06

2.2. Surface Micro-Hardness

The mean micro-hardness ratios (MHR) in each group, as a function of testing round k, are shown in Figure 1. In general, the MHR decreased with the number of drug immersion in all experimental groups despite variations in the magnitude. In the control group, only a small fluctuation (<6%) on MHR was observed after 20 rounds of immersion. However, there were drastic decreases of around 15% in the MHR in both the GC and GD groups, whilst the GB group only exhibited a 7% decrease in MHR. One-way ANCOVA revealed that test groups collectively have statistically significant differences from one another (Table 2), and the control group has a statistically significantly different regression slope from all others ($p < 0.001$), whilst GA, GC and GD has no statistical significant difference between each other ($p > 0.05$) (Table 3).

Table 2. One-way ANCOVA results of micro-hardness ratios (MHR).

	Dependent Variable: MHR							
Source	Type III Sum of Squares	df	Mean Square	F	Sig.	Partial Eta Squared	Noncent. Parameter	Observed Power [b]
Corrected Model	0.158 [a]	5	0.032	119.792	0.000	0.858	598.961	1.000
Intercept	27.991	1	27.991	106,059.503	0.000	0.999	106,059.503	1.000
Round	0.093	1	0.093	354.279	0.000	0.782	354.279	1.000
Drug Type	0.064	4	0.016	60.926	0.000	0.711	243.706	1.000
Error	0.026	99	0.000					
Total	94.592	105						
Corrected Total	0.184	104						

[a] R Squared = 0.858 (Adjusted R Squared = 0.851); [b] Computed using alpha = 0.05.

Table 3. One-way ANCOVA pairwise comparisons.

(I) Drug Type	(J) Drug Type	Mean Difference (I–J)	Std. Error	Sig. [b]	95% Confidence Interval for Difference [b]	
					Lower Bound	Upper Bound
GA	GB	−0.033 *	0.005	0.000	−0.043	−0.023
	GC	0.004	0.005	0.422	−0.006	0.014
	GD	0.007	0.005	0.180	−0.003	0.017
	GE	−0.056 *	0.005	0.000	−0.066	−0.046
GB	GA	0.033 *	0.005	0.000	0.023	0.043
	GC	0.037 *	0.005	0.000	0.027	0.047
	GD	0.039 *	0.005	0.000	0.030	0.049
	GE	−0.023 *	0.005	0.000	−0.033	−0.013
GC	GA	−0.004	0.005	0.422	−0.014	0.006
	GB	−0.037 *	0.005	0.000	−0.047	−0.027
	GD	0.003	0.005	0.604	−0.007	0.013
	GE	−0.060 *	0.005	0.000	−0.070	−0.050
GD	GA	−0.007	0.005	0.180	−0.017	0.003
	GB	−0.039 *	0.005	0.000	−0.049	−0.030
	GC	−0.003	0.005	0.604	−0.013	0.007
	GE	−0.063 *	0.005	0.000	−0.073	−0.053
GE (Control)	GA	0.056 *	0.005	0.000	0.046	0.066
	GB	0.023 *	0.005	0.000	0.013	0.033
	GC	0.060 *	0.005	0.000	0.050	0.070
	GD	0.063 *	0.005	0.000	0.053	0.073

Based on estimated marginal means

*. The mean difference is significant at the 0.05 level; [b] Adjustment for multiple comparisons: Least Significant Difference (equivalent to no adjustments).

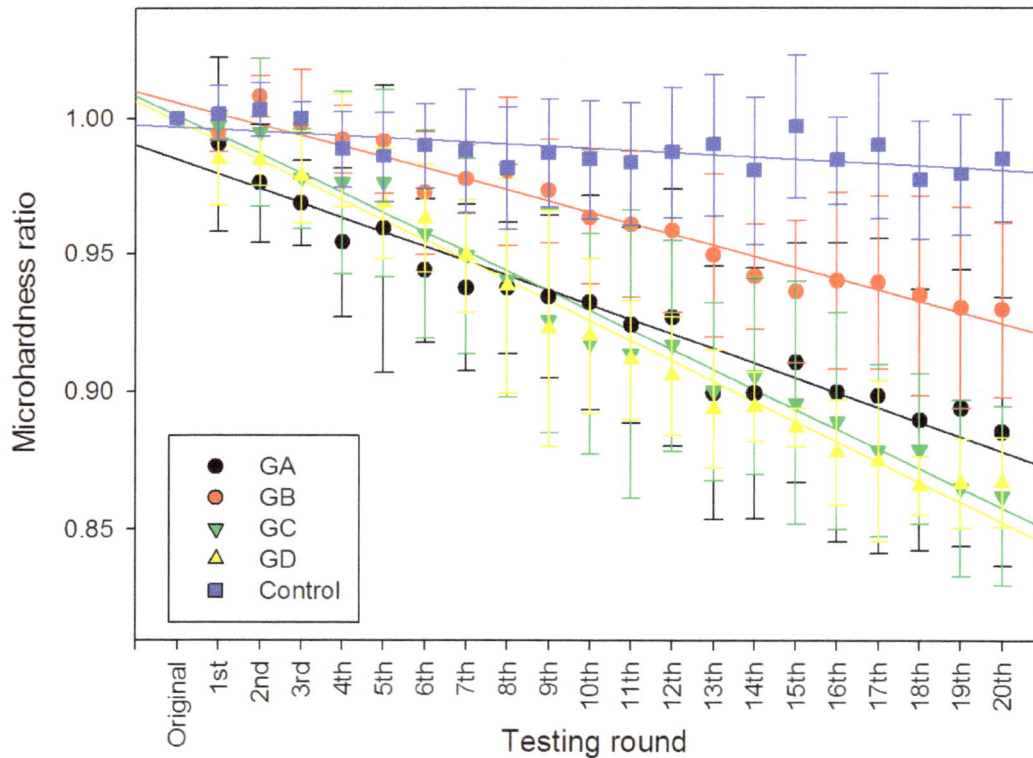

Figure 1. The relationship between mean micro-hardness ratio and standard deviation vs. testing rounds. GA and GB groups contain paracetamol, GC and GD groups contain chlorpheniramine, GE is the control group which is deionised water.

2.3. Scanning Electron Microscope (SEM) / Energy Dispersive X-Ray Spectrometry (EDS) Analysis

The median values for the three repeated EDS measurements in each sample before and after the experiment were calculated and analysed in the Kruskal–Wallis test (Table 4). Generally, the Ca/C ratio decreased after the drug immersion, while the Ca/P ratio and Mg, Na weight percentages mostly remained stable. However, no statistically significant differences have been found. Moreover, the data revealed that, before the immersion, all enamel surfaces appeared to be flat (Figure 2). After the twenty rounds of immersion, the surfaces of the GA group displayed a distinctive enamel loss with irregular craters. The surfaces of the GB group showed a corroded surface and the fracture lines were along the border of prism heads. In group GC, the surfaces presented a remarkable acid-etched prism-sheath structure of enamel, with the prisms surrounded by a wide sheath region. Group GD also exhibited disorganised enamel loss with increased porosity on the surface. No distinctive microstructure loss was observed in control group (group GE).

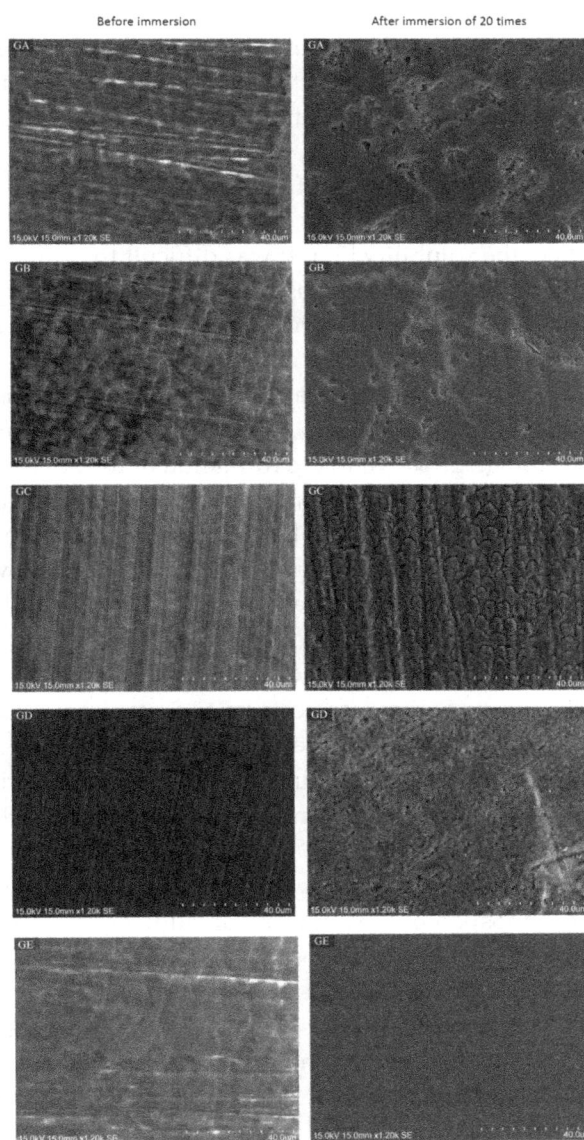

Figure 2. Scanning electron microscope (SEM) micrographs (×1200) of deciduous enamel before and after immersion 20 times in drugs containing paracetamol (groups GA and GB), chlorpheniramine (groups GC and GD), or deionized water (Control group).

Table 4. Energy dispersive x-ray spectrometry (EDS) measurements of Ca/P and Ca/C ratios, and Mg and Na wt % in the test groups before immersion and after 20 rounds of immersion. Kruskal–Wallis test revealed no statistical significance before and after the immersion for each group at $\alpha = 0.05$.

	Ca/P		Ca/C		Mg (wt %)		Na (wt %)	
	Before Immersion	After 20 Rounds	Before Immersion	After 20 Rounds	Before Immersion	After 20 Rounds	Before Immersion	After 20 Rounds
GA	1.95	1.96	10.45	8.26	1.32	1.56	2.10	2.10
GB	1.99	1.92	10.65	8.71	1.26	1.48	2.02	2.00
GC	1.97	1.98	10.21	9.13	1.50	1.41	2.09	1.83
GD	1.94	1.94	9.79	8.63	1.46	1.55	2.10	1.95
GE (control)	1.80	1.76	7.85	6.76	1.62	1.52	2.46	2.25

3. Discussion

In this in vitro study, we found that the OTC paediatric oral liquids could significantly lower the Vickers micro-hardness of enamel, i.e., had a softening effect, causing damage on the surface of enamel as seen from SEM after successive immersion cycles. It seems that the enamel of deciduous teeth is susceptible to acid erosion caused by the oral liquids, while the presence of sugar or pH of the oral liquids were not the major factors.

Three of the tested medicines showed a pH lower than the "critical pH of enamel", i.e., 5.5. However, impurities in the dental mineral may increase its solubility, thus the relative rates of dissolution do not truly reflect the solubility [25]. It was difficult to evaluate the solubility products based on the actual mineral composition, since it has been demonstrated that the minerals in biological samples were heterogeneous [26]. Accordingly, the critical pH for enamel was typically considered to be in a range of 4.5 to 5.5 [27]. Even so, the current study confirmed that liquid medication with an endogenous pH of 5.7 might also cause erosive damage to the enamel surface. In fact, the rate of dissolution of enamel is strongly influenced by other physical factors (e.g., temperature, consumption frequency) and biological factors (e.g., saliva in the formation of the acquired pellicle, as a lubricant, buffer and ion reservoir). For example, solubility is dependent on temperature and heat is required to break the bonds holding the molecules in a solid [28]. Thus, erosion is predicted to be more severe at high temperatures and less at low temperatures, which has been shown by Banan et al. that dairy beverages caused less decrease of pH in plaque and saliva at temperatures lower than room temperature [29,30].

In addition, from a biological perspective, the presence of saliva is greatly beneficial to an oral cavity under erosive attack. Saliva is required to form the acquired pellicle, which is defined as a proteinaceous layer on all solid surfaces exposed to the oral cavity [31–33]. It is an organic film composed of glycoproteins and proteins, including several enzymes, without the involvement of bacteria [31,32]. It works as a protective membrane to prevent direct attack from acidic substances, thus lowering the rate of demineralisation [33]. Furthermore, bicarbonate is the most important component in saliva to protect against acidic products generated by dental plaque or extrinsic acids [34]. The presence of calcium and phosphate, as well as an alkaline or neutral environment is essential for remineralisation. Preserving calcium and phosphate in saliva allows them to penetrate into the minerals of enamel, slowing down the rate of mineral dissolution [35]. One research study has shown that salivary proteins would bind to demineralised sites and cover exposed crystals by a specific adsorption mechanism [36]. In the oral cavity, the contact of the enamel with acidic substances is usually only transient before clearance by saliva. Consequently, under in vivo conditions, an early stage of erosion is limited to a very insignificant loss of mineral and erosive craters on a nanometer scale or even near atomic level [37]. In this sense, there might be discrepancies between the current in vitro study and other in vivo studies.

Since there was no involvement of saliva in this study, it is possible that the erosive potential of medications was overestimated. For example, we have not included the buffer capacity of saliva which could alter the final pH in the oral cavity and hence lower the dissolution rate of enamel [38], possibly due to the high bicarbonate concentration in saliva [39]. Nevertheless, significantly different buffering capacities have been found between genders (e.g., male and female), as well as the method of collection (e.g., unstimulated or stimulated) [38]. Thus, in most of the in vitro studies, various formulations of artificial saliva were employed. However, most simple simulated saliva compositions have no proteins and do not form acquired pellicles, which play an important protective role against erosion. Moreover, collection of natural saliva in a restricted time frame is not a simple task, particularly with the quick deterioration of saliva [40]. Therefore, more in vivo studies are necessary to reliably evaluate the erosive effect under the influence of saliva and masticatory activities.

Deciduous tooth enamel is softer than permanent tooth enamel. A study has found that deciduous teeth had a lower prismatic density, which meant a smaller number of prisms per unit area, and a shorter prismatic diameter compared to permanent teeth despite having the same morphology [41]. The higher percentage of minerals makes the enamel more resistant to masticatory forces, but its extreme hardness makes it more prone to fractures and more reliant on the presence of the dentine—which is more resilient—to maintain its integrity [42]. Nevertheless, some investigators found that deciduous enamel was softer and more prone to fracture than permanent enamel [43]. Furthermore, the lessened mineralisation and the smaller thickness in deciduous enamel make primary teeth more prone to erosion and decay [44–46]. Generally speaking, the erosive potential of primary enamel is greater and its weaker mechanical properties could be explained by the reduced mineralisation in deciduous enamel tissue.

In the current study, the deciduous teeth were challenged by 20 rounds of 15 s drug immersion time. Fifteen seconds was chosen for the immersion time so as to reflect the drug taking habits of children and the residence time of drugs on enamel. The twenty rounds were to mimic the times of consumption (*quater die sumendus* for five days). In addition, since the initial values of micro-hardness differed among the specimens, ratios (MHR) were calculated instead and corresponding trend lines were drawn in order to allow for better data comparison among the groups.

Liquid formulations are usually complex compositions containing many other components besides the main active ingredients; the additives include bulk materials, flavourings, sweeteners, buffers, preservatives and colouring agents [12]. Although we do not know the exact formulation of the purchased medicinal liquids, acidic contents were common to all the liquids and acted as buffering agents, and they were responsible for improving palatability, maintaining chemical stability, controlling tonicity and ensuring the physiological compatibility [13]. For example, citric acid was the most frequently added acid, yet it has been linked to tooth erosion due to its ability to dissolve the hydroxyapatite of tooth enamel and dentine [47]. It has been found that citric acid acts as a chelator that binds to the minerals of the hydroxyapatite, reduces saliva supersaturation and increases the dissolution rate of hydroxyapatite crystals [48]. Other acids have also demonstrated various erosive effects on enamel; it has been reported that lactic acid at low pH was more erosive than both citric and maleic acids [49].

In the chlorpheniramine groups, a sugar-free formulation group GD having a higher pH value exhibited a similar micro-hardness decreasing trend as group GC. It might be due to the addition of "sugar-free" excipients, i.e. artificial sweeteners, are acidic or chemically stable under acidic environment [50]. This result was further confirmed by another study of comparing the erosive potential between sugar-free medicine and sugar-containing ones. They found that the sugar-free medications still carried a similar erosive potential as the sugar-containing syrups [13]. In addition, the active ingredient of these two drugs was chlorpheniramine maleate, which in fact would be dissociated into chlorpheniramine free base and maleic acid in aqueous conditions [51]. Indeed, despite maleic acid being a weak acid, it has the potential to etch [52] or chemisorb [53] on enamel, so much so that it could be utilised for bonding orthodontic brackets onto enamel [54]. It seems to be that simply shifting to sugar-free medications is not as beneficial as once thought, and a fundamental understanding of the formulation science and chemistry is essential.

With respect to the elemental analysis by EDS, semi-quantitative data were presented to show the chemical changes of enamel surface after liquid medicine immersion. A previous study has examined the Ca/P and Ca/C ratio to compare the elemental difference before and after demineralisation, since it was thought that the ratios were altered from calcium hydroxyapatite due to the alteration or substitution of mineral phase [55]. However, in the present study, the Ca/P ratio before drug immersion determined by using the EDS was found to be around 1.9, which was not significantly different from that of enamel which experienced drug immersion. Accordingly, we speculate that the components of Ca and P change together (i.e., dissolved in the oral liquids) in the same direction. Besides, several other studies were unable to demonstrate any significant difference in the Ca/P ratio in compromised enamel [55,56]. Multiple studies on developing enamel have shown that the Ca/P ratio was constant during tooth development despite variations among individuals [57,58]. Nevertheless, Jälevik and co-workers did find that median Ca/P ratio of hypo-mineralised enamel was significantly lower than sound enamel [59]. Therefore, the teeth collected in various stages in different countries might have high variations which eventually led to the scattering of results.

One study also revealed a relation between micro-hardness and the Ca/C ratio in demineralised enamel [56]. As the crystals were dissolved with more organic components exposed, it seemed plausible that the Ca/C ratio would increase. However, in this study, despite a Ca/C ratio decrease after drug challenge, the difference had no statistical significance. The limited sample size in this study and variations among individuals could contribute to the contrasting result.

Given the findings of this study, paediatricians and patients should realise the risk of erosion during the consumption of liquid medicines by children. Dentists should not overlook the early stages of erosion, regarding minor tooth surface loss as a normal occurrence of daily life, since early diagnosis and appropriate intervention are seldom reached in time [60]. Children should also visit dentists regularly and oral hygiene education in preschool is necessary. Other methods such as an adequate use of fluoride-containing mouth-rinses, toothpastes, tablets and lozenges have been demonstrated to remineralise enamel effectively [61]. In future, more clinical studies or in vivo studies are needed, since the limits of in vitro studies do not allow simulation of all the complex biological effects. We anticipate this study could raise awareness of the erosion susceptibility from paediatric OTC oral liquids.

4. Materials and Methods

This study was approved by the Institutional Review Board of Hong Kong (IRB UW15-172). The procedure has been illustrated as a flowchart in Figure 3.

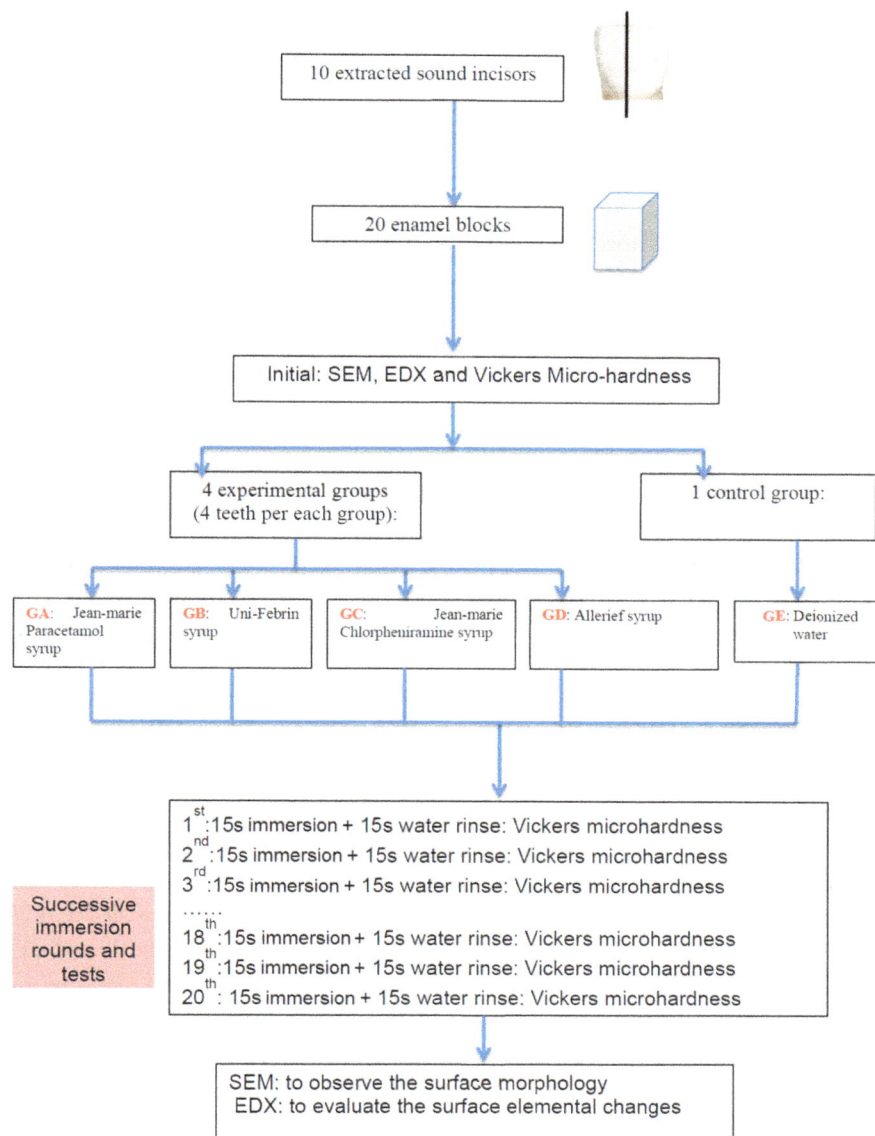

Figure 3. The flowchart of experimental design.

4.1. Teeth and Specimen Preparation

Twenty sectioned enamel blocks, with 2×2 mm^2 buccal enamel surface, were obtained from ten sound extracted primary incisors. The incisors were stored in distilled water at 4 °C prior to use for no longer than one week. Each incisor was sliced longitudinally parallel to its long axis to get two enamel blocks by a cutting machine under running water. All enamel blocks were embedded in light-cured resin (Filtek Z250, 3M ESPE) onto an acrylic plate. The buccal surfaces were faced upwards to make sure most regions of the surface are parallel to the plate.

After embedding the enamel into the resin, the buccal surfaces of the enamel were polished using 1000- and 2000-grit SiC abrasive paper by a manually water-cooled low-speed polishing machine to obtain a flat surface without dentine exposure, and the specimen underwent ultrasonic washing in deionised water before and after polishing. Then, the twenty blocks were randomly divided into five groups (four experimental groups GA, GB, GC, GD, and one control group GE; see Table 1), i.e., four blocks in one group, to immerse into the oral liquids or deionised water.

4.2. Oral Liquids

As the most commonly used paediatric OTC drugs to relieve respiratory symptoms were usually for acute occasions [9], two commonly-used single component formulations, i.e., paracetamol and chlorpheniramine, were used (Table 1). Paracetamol (in US: acetaminophen) is a major ingredient in numerous cold and flu remedies and it is also classified as a mild analgesic to relieve headaches, fever and other minor aches and pains. Chlorpheniramine is an antihistamine used to relieve the symptoms of allergic conditions and the common cold, such as rhinorrhoea. Two different brands of paediatric OTC oral liquids containing one of each of the drugs were selected to make a comparison. In the chlorpheniramine group, the Jean-Marie brand contains sugar, while the Allerief belongs to a sugar-free type. All of the OTC drugs were purchased from local pharmacies and no further information from manufacturers was acquired.

4.3. pH Measurement

The endogenous pH of the testing medications was determined at room temperature by using a digital pH meter (CyberScan pH500, Eutech Instruments, UK) in triplicate to get a mean value. The pH meter was calibrated before measurement according to the manufacturer's instructions, using buffer standards of pH 4 and pH 7. Then, 10 mL of the testing medicine was placed in one beaker, the probe of the pH meter was immersed directly into the syrup and the value was recorded with the precision of 0.01.

4.4. Micro-Hardness Measurement

To evaluate and compare the erosive potentials of four medications on a continuous scale, each specimen was subjected to twenty rounds of immersion in one of the drugs, followed by micro-hardness measurements. To set a baseline of the mean initial micro-hardness (MH_0), each enamel block was immersed into deionised water (DI) for 15 s, and then five random spots were picked and tested using a micro-hardness tester (Leica DC 300, Leitz, Germany) with a Vickers tip and load of 200 g (1.962 N) lasting for 15 s. Then, in each round k, the enamel block was immersed into 10 mL of the corresponding test group for 15 s and followed by rinsing with DI water for 15 s. Again, the average micro-hardness values (MH_k) of the enamel surfaces were measured immediately from five random spots using the same micro-hardness tester and parameters. The same immersion and measuring procedures were repeated for twenty rounds (i.e., k = 1–20). Fresh drug or DI water was used for each new round of immersion. As a whole, each sample experienced 21 (one initial + twenty after drug immersion) micro-hardness measurements. All the values were then plotted as the ratio (MHR) vs. round of immersion to give a trend (Figure 1) on how the surface hardness changes following a continuous drug attack, i.e.,:

$$MHR = MH_k/MH_0 \tag{1}$$

where MH_k is the mean micro-hardness at k = 0–20 rounds, and MH_0 is the mean initial micro-hardness. The MHR and slope of regression lines of Figure 1 was statistically analysed by one-way ANCOVA at α = 0.05 (SPSS v.22, IBM, New York, NY, USA).

4.5. Scanning Electron Microscope Analysis

The surface topography of the enamel specimens at 1200× magnification was studied under a scanning electron microscope (Hitachi SU-1510 Variable Pressure SEM, Hitachi Ltd., Tokyo, Japan) at 15 kV in high-vacuum mode. The SEM micrographs of all enamel blocks were taken on two occasions: (1) before the immersion procedures, where the enamel blocks were mounted onto an aluminium stub separately to assess their surface topography without coating, and (2) after 20 rounds of immersion, where all the specimens were sputter-coated with carbon at 15 kV and the entire buccal surface was scanned. The SEM micrographs provided visual and illustrative comparisons of the surface morphologic changes of specimens before and after the drug/water challenge.

4.6. Energy Dispersive X-Ray Spectrometry Analysis

The same samples that had been observed in SEM were also used for the EDS analysis on the same occasions, except the EDS was done prior to the coating. The EDS system comprised of an X-ray detector system (Model 550i, IXRF-Systems, Austin, TX, USA) attached to the SEM operated at 15 kV with a spot size of 5 nm, specimen tilt of 35°, working distance of 15 mm and a counting time of 20 s. Three counts from each enamel sample were measured to give a mean weight percentage of calcium (Ca), phosphorus (P), sodium (Na), magnesium (Mg), carbon (C) and oxygen (O). The mean wt % ratios of Ca/P and Ca/C, and the wt % of Mg and Na before and after tests were statistically evaluated by Kruskal–Wallis test at $\alpha = 0.05$ (SPSS v.22).

5. Conclusions

Within the limitations of this laboratory study, the four tested paediatric OTC oral liquids were found to significantly soften enamel of primary teeth and deem them susceptible to caries. There is a possible association between drug formulations and their erosive potentials.

Acknowledgments: The authors deny any conflicts of interest related to this study. This work was done in partial fulfilment of the requirements of the degree of MSc (DMS) for the first author at the Faculty of Dentistry, The University of Hong Kong. We thank Madeline J.Y. Yon for proofreading the article.

Author Contributions: D.Z. and J.K.-H.T. conceived and designed the experiments; D.Z. performed the experiments; D.Z., J.K.-H.T. and J.P.M. analysed the data; H.M.W. and C.H.C. contributed reagents/materials/ analysis tools; D.Z., J.K.-H.T., H.M.W., C.H.C. and J.P.M. wrote the paper.

References

1. Bahal, P.; Djemal, S. Dental erosion from an excess of vitamin C. *Case Rep. Dent.* **2014**, *2014*, 5. [CrossRef] [PubMed]
2. Bartlett, D.; Dugmore, C. Pathological or physiological erosion—Is there a relationship to age? *Clin. Oral Investig.* **2008**, *12*, 27–31. [CrossRef] [PubMed]
3. Scheutzel, P. Etiology of dental erosion–intrinsic factors. *Eur. J. Oral Sci.* **1996**, *104*, 178–190. [CrossRef] [PubMed]
4. Lussi, A.; Schlueter, N.; Rakhmatullina, E.; Ganss, C. Dental erosion—An overview with emphasis on chemical and histopathological aspects. *Caries Res.* **2011**, *45*, 2–12. [CrossRef] [PubMed]
5. Dawes, C. What is the critical ph and why does a tooth dissolve in acid? *Can. Dent. Assoc.* **2003**, *69*, 722–724.
6. Zhang, S.; Chau, A.M.H.; Lo, E.C.M.; Chu, C.-H. Dental caries and erosion status of 12-year-old Hong Kong children. *BMC Public Health* **2014**, *14*, 7. [CrossRef] [PubMed]
7. Tahmassebi, J.F.; Duggal, M.S.; Malik-Kotru, G.; Curzon, M.E.J. Soft drinks and dental health: A review of the current literature. *J. Dent.* **2006**, *34*, 2–11. [CrossRef] [PubMed]
8. Mantonanaki, M.; Koletsi-Kounari, H.; Mamai-Homata, E.; Papaioannou, W. Dental erosion prevalence and associated risk indicators among preschool children in Athens, Greece. *Clin. Oral Investig.* **2013**, *17*, 585–593. [CrossRef] [PubMed]
9. Sturkenboom, M.; Verhamme, K.; Nicolosi, A.; Murray, M.; Neubert, A.; Caudri, D.; Picelli, G.; Sen, E.; Giaquinto, C.; Cantarutti, L.; et al. Drug use in children: Cohort study in three European countries. *Br. Med. J.* **2008**, *337*, 1338–1341. [CrossRef] [PubMed]
10. Lussi, A.; Schaffner, M.; Jaeggi, T. Dental erosion-diagnosis and prevention in children and adults. *Int. Dent. J.* **2007**, *57*, 385–398. [CrossRef]
11. Neves, B.G.; Farah, A.; Lucas, E.; de Sousa, V.P.; Maia, L.C. Are paediatric medicines risk factors for dental caries and dental erosion? *Commun. Dent. Health* **2010**, *27*, 46–51.
12. Mennella, J.A.; Spector, A.C.; Reed, D.R.; Coldwell, S.E. The bad taste of medicines: Overview of basic research on bitter taste. *Clin. Ther.* **2013**, *35*, 1225–1246. [CrossRef] [PubMed]

13. Maguire, A.; Baqir, W.; Nunn, J.H. Are sugars-free medicines more erosive than sugars-containing medicines? An in vitro study of paediatric medicines with prolonged oral clearance used regularly and long-term by children. *Int. J. Paediatr. Dent.* **2007**, *17*, 231–238. [CrossRef] [PubMed]

14. Liem, D.G.; Mennella, J.A. Heightened sour preferences during childhood. *Chem. Senses* **2003**, *28*, 173–180. [CrossRef] [PubMed]

15. Marquezan, M.; Pozzobon, R.; Oliveira, M. Medicines used by pediatric dentistry patients and its cariogenic potential. *RPG Rev. Pos. Grad.* **2007**, *13*, 334–339.

16. Durward, C.; Thou, T. Dental caries and sugar-containing liquid medicines for children in new zealand. *N. Z. Dent. J.* **1997**, *93*, 124–129. [PubMed]

17. Feigal, R.J.; Jensen, M.E.; Mensing, C.A. Dental caries potential of liquid medications. *Pediatrics* **1981**, *68*, 416–419. [PubMed]

18. Babu, K.L.; Doddamani, G.M.; Naik, L.R.; Jagadeesh, K.N. Pediatric liquid medicaments—Are they cariogenic? An in vitro study. *J. Int. Soc. Prev. Commun. Dent.* **2014**, *4*, 108–112. [CrossRef] [PubMed]

19. Arora, R.; Mukherjee, U.; Arora, V. Erosive potential of sugar free and sugar containing pediatric medicines given regularly and long term to children. *Indian J. Pediatr.* **2012**, *79*, 759–763. [CrossRef] [PubMed]

20. Babu, K.L.G.; Rai, K.; Hedge, A.M. Pediatric liquid medicaments—Do they erode the teeth surface? An in vitro study: Part I. *J. Clin. Pediatr. Dent.* **2008**, *32*, 189–194. [CrossRef] [PubMed]

21. Sahgal, J.; Sood, P.B.; Raju, O.S. A comparison of oral hygiene status and dental caries in children on long term liquid oral medications to those not administered with such medications. *J. Indian Soc. Pedod. Prev. Dent.* **2002**, *20*, 144–151. [PubMed]

22. Cavalcanti, A.; de Oliveira, K.; Xavier, A.; Pinto, D.; Vieira, F. Evaluation of total soluble solids content (TSSC) and endogenous ph in antimicrobials of pediatric use. *Indian J. Dent. Res.* **2013**, *24*, 498–501. [CrossRef] [PubMed]

23. Strickley, R.G.; Iwata, Q.; Wu, S.; Dahl, T.C. Pediatric drugs-a review of commercially available oral formulations. *J. Pharm. Sci.* **2008**, *97*, 1731–1774. [CrossRef] [PubMed]

24. Donaldson, M.; Goodchild, J.H.; Epstein, J.B. Sugar content, cariogenicity, and dental concerns with commonly used medications. *J. Am. Dent. Assoc.* **2015**, *146*, 129–133. [CrossRef] [PubMed]

25. Featherstone, J.; Lussi, A. Understanding the chemistry of dental erosion. *Dent. Eros.* **2006**, *20*, 66–76.

26. Shellis, R.P. A scanning electron-microscopic study of solubility variations in human enamel and dentine. *Arch. Oral Biol.* **1996**, *41*, 473–484. [CrossRef]

27. Axelsson, P.D.D.S. *Diagnosis and Risk Prediction of Dental Caries*; Quintessence Publishing: Chicago, IL, USA, 2000.

28. Pinto, S.C.S.; Batitucci, R.G.; Pinheiro, M.C.; Zandim, D.L.; Spin-Neto, R.; Sampaio, J.E.C. Effect of an acid diet allied to sonic toothbrushing on root dentin permeability: An in vitro study. *Braz. Dent. J.* **2010**, *21*, 390. [CrossRef] [PubMed]

29. Ferreira, F.V.; Pozzobon, R.T. Processed dairy beverages ph evaluation: Consequences of temperature variation. *J. Clin. Pediatr. Dent.* **2009**, *33*, 319. [CrossRef] [PubMed]

30. Banan, L.K.; Hegde, A.M. Plaque and salivary ph changes after consumption of fresh fruit juices. *J. Clin. Pediatr. Dent.* **2005**, *30*, 9. [CrossRef] [PubMed]

31. Hannig, C.; Hannig, M.; Attin, T. Enzymes in the acquired enamel pellicle. *Eur. J. Oral Sci.* **2005**, *113*, 2–13. [CrossRef] [PubMed]

32. Lendenmann, U.; Grogan, J.; Oppenheim, F.G. Saliva and dental pellicle—A review. *Adv. Dent. Res.* **2000**, *14*, 22–28. [CrossRef] [PubMed]

33. Hannig, M.; Balz, M. Influence of in vivo formed salivary pellicle on enamel erosion. *Caries Res.* **1999**, *33*, 372–379. [CrossRef] [PubMed]

34. Edgar, W.M.; Dawes, C.; Mullane, D.M. *Saliva and Oral Health*; British Dental Association: London, UK, 2004.

35. Meurman, J.H.; Ten Cate, J.M. Pathogenesis and modifying factors of dental erosion. *Eur. J. Oral Sci.* **1996**, *104*, 199–206. [CrossRef] [PubMed]

36. Voegel, J.C.; Belcourt, A.; Gillmeth, S. Dissolution of hydroxyapatites treated with salivary glycoproteins and fluoride. *Caries Res.* **1981**, 243–249. [CrossRef]

37. Attin, T.; Wegehaupt, F.J. *Methods for Assessment of Dental Erosion*; Karger: Basel, Switzerland, 2014.

38. Gittings, S.; Turnbull, N.; Henry, B.; Roberts, C.J.; Gershkovich, P. Characterisation of human saliva as a platform for oral dissolution medium development. *Eur. J. Pharm. Biopharm.* **2015**, *91*, 16–24. [CrossRef] [PubMed]

39. Izutsu, K.T. Theory and measurement of the buffer value of bicarbonate in saliva. *J. Theor. Biol.* **1981**, *90*, 397–403. [CrossRef]

40. Amaechi, B.T.; Higham, S.M. Eroded enamel lesion remineralization by saliva as a possible factor in the site-specificity of human dental erosion. *Arch. Oral Biol.* **2001**, *46*, 697–703. [CrossRef]

41. Gentile, E.; Di Stasio, D.; Santoro, R.; Contaldo, M.; Salerno, C.; Serpico, R.; Lucchese, A. In vivo microstructural analysis of enamel in permanent and deciduous teeth. *Ultrastruct. Pathol.* **2015**, *39*, 131–134. [CrossRef] [PubMed]

42. Low, I.M.; Duraman, N.; Davies, I.J. Microstructure-property relationships in human adult and baby canine teeth. *Key Eng. Mater.* **2006**, *309*, 23–26. [CrossRef]

43. De Menezes Oliveira, M.A.H.; Torres, C.P.; Gomes-silva, J.M.; Chinelatti, M.A.; De Menezes, F.C.H.; Palma-dibb, R.G.; Borsatto, M.C. Microstructure and mineral composition of dental enamel of permanent and deciduous teeth. *Microsc. Res. Tech.* **2010**, *73*, 572–577. [CrossRef] [PubMed]

44. Wang, L.J.; Tang, R.; Bonstein, T.; Bush, P.; Nancollas, G.H. Enamel demineralization in primary and permanent teeth. *J. Dent. Res.* **2006**, *85*, 359. [CrossRef] [PubMed]

45. Johansson, A.K.; Sorvari, R.; Birkhed, D.; Meurman, J.H. Dental erosion in deciduous teeth—An in vivo and in vitro study. *J. Dent.* **2001**, *29*, 333–340. [CrossRef]

46. Hunter, M.L.; West, N.X.; Hughes, J.A.; Newcombe, R.G.; Addy, M. Erosion of deciduous and permanent dental hard tissue in the oral environment. *J. Dent.* **2000**, *28*, 257–263. [CrossRef]

47. Grenby, T.H.; Phillips, A.; Desai, T.; Mistry, M. Laboratory studies of the dental properties of soft drinks. *Br. J. Nutr.* **1989**, *62*, 451–464. [CrossRef] [PubMed]

48. Lussi, A.; Jaeggi, T. Erosion—Diagnosis and risk factors. *Clin. Oral Investig.* **2008**, *12*, 5–13. [CrossRef] [PubMed]

49. Hughes, J.A.; West, N.X.; Parker, D.M.; van den Braak, M.H.; Addy, M. Effects of ph and concentration of citric, malic and lactic acids on enamel, in vitro. *J. Dent.* **2000**, *28*, 147–152. [CrossRef]

50. Chattopadhyay, S.; Raychaudhuri, U.; Chakraborty, R. Artificial sweeteners–a review. *J. Food Sci. Technol.* **2014**, *51*, 611–621. [CrossRef] [PubMed]

51. Pandit, N.K. *Introduction to the Pharmaceutical Sciences An Integrated Approach*; Soltis, R.P., Ed.; Lippincott Williams and Wilkins: Baltimore, MD, USA, 2012.

52. Hermsen, R.J.; Vrijhoef, M.M. Loss of enamel due to etching with phosphoric or maleic acid. *Dent. Mater.* **1993**, *9*, 332–336. [CrossRef]

53. Fu, B.P.; Yuan, J.; Qian, W.X.; Shen, Q.Y.; Sun, X.M.; Hannig, M. Evidence of chemisorption of maleic acid to enamel and hydroxyapatite. *Eur. J. Oral Sci.* **2004**, *112*, 362–367. [CrossRef] [PubMed]

54. Olsen, M.E.; Bishara, S.E.; Damon, P.; Jakobsen, J.R. Evaluation of scotchbond multipurpose and maleic acid as alternative methods of bonding orthodontic brackets. *Am. J. Orthod. Dentofac. Orthop.* **1997**, *111*, 498–501. [CrossRef]

55. Mahoney, E.K.; Rohanizadeh, R.; Ismail, F.S.M.; Kilpatrick, N.M.; Swain, M.V. Mechanical properties and microstructure of hypomineralised enamel of permanent teeth. *Biomaterials* **2004**, *25*, 5091–5100. [CrossRef] [PubMed]

56. Fagrell, T.G.; Dietz, W.; Jälevik, B.; Norén, J.G. Chemical, mechanical and morphological properties of hypomineralized enamel of permanent first molars. *Acta Odontol. Scand.* **2010**, *68*, 215. [CrossRef] [PubMed]

57. Kodaka, T.; Debari, K.; Kuroiwa, M. Mineral content of the innermost enamel in erupted human teeth. *J. Electron. Microsc.* **1991**, *40*, 19–23.

58. Sasaki, T.; Debrari, K.; Garant, P.R. Ameloblast modulation and changes in the Ca, P, and S content of developing enamel matrix revealed by SEM-EDX. *J. Dent. Res.* **1987**, *66*, 778–786. [CrossRef] [PubMed]

59. Jälevik, B.; Odelius, H.; Dietz, W.; Norén, J. Secondary ion mass spectrometry and X-ray microanalysis of hypomineralized enamel in human permanent first molars. *Arch. Oral Biol.* **2001**, *46*, 239–247. [CrossRef]

60. Larsen, M.J. Chemical events during tooth dissolution. *J. Dent. Res.* **1990**, *69*, 575–580. [CrossRef] [PubMed]

61. Edgar, W.M. Sugar substitutes, chewing gumand dental caries-a review. *Br. Dent. J.* **1998**, *184*, 29–32. [CrossRef] [PubMed]

4

Weight Status and Dental Problems in Early Childhood: Classification Tree Analysis of a National Cohort

Michael Crowe [1],* , Michael O' Sullivan [1] , Oscar Cassetti [1] and Aifric O' Sullivan [2]

[1] Division of Restorative Dentistry & Periodontology, Dublin Dental University Hospital, Trinity College Dublin, Dublin, Dublin 2, Ireland; michael.osullivan@dental.tcd.ie (M.O.S.); oscar.getstring@gmail.com (O.C.)

[2] UCD Institute of Food and Health, 2.05 Science Centre, South, UCD, Belfield, Dublin, Dublin 4, Ireland; aifric.osullivan@ucd.ie

* Correspondence: michael.crowe@dental.tcd.ie;

Abstract: A poor quality diet may be a common risk factor for both obesity and dental problems such as caries. The aim of this paper is to use classification tree analysis (CTA) to identify predictors of dental problems in a nationally representative cohort of Irish pre-school children. CTA was used to classify variables and describe interactions between multiple variables including socio-demographics, dietary intake, health-related behaviour, body mass index (BMI) and a dental problem. Data were derived from the second (2010/2011) wave of the 'Growing Up in Ireland' study (GUI) infant cohort at 3 years, $n = 9793$. The prevalence of dental problems was 5.0% ($n = 493$). The CTA model showed a sensitivity of 67% and specificity of 58.5% and overall correctly classified 59% of children. Ethnicity was the most significant predictor of dental problems followed by longstanding illness or disability, mother's BMI and household income. The highest prevalence of dental problems was among children who were obese or underweight with a longstanding illness and an overweight mother. Frequency of intake of some foods showed interactions with the target variable. Results from this research highlight the interconnectedness of weight status, dental problems and general health and reinforce the importance of adopting a common risk factor approach when dealing with prevention of these diseases.

Keywords: body mass index; diet; dental problem; classification tree

1. Introduction

Early childhood caries (ECC) is a disease defined by the presence of one or more decayed, missing (due to caries), or filled tooth surfaces in any primary tooth in a child < 71 months old [1]. ECC is the most prevalent dental problem in pre-schoolers [2], one of the most common causes of hospital admission and the most common cause of dental extractions under general anaesthesia [1,2]. Obesity, defined as an excess of body fat [3], is another growing concern among preschool children. Body mass index (BMI) is frequently used to classify adults as overweight or obese; however, classifying overweight and obesity in children is complicated by age and gender specific differences [3,4]. For this reason, the International Obesity Task Force (IOTF) defines childhood weight status based on BMI centile curves that correspond to adult criteria from 2 to 18 years for males and females [5]. In Europe, 12%–15% of preschool children are classified as overweight or obese based on IOTF criteria [6]. Concerns around EEC and childhood obesity are heightened by the fact that both are strong predictors of these respective conditions throughout the life-course [7,8].

The preschool age is a particularly important period to minimise the risks for dental caries and obesity [9] and the primary caregiver (PCG) plays a key role in facilitating prevention through feeding patterns and other behaviours [1,8,10]. Obesity and dental caries share some common risk factors including food choice, dietary intake patterns, diet quality and socioeconomic factors such as PCG education and household income [11–13]. Given the associations that exist between oral health and general health interest is growing in using a common risk factor approach to investigate the multidimensional causes of dental and weight-status problems, particularly in preschool children [14–17]. Although some studies have shown a positive relationship between BMI and dental caries, others suggest that they are weakly correlated, inverse or even U-shaped and that different predictors may be associated with dental caries at both high and low BMI levels [11,12,14,17]. Indeed, very few studies report the oral health status of underweight children and often group underweight and normal weight without considering differences in risk [14,18].

Data-driven methods are being increasingly proposed to empirically derive dietary patterns associated with chronic disease [19]. Methods that aim to uncover the relationship between independent variables and a dependent variable are described as supervised learning. The discovered relationship is typically presented as a classification or regression model [20]. Thus, in Classification and Regression Tree Analysis (CART) when the target (dependent) variable is continuous a regression analysis is performed and when the target variable is categorical a classification tree analysis (CTA) is carried out. Data mining techniques are invaluable when analysing multidimensional data from large-scale survey microdata files as they provide a means to identify novel diet-disease relationships and can help establish inter-relationships between causal factors [20].

With a few exceptions, most national dental surveys tend to focus on children aged 5 and older. While nationally representative studies of obesity prevalence in older Irish children are well documented [21] there are few, apart from a National Preschool Nutrition Survey [22] that relate to pre-schoolers. The research in this secondary analysis proposed to use a flexible analytical approach (CTA) to explore the multilevel relations between weight status and dental problems in a large, nationally representative cohort of 3-year old children from the 'Growing Up in Ireland' study (GUI).

2. Methods

2.1. Data Collection and Participants

The aim of the GUI infant survey is to determine the individual, family and wider social and environmental factors that affect the development of children. GUI is a nationally representative longitudinal study that collected data from infants at 9 months (Wave-1) and followed up when children were 3-years old (Wave-2) providing the data file used in this study with 9793 cases. Between December 2007 and June 2008 GUI selected a random sample on a systematic basis, pre-stratified by marital status, county of residence, nationality and number of children from the National Child Benefits Register which is a universal welfare entitlement in the Republic of Ireland [23]. The sampling fraction was 0.42 with an overall response of 64.5% providing 11,134 families in Wave 1. Follow-up interviews for Wave-2 occurred between December 2010 and July 2011 and 91% of families responded while 3.8% emigrated or deceased and the remainder either refused or were not contactable. The PCG was interviewed in the family home using a questionnaire after written informed consent was obtained [23].

2.2. Anthropometric Measurements

A standard (Leicester) portable height stick was used to measure height of PCGs and children. The weight of the children was recorded using a digital scales (SECA 835, Hamburg, Germany). Data for height and weight of the PCGs were used from Wave-1 measurements and only taken at Wave-2 if they were missing or required rechecking. PCG weight was recorded using a flat mechanical scale (SECA 761, Hamburg, Germany).

BMI was calculated as weight divided by height squared (kg/m^2) and, for children, classified as overweight, obese, normal weight or thinness according to the IOTF age and gender specific cut-offs for 3-year olds [5,24]. For simplicity, the classification of thinness (low BMI for age) is also described as underweight in this paper although the latter strictly means low weight for age in children. Overweight and obesity for children was also classified using the UK adaptation of percentile cut-offs from the WHO Multicentre Growth Reference Study (MGRS) with overweight criteria defined as a BMI between the 91st and 98th percentile while obesity was defined as a BMI on or greater than the 98th percentile [25]. PCG BMI was categorised into underweight (BMI < 18.5), normal (BMI 18.5–24.9), overweight (BMI 25–29.9) and obese (BMI > 30).

2.3. CTA Target Variable

The dichotomous target variable was a PCG reported dental problem. The question asked was: Has <child> been to visit the dentist because of a problem with his/her teeth?

2.4. CTA Predictor Variables

Attributes (independent variables) that were relevant to the target variable (dependent variable) were selected for inclusion in the model based on findings from previous research. The demographic and socioeconomic variables selected were child gender, PCG age and gender, ethnicity, PCG education level, family social class and annual equivalised household income [1,14–16,26,27]. Ethnicity was defined as Irish, Any other White background, Black, Asian or Other. The highest education level attained by the PCG was one of thirteen categories ranging from no formal education to doctorate level which was collapsed to five groups for descriptive analysis. Family social class was measured using the Irish Central Statistics Office's classification based on occupation, categorising families into one of seven groups which was collapsed to four groups for descriptive analysis. Annual disposable household income was calculated by using an equivalence scale to "weight" each household for differences in size and composition with respect to number of adults and children [23]. Markers of health status [12,13,26,28] included PCG reported child illness, disability, allergies and injuries, as well as TV-viewing hours, tooth-brushing, soother/thumb-sucking, and breastfeeding as markers of health behaviour [9,14,26,29]. Dietary intake [9,11,26] was assessed using a modified version of the Sallis-Amherst Food Frequency Questionnaire from the Longitudinal Study of Australian Children (LSAC) [30]. PCG reported the child's frequency of consumption of 15 food categories (e.g., 'sweets', 'fizzy drinks/minerals/cordials') over the previous 24-h as once, more than once or none at all.

2.5. Data Analysis

Wave-1 GUI data were statistically re-weighted to represent the population. Wave-2 data was weighted for attrition between waves and emigration combined with the Wave-1 weight [31].

Classification tree analysis (CTA) is based on recursive partitioning whereby the algorithm repeatedly creates splits in the sample based on the most significant predictor variable. The root node contains the entire sample and each subsequent split results in child nodes with the proportion of the classes displayed together with an adjusted P value. For this analysis the following parameters were selected in either SPSS (v. 20.0: SPSS, Chicago, IL, USA) or SPSS modeller (IBM SPSS Modeler v. 14.2: Chicago, IL, USA) using the Chi-squared Automatic Interaction Detection (CHAID) algorithm [32]: maximum tree depth = 5, parent node = 100, child node = 50 and bonferroni-adjusted chi-square statistic, significance < 0.05. A 10-fold cross-validation assessed model performance and produced an average misclassification risk. Details of the analysis methods were previously reported [33]. The degree of missing cases in the 3-year old GUI infant cohort was small except for the PCG BMI (5.2%), equivalised annual income (5.5%) and child BMI (2.6%), as previously reported [29]. The CHAID algorithm handles missing values by defining a separate category and treating them as a single category so that they are not excluded in the analysis [34]. A binary logistical regression analysis (*forward-wald*) was also conducted to compare findings with those generated by the classification tree output. A confusion matrix for a binary classifier provided estimation of selected performance metrics.

3. Results

3.1. Cohort Profile

Five percent of 3-year olds had a dental problem. As is common in investigations of health outcome the class distribution of the dataset was imbalanced. The minority class was the positive instances of having 'a dental problem' and the negative response was the majority class.

Table 1 describes the cohort characteristics, including anthropometric measurements, child health and behaviours. Almost all of the self-identified PCGs were female and the biological parent of the study child. Eighty five percent were 'Irish'. Using the IOTF cut-offs [5] the prevalence of thinness and obesity were 5.7% each with an additional ~18% of children being overweight. Using the WHO growth charts and BMI cut-offs, the prevalence of overweight was 18.5% and obesity was 12.8%.

Table 1. Weighted [a] Sample Characteristics, Growing Up in Ireland infant cohort participants 2010/11 (Child 3-years of age).

	Child		PCG	
			Mean	SD
Age (years)			29.6	(6.1)
Gender	*n*	%	*n*	%
Male	5024	51.3	161	1.6
Female	4769	48.7	9632	98.4
Anthropometrics	**Mean**	**SD**	**Mean**	**SD**
Weight (Kg)	15.27	(2.02)		
Height (m)	95.48	(3.92)		
Body Mass Index (Kg/m^2)				
Total	16.71	(1.61)	25.99	(5.16)
Male	16.99	(1.52)	26.98	(5.59)
Female	16.71	(1.61)	25.97	(5.15)
BMI Categories	*n*	%	*n*	%
Thinness IOTF	557	5.7	166	1.7
Normal IOTF	6685	68.3		
Normal WHO	6464	66.0	4523	46.2
Overweight IOTF	1737	17.7		
Overweight WHO	1815	18.5	2941	30.0
Obese IOTF	559	5.7		
Obese WHO	1257	12.8	1655	16.9
Missing	256	2.6	508	5.2
Child Health and Behaviours	*n*	%		
Dental Problems (in last 12 months)	493	5		
Longstanding illness or disability	1543	15.8		
Hospital admission (ever)	1569	16.1		
Tooth brushing 2 or more per day	5107	52.2		
Tooth brushing <2 per day	4685	47.8		
Thumb sucking	765	7.8		
Soother	3163	32.3		
TV viewing time (min/day)	1133	(72.0)		
TV viewing 1 hour or less per day	3569	36.4		
TV viewing 2 hours or less per day	3587	36.6		
TV viewing 2 hours or more per day	2630	26.9		

Table 1. *Cont.*

Child	PCG	
	Mean	SD
Socio-Demographics	*n*	%
Ethnicity		
Irish	8261	84.4
Non-Irish white	1018	10.4
Black	252	2.6
Asian	202	2.1
Other	54	0.6
Family Social Class		
Professional/Managerial	4553	46.5
Other non-manual/Skilled manual	3233	33.0
Semi-skilled/Unskilled	1061	10.8
Unclassified	947	9.7
Highest Education Level		
Lower secondary or less	1361	13.9
Upper secondary	3192	32.6
Non-degree	2080	21.2
Third level	3144	32.1
	Mean	SD
Equivalised Annual Income (€)	18,004	(10,997)

Data presented as mean and standard deviation (SD) or n and percentage. [a] Sample weighting factors applied to statistically adjust the data to be more representative of the population. IOTF, International Obesity Task Force; WHO, World Health Organisation.

The frequency of food items consumed are reported in Figure 1. The majority of children consumed water' (~83.0%), 'full-fat milk/cream' (~84.5%), 'full-fat cheese/yoghurt' (~85.0%), 'cooked veg' (~85.0%), 'fresh fruit' (~89%), and 'biscuits/doughnuts/cake/chocolate' (~74%) once or more than once in the previous 24-h. Of interest, a considerable proportion of 3-year olds consumed "un-healthy" foods including 'crisps' (~47%), "hot-chips" (~28%), sugar containing drinks (~30%), and sweets (~49%).

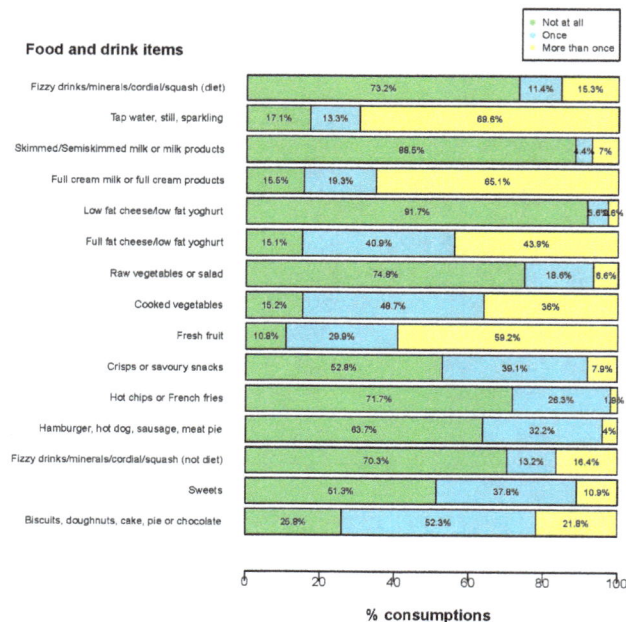

Figure 1. Food and drink items consumed in previous 24 h by the Growing Up in Ireland infant cohort at 3-years of age.

3.2. Classification Tree Analysis

CHAID analysis generated a CTA output as depicted in Figure 2 with 30 nodes, including 17 terminal nodes. Each node contains the number and percentage of infants in each category for the dependant variable (dental problem), the categories chosen by CHAID for the predictor variable and the cut-off points for continuous variables. PCG ethnicity was the most important predictor of the 3-year old child having a dental problem splitting the root node. Twelve predictor variables were included in the final tree (Bonferroni-adjusted $p < 0.05$). Two predictors appeared twice in the output, PCG BMI (nodes 2 and 5) and equivalised household annual income (nodes 3 and 4). A confusion matrix (Table 2) produced performance metrics for the classification tree: sensitivity 66.8%, specificity 58.5% and overall accuracy 58.9%.

The ethnic subgroups were split into 3 nodes with the highest prevalence of dental problems (8.4%) among those children from a "non-Irish white" background (Node-3). Node-1 contained almost 87% of the sample (Irish and Asian ethnicity) with a 4.7% prevalence of dental problems. The tree output from node-1 to nodes 22–24 delineated subgroups linking child BMI categories with dental problems by the following predictors: PCG from an Irish/Asian background (node-1), the presence of a longstanding illness or disability in the child (node-5) and an overweight mother (node-13). The final predictor at node-13 was BMI classification of the child which split into three terminal nodes resulting in normal, overweight/missing and obese/underweight subgroups. The highest dental problem prevalence (19%, $n = 17$) was in those children in this final subgroup who were obese or underweight (node-24). Also, the subgroup at node-1 who had a longstanding illness or disability had a reported dental problem prevalence of 7.0% while those with no illness or disability had a prevalence of 4.3% (node-4). The food variables included in the tree output were 'water' (level-3), 'low-fat cheese/yoghurt' (level-4) and 'raw vegetables/salad', 'fresh fruit' and 'hot chips'.

Logistic regression failed to generate a significant model (chi-square (6) = 9.38, $p = 0.15$).

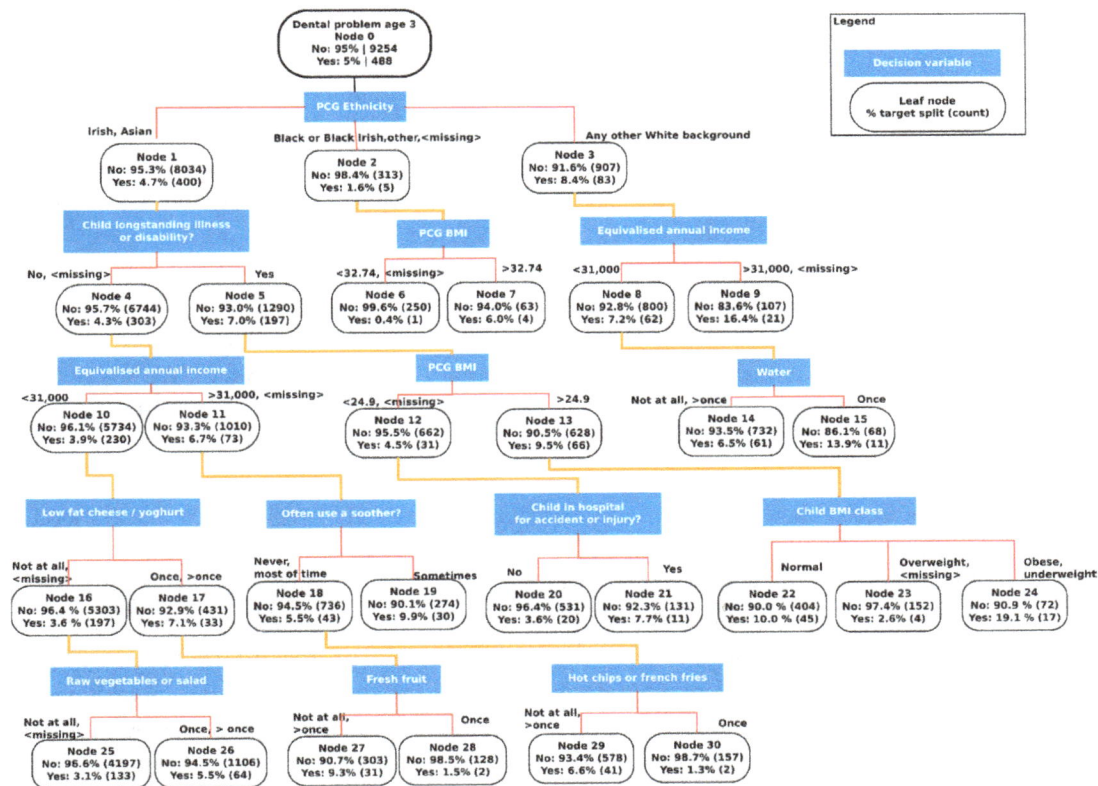

Figure 2. Prevalence of reported dental problems by the Growing Up in Ireland infant cohort at 3-years of age among classification tree subgroups, percentage (%) and number (n) in each class.

Table 2. Confusion matrix showing selected performance measures for Classification tree analysis of dental problem prevalence in the Growing Up in Ireland infant cohort at 3-years of age.

Observed		Predicted Dental Problem		Percentage Correct	Measure
		Yes	No		
Dental problem	Yes	326	162	66.8%	Sensitivity [a]
	No	3839	5415	58.5%	Specificity [b]
Overall percentage				58.9%	Accuracy [c]

[a] Sensitivity = True Positive Rate = Number of True Positives/(Number of True Positives + Number of False Negatives); [b] Specificity = True Negative Rate = Number of True Negatives/(Number of True Negatives + Number of False Positives); [c] Accuracy = (True Positives + True Negatives)/(True Positives + False Positives + False Negatives + True Negatives)

4. Discussion

This study used a CHAID classification tree as a method to classify the dataset and identify relationships between the predictor variables selected and the target variable (a PCG-reported dental problem requiring a visit to the dentist). PCG ethnicity was the most significant predictor of dental problems in the CTA model and the highest prevalence of dental problems in this study was among children who were obese or underweight with a longstanding illness and an overweight PCG.

This analysis was carried out using data from a nationally representative cohort of 3-year old children, the largest child population study ever carried out in Ireland, which includes a wide range of PCG and child health and development characteristics. CTA is a non-parametric method which handles nominal and numeric input and classification trees are ideal for representing complex interactions [20]. The output produces a visualisation of all the significant interactions with the target variable at multiple levels and can, potentially, uncover subgroups that might not be discovered using other data methods [34]. The partitioning variable at the first level of the classification tree was PCG ethnicity while at the next level the most significant predictors of dental problems were the child having a longstanding illness, PCG BMI and household income. It has been reported that trends in overweight and obesity differ among different ethnic groups, even at the early preschool age, and that this cannot be explained by variations in household income [35]. Similarly, the disparities in dental caries prevalence between different ethnic groups is not fully explained by social inequalities [27]. Surprisingly, ethnicity has been used as a variable in relatively few studies of dental caries in children while the PCG education level, although it was not a significant predictor in our CTA model, has been consistently shown to be an important risk factor for caries in children [26].

While the results of our CTA are exploratory they identify certain characteristics previously suggested as risk factors or risk indicators for both obesity and dental caries [14,26,36]. The study supports recent views that data driven-outcome dependant methods such as CTA are potentially useful for investigating dietary components or patterns most associated with a health outcome and are a valid, non-parametric, alternative to logistic regression analysis [19]. The results of this analysis must be cautiously interpreted by gauging the model performance (Table 2) and understanding the limitations of both the data structure and classification tree algorithms. An imbalanced class distribution has been characterised as "one that has many more instances of some classes than others [37]. CTA of imbalanced data sets tends to result in high predictive accuracy for the majority class and low accuracy for the minority class [34]. In most health outcome investigations, including dental problems, the correct classification of the minority class is of greater interest or value than that of the majority class. The confusion matrix (Table 2) shows the results of the actual and predicted classifications carried out by CTA. The metrics calculated include sensitivity or recall (66.8%) which is the proportion of actual positive cases correctly predicted by the model and specificity (58.5%) which is the proportion of actual negative cases correctly identified by the model. The overall accuracy (58.9%) indicated the proportion of the total number of correct predictions. Logistic regression did not perform well as a classifier and none of the same input variables were significant in the final regression model. This may be due to inherent differences in the way CTA captures the division of the classes by partitioning the space using multiple decision boundaries whereas logistic regression uses a single linear decision boundary [34]. To be suitable as a prediction model for targeting risk it has been suggested that both sensitivity and specificity should be 80% or the sum be at least 160% [38].

While overweight and obesity dominate the focus of recent research with children, it is important to consider underweight (thinness) in early childhood as a condition related to poor health outcomes also. There is some evidence to suggest that dental caries may be associated with children who are underweight and suffer with slow growth due to pain on mastication [15,18,28]. The results (Table 1) shows a similar prevalence of underweight and obese children. A small subgroup (node-24) of children which combined obese and underweight categories had the highest prevalence of dental problems (19%) in the sample. This group were predominantly Irish with a longstanding illness and had an overweight PCG. It should also be noted that normal weight children (node-22) in this group had a dental problem prevalence of 10% approximately half that of the obese/underweight group, but double that of the overall sample. This finding of itself highlights the interconnectedness of weight status, dental problems and general health and reinforces the importance of adopting a common risk factor approach when dealing with prevention of these diseases [13,39]. However, while of interest in classifying this dataset, it is important to be cautious when interpreting these subgroups identified by CTA as hierarchical splitting means that they are mutually exclusive. Furthermore, successful targeting of high risk population subgroups for problems with both weight status and dental health would require a risk prediction model with both high sensitivity and specificity.

The prevalence of PCG-reported dental problems requiring a visit to the dentist was 5% which may be an under-estimate given that dental problems are often not treated unless symptomatic in the preschool years [28]. This age is a pivotal period for development of both obesity and dental caries as patterns of eating behaviour that predispose to later development of these conditions are established [8,10,15]. The prevalence of overweight or obesity in 3-year old children determined by IOTF cut-offs was approximately 23% which was similar to previous reports [22]. Almost 47% of PCG's were overweight or obese and it is well established that parental overweight and obesity increases the risk of a child becoming overweight [39]. There are limitations in using BMI as an indirect measure of "fatness" particularly with respect to children [4] and it is important to note that there is no reference population in Ireland for grading BMI. In the CTA, we used the IOTF classification as the more conservative estimate of obese children with a higher cut-off threshold. The FFQ adopted for the GUI survey was a modified dietary screening recall and provided an indication of types and frequency of foods consumed. While PCG-reported measures of foods consumed on a single occasion may be useful in differentiating patterns of food intake it does not provide a good estimate of usual daily consumption and cannot accurately capture total energy or total nutrient intake [40]. Preschool children with unhealthy eating habits have an increased likelihood of experiencing dental caries [10]. While obesity and dental caries are both diet-mediated diseases it is clear that sugars are required in the diet for dental caries to occur [41] whereas a high consumption of energy dense foods including sugars and saturated fats are linked with obesity [16,39]. Fundamentally, obesity occurs due to an energy imbalance between calories consumed versus those expended over a period of time [11,39]. Approximately 74% of the children in GUI consumed biscuits, doughnuts, cake, pie or chocolate at least once or more than once in a 24-h period (Figure 1). Almost 49% of children ate sweets and 30% drank non-diet fizzy drinks, minerals, cordials or squash at least once or more than once. Dietary interventions aimed at reducing the intake of these unhealthy food groups may help impact on both obesity and dental caries but further investigation of these factors in longitudinal studies is still required, especially given the temporal and cumulative aspects of both conditions.

The results of this data analysis may help raise awareness among clinicians and nutrition researchers of the interrelations between weight status and dental problems, even before the primary dentition is complete. Classification tree analysis visually demonstrates how factors, such as the BMI of the primary caregiver (PCG), can interact at multiple levels and affect different subgroups of the child population. Future intervention strategies for oral health should involve consideration of the weight of both the young child and PCG at both the patient and population level. This approach has been advocated recently as both obesity and dental caries may be more likely to occur in the same populations [17]. Given the increasing public health implications of these conditions adopting a more interdisciplinary approach to shared risk factors may assist in the reduction of both problems.

A limitation of CTA is that the hierarchical nature of recursive partitioning has an inherent instability to small changes in the learning data [34]. Overfitting of the model is a known problem and this can be guarded against by using cross-validation which splits the dataset into a training portion and test portion before estimating an average misclassification risk [20]. While dental caries is the most common dental problem at this age the survey did not include a report of the outcome of the dental visit. However, it has been shown that dental disease and treatment need of young children are associated with parents' perceptions of their children's oral health status [42]. Also, it is important to note that this study was based on a cross sectional rather than longitudinal analysis of the infant cohort from the GUI survey. The data is reliant on PCG reporting and this is subject to recall bias and social desirability, particularly in relation to reporting of food and drink perceived as 'healthy' or 'unhealthy'. Further research is focussed on maximising the quality of food intake data by augmenting the GUI survey data with more reliable dietary intake values from a national nutritional database [43] and using the longitudinal aspect of the next wave of the GUI infant cohort. Inclusion of more detailed oral health measures should also be considered.

5. Conclusions

The highest prevalence of dental problems in this study was among children who were obese or underweight with a longstanding illness and an overweight PCG. Societal changes may require renewed focus on oral health policies to focus on minority groups and CTA is a novel approach for exploring large survey data and health-related outcomes. The common risk factor approach may be a pragmatic means of developing shared modifiable strategies for prevention of both dental and weight problems.

Acknowledgments: Data have been collected under the Statistics Act, 1993, of the Central Statistics Office. The GUI survey has been designed and carried out by the ESRI-TCD Growing up in Ireland team.

Author Contributions: All authors contributed equally to this work.

References

1.   Gussy, M.G.; Waters, E.G.; Walsh, O.; Kilpatrick, N.M. Early childhood caries: Current evidence for aetiology and prevention. *J. Paediatr. Child Health* **2006**, *42*, 37–43. [CrossRef] [PubMed]

2.   Public Health England. *National Dental Epidemiology Programme for England: Oral Health Survey of Five-Year-Old Children 2012*; A Report on the Prevalence and Severity of Dental Decay; Public Health England: London, UK, 2013. Available online: http://www.nwph.net/dentalhealth/survey-results5.aspx?id=1 (accessed on 20 February 2017).

3.   Flegal, K.M.; Ogden, C.L. Childhood obesity: Are we all speaking the same language? *Adv. Nutr.* **2011**, *2*, 159S–166S. [CrossRef] [PubMed]

4.   Rolland-Cachera, M.F. Childhood obesity: Current definitions and recommendations for their use. *Int. J. Pediatr. Obes.* **2011**, *6*, 325–331. [CrossRef] [PubMed]

5.   Cole, T.J.; Bellizzi, M.C.; Flegal, K.M.; Dietz, W.H. Establishing a standard definition for child overweight and obesity worldwide: International survey. *BMJ* **2000**, *320*, 1240. [CrossRef] [PubMed]

6.   Ahrens, W.; Pigeot, I.; Pohlabeln, H.; de Henauw, S.; Lissner, L.; Molnár, D.; Moreno, L.; Tornaritis, M.; Veidebaum, T.; Siani, A. Prevalence of overweight and obesity in European children below the age of 10. *Int. J. Obes.* **2014**, *38*, S99–S107. [CrossRef] [PubMed]

7.   Dye, B.A.; Hsu, K.L.; Afful, J. Prevalence and measurement of dental caries in young children. *Pediatr. Dent.* **2015**, *37*, 200–216. [PubMed]

8. Wake, M.; Hardy, P.; Sawyer, M.G.; Carlin, J.B. Comorbidities of overweight/obesity in australian preschoolers: A cross-sectional population study. *Arch. Dis. Child.* **2008**, *93*, 502–507. [CrossRef] [PubMed]

9. Chaffee, B.W.; Feldens, C.A.; Rodrigues, P.H.; Vitolo, M.R. Feeding practices in infancy associated with caries incidence in early childhood. *Commun. Dent. Oral Epidemiol.* **2015**, *43*, 338–348. [CrossRef] [PubMed]

10. Dye, B.A.; Shenkin, J.D.; Ogden, C.L.; Marshall, T.A.; Levy, S.M.; Kanellis, M.J. The relationship between healthful eating practices and dental caries in children aged 2–5 years in the united states, 1988–1994. *J. Am. Dent. Assoc.* **2004**, *135*, 55–66. [CrossRef] [PubMed]

11. Marshall, T.A.; Eichenberger-Gilmore, J.M.; Broffitt, B.A.; Warren, J.J.; Levy, S.M. Dental caries and childhood obesity: Roles of diet and socioeconomic status. *Commun. Dent. Oral Epidemiol.* **2007**, *35*, 449–458. [CrossRef] [PubMed]

12. Kantovitz, K.R.; Pascon, F.M.; Rontani, R.M.P.; Gaviao, M.B.D. Obesity and dental caries—A systematic review. *Oral Health Prev. Dent.* **2006**, *4*, 137–144. [PubMed]

13. Sheiham, A.; Watt, R.G. The common risk factor approach: A rational basis for promoting oral health. *Commun. Dent. Oral Epidemiol.* **2000**, *28*, 399–406. [CrossRef]

14. Hooley, M.; Skouteris, H.; Boganin, C.; Satur, J.; Kilpatrick, N. Body mass index and dental caries in children and adolescents: A systematic review of literature published 2004 to 2011. *Syst. Rev.* **2012**, *1*, 57. [CrossRef] [PubMed]

15. Hooley, M.; Skouteris, H.; Millar, L. The relationship between childhood weight, dental caries and eating practices in children aged 4–8 years in australia, 2004–2008. *Pediatr. Obes.* **2012**, *7*, 461–470. [CrossRef] [PubMed]

16. Hayden, C.; Bowler, J.O.; Chambers, S.; Freeman, R.; Humphris, G.; Richards, D.; Cecil, J.E. Obesity and dental caries in children: A systematic review and meta-analysis. *Commun. Dent. Oral Epidemiol.* **2012**, *41*, 289–308. [CrossRef] [PubMed]

17. Public Health England. *The Relationship between Dental Caries and Obesity in Children: An Evidence Summary*; Public Health England: London, UK, 2015. Available online: https://www.gov.uk/government/publications/dental-caries-and-obesity-their-relationship-in-children (accessed on 5 March 2017).

18. Tramini, P.; Molinari, N.; Tentscher, M.; Demattei, C.; Schulte, A.G. Association between caries experience and body mass index in 12-year-old french children. *Caries Res.* **2009**, *43*, 468–473. [CrossRef] [PubMed]

19. Krebs-Smith, S.M.; Subar, A.F.; Reedy, J. Examining dietary patterns in relation to chronic disease: Matching measures and methods to questions of interest. *Circulation* **2015**, *132*, 790–793. [CrossRef] [PubMed]

20. Yoo, I.; Alafaireet, P.; Marinov, M.; Pena-Hernandez, K.; Gopidi, R.; Chang, J.F.; Hua, L. Data mining in healthcare and biomedicine: A survey of the literature. *J. Med. Syst.* **2012**, *36*, 2431–2448. [CrossRef] [PubMed]

21. Keane, E.; Kearney, P.M.; Perry, I.J.; Kelleher, C.C.; Harrington, J.M. Trends and prevalence of overweight and obesity in primary school aged children in the republic of ireland from 2002–2012: A systematic review. *BMC Public Health* **2014**, *14*, 974. [CrossRef] [PubMed]

22. Walton, J. *National Pre-School Nutrition Survey*; Summary Report on: Food and Nutrient Intakes, Physical Measurements and Barriers to Healthy Eating; Irish Universities Nutrition Alliance: Dublin, Ireland, 2012. Available online: http://www.iuna.net/ (accessed on 11 March 2017).

23. Murray, A.; Quail, A.; McCrory, C.; Williams, J. *A Summary Guide to Wave 2 of the Infant Cohort (at 3 Years) of Growing up in Ireland*; The Economic and Social Research Institute: Dublin, Ireland, 2013.

24. Cole, T.J.; Flegal, K.M.; Nicholls, D.; Jackson, A.A. Body mass index cut offs to define thinness in children and adolescents: International survey. *BMJ* **2007**, *335*, 194. [CrossRef] [PubMed]

25. Cole, T.J.; Wright, C.M.; Williams, A.F.; Group, R.G.C.E. Designing the new uk-who growth charts to enhance assessment of growth around birth. *Arch. Dis. Child. Fetal Neonatal Ed.* **2012**, *97*, F219–F222. [CrossRef] [PubMed]

26. Harris, R.; Nicoll, A.D.; Adair, P.M.; Pine, C.M. Risk factors for dental caries in young children: A systematic review of the literature. *Commun. Dent. Health* **2004**, *21*, 71–85.

27. Van der Tas, J.T.; Kragt, L.; Veerkamp, J.J.; Jaddoe, V.W.; Moll, H.A.; Ongkosuwito, E.M.; Elfrink, M.E.; Wolvius, E.B. Ethnic disparities in dental caries among six-year-old children in the netherlands. *Caries Res.* **2016**, *50*, 489–497. [CrossRef] [PubMed]

28. Sheiham, A. Dental caries affects body weight, growth and quality of life in pre-school children. *Br. Dent. J.* **2006**, *201*, 625–626. [CrossRef] [PubMed]

29. Layte, R.; Bennett, A.; McCrory, C.; Kearney, J. Social class variation in the predictors of rapid growth in infancy and obesity at age 3 years. *Int. J. Obes.* **2014**, *38*, 82–90. [CrossRef] [PubMed]

30. Sallis, J.F.; Taylor, W.C.; Dowda, M.; Freedson, P.S.; Pate, R.R. Correlates of vigorous physical activity for children in grades 1 through 12: Comparing parent-reported and objectively measured physical activity. *Pediatr. Exer. Sci.* **2002**, *14*, 30. [CrossRef]

31. Quail, A.; Williams, J.; McCrory, C.; Murray, A.; Thornton, M. *Sample Design and Response in Wave 1 of the Infant Cohort (at 9 months) of Growing up in Ireland*; Department of Health and Children: Dublin, Ireland, 2011.

32. Kass, G.V. An exploratory technique for investigating large quantities of categorical data. *Appl. Stat.* **1980**, *29*, 119–127. [CrossRef]

33. Crowe, M.; O'Sullivan, A.; McGrath, C.; Cassetti, O.; Swords, L.; O'Sullivan, M. Early childhood dental problems classification tree analyses of 2 waves of an infant cohort study. *JDR Clin. Trans. Res.* **2016**, *1*, 275–284. [CrossRef]

34. Maimon, O.; Rokach, L. Classification trees. In *Data Mining and Knowledge Discovery Handbook*; Maimon, O., Rokach, L., Eds.; Springer: New York, NY, USA, 2005; Volume 2, pp. 149–174.

35. Karlsen, S.; Morris, S.; Kinra, S.; Vallejo-Torres, L.; Viner, R.M. Ethnic variations in overweight and obesity among children over time: Findings from analyses of the health surveys for england 1998–2009. *Pediatr. Obes.* **2014**, *9*, 186–196. [CrossRef] [PubMed]

36. De Onis, M.; Lobstein, T. Defining obesity risk status in the general childhood population: Which cut-offs should we use? *Int. J. Pediatr. Obes.* **2010**, *5*, 458–460. [CrossRef] [PubMed]

37. Sun, Y.; Kamel, M.S.; Wong, A.K.C.; Wang, Y. Cost-sensitive boosting for classification of imbalanced data. *Pattern Recognit.* **2007**, *40*, 3358–3378. [CrossRef]

38. Hausen, H. Caries prediction–state of the art. *Commun. Dent. Oral Epidemiol.* **1997**, *25*, 87–96. [CrossRef]

39. Lobstein, T.; Jackson-Leach, R.; Moodie, M.L.; Hall, K.D.; Gortmaker, S.L.; Swinburn, B.A.; James, W.P.T.; Wang, Y.; McPherson, K. Child and adolescent obesity: Part of a bigger picture. *Lancet* **2015**, *385*, 2510–2520. [CrossRef]

40. Magarey, A.; Watson, J.; Golley, R.K.; Burrows, T.; Sutherland, R.; McNaughton, S.A.; Denney-Wilson, E.; Campbell, K.; Collins, C. Assessing dietary intake in children and adolescents: Considerations and recommendations for obesity research. *Int. J. Pediatr. Obes.* **2011**, *6*, 2–11. [CrossRef] [PubMed]

41. Peres, M.A.; Sheiham, A.; Liu, P.; Demarco, F.F.; Silva, A.E.; Assuncao, M.C.; Menezes, A.M.; Barros, F.C.; Peres, K.G. Sugar consumption and changes in dental caries from childhood to adolescence. *J. Dent. Res.* **2016**, *95*, 388–394. [CrossRef] [PubMed]

42. Talekar, B.S.; Rozier, R.G.; Slade, G.D.; Ennett, S.T. Parental perceptions of their preschool-aged children's oral health. *J. Am. Dent. Assoc.* **2005**, *136*, 364–372. [CrossRef] [PubMed]

43. Crowe, M.; O'Sullivan, M.; Cassetti, O.; McGrath, C.; O'Sullivan, A. Data mapping to augment dietary intake values from a nutritional database to a national cohort survey: Protocols to improve quality of reported food intake. *Proc. Nutr. Soc.* **2016**, *75*. [CrossRef]

5

The Use of Pit and Fissure Sealants

Reem Naaman [1]**, Azza A. El-Housseiny** [1,2] **and Najlaa Alamoudi** [1,*]

[1] Pediatric Dentistry Department, Faculty of Dentistry, King Abdulaziz University, 21589 Jeddah, Saudi Arabia; dr.reem.naaman@hotmail.com or rnouman@stu.kau.edu.sa (R.N.); aalhosseiny@kau.edu.sa or ahussini@hotmail.com or azza.elhousseiny@dent.alex.edu.eg (A.A.E.-H.)

[2] Pediatric Dentistry Department, Faculty of Dentistry, Alexandria University, 21526 Alexandria, Egypt

[*] Correspondence: nalamoudi2011@gmail.com or nalamoudi@kau.edu.sa;

Abstract: This paper reviews the literature and discusses the latest updates on the use of pit and fissure sealants. It demonstrates the effectiveness of pit and fissure sealants in preventing caries and the management of early carious lesions. It compares the use of different sealant materials and their indications. It describes the application technique for sealants. It also reviews the cost-effectiveness of sealants as a preventive strategy. From this review and after the discussion of recently published studies on pit and fissure sealants, it is evident that sealants are effective in caries prevention and in preventing the progression of incipient lesions. It is therefore recommended that pit and fissure sealant be applied to high-caries-risk children for optimum cost-effectiveness. It is a highly sensitive technique that needs optimum isolation, cleaning of the tooth surface, etching, and the application of a thin bonding layer for maximum benefit. Recall and repair, when needed, are important to maximize the effectiveness of such sealant use.

Keywords: pit and fissure sealants; caries prevention; resin-based sealants

1. Introduction

Dental caries is a multifactorial disease caused by alteration in the composition of the bacterial biofilm, leading to an imbalance between the demineralization and remineralization processes and manifested by the formation of caries lesions in primary and permanent dentitions [1]. The National Health and Nutrition Examination Survey (NHANES) 2011–2012 data showed that 37% of children, aged 2–8 years old, were diagnosed with dental caries in primary teeth, and 21% of children, aged 6–11, and 58% of children, aged 12–19, were diagnosed with dental caries in their permanent teeth. When comparing this data to the earlier survey of 1999–2004, an overall decline in the prevalence of caries in primary teeth and a slight decrease in the caries percentage in permanent teeth was noticed [2,3] (Table 1). However, this decrease was not found to be uniform across different age groups or consistent with sociodemographic status and different tooth surface sites. Instead, it was found that the greatest decrease in caries was among smooth surfaces rather than pits and fissures [4,5]. Pit and fissure caries accounts for about 90% of the caries of permanent posterior teeth and 44% of caries in the primary teeth in children and adolescents [6]. The use of caries preventive approaches, such as community water fluoridation, topical fluoride therapy, plaque control, and dietary sugar control, has been generally seen to be the cause of the overall decline of caries prevalence, which in turn has had a greater effect on smooth surface carious lesion reduction. The plaque retentive nature of pits and fissures make them difficult to clean, thereby causing them to be more susceptible to caries than smooth surfaces and possibly not to be protected by fluoride administration [7].

Table 1. Summary of data reported by NHANES [1] on the prevalence of caries and sealants.

Epidemiology	NHANES 1999–2004	NHANES 2011–2012
Dental Caries Experience		
Total% in Primary Teeth	42%	37%
Age group 2–5	28%	23%
Age group 6–8	51%	56%
Total% in Permanent Teeth in Children	21%	21%
Age group 6–8	10%	14%
Age group 9–11	31%	29%
Total% in Permanent Teeth in Adolescents		
Age group 12–19	59% permanent teeth	58% permanent teeth
Untreated Dental Caries (Primary Teeth)		
Age group 2–5	19%	10%
Age group 6–8	25.5%	20%
Untreated Dental Caries (Permanent Teeth)		
Age group 6–8	4%	3.3%
Age group 9–11	11%	8%
Age group 12–19	19.6	15%
Sealant Prevalence (Had At Least One Sealed Permanent Tooth)		
Age group 6–8	20%	31%
Age group 9–11	40%	49%
Age group 12–19	37%	43%

[1] NHANES: national health and nutrition examination survey.

More effective measures are necessary to protect pits and fissures; these include the use of pit and fissure sealants. Sealant application is a preventive conservative approach involving the introduction of sealants into the pits and fissures of caries prone teeth; this sealant then bonds to the tooth micromechanically, providing a physical barrier that keeps bacteria away from their source of nutrients [8]. Despite the overall increases in sealant use, they are still considered to be underused worldwide although the efficacy and caries-preventive effect of pit and fissure sealants has been well documented in the literature.

Data from NHANES in 2011–2012, when compared to that from a previous survey in 1999–2004, showed an increase in the use of sealants in permanent teeth. About 31% of children, aged 6–8 years old, 49% of children, aged 9–11, and 43% of adolescents, aged 12–19, had at least one sealed permanent tooth [2,3,6] (Table 1).

In Europe, sealant prevalence in adolescents was found to be about 58.8% in Portugal and 8% in Greece [9,10]. In the Middle East, in Saudi Arabia, it was found that only 9% had a minimum of one permanent molar sealed [11].

The aim of this paper was to review the literature regarding the latest updates on the use of pit and fissure sealants on primary and permanent molars in children and adolescents.

2. History of Fissure Sealant Development

In the past, several attempts were made to protect pits and fissures from becoming carious; approaches, such as enamel fissure eradication, were used. This involved the widening of the fissures, or so-called fissurotomy, to transform deep fissures into cleansable ones [12]. Another method was to treat pits and fissures with ammoniacal silver nitrate [13]. None of these approaches, however, had a great measure of success. A more invasive approach was introduced by Hyatt in 1923 and this involved the preparation of a class I cavity that included all deep pits and fissures and the placement of a prophylactic restoration. In fact, this approach remained the treatment of choice until the 1970s [14]. In 1955, Buonocore published his classic study, documenting the method of bonding of acrylic resin to previously etched dental enamel. He described the technique of acid etching, using 85% phosphoric acid for 30 s, as a tool to increase the adhesion of self-curing methyl methacrylate resin materials to dental enamel. This study was indeed the beginning of a revolution in dental clinical practice [15]. In the mid-1960s, Cueto generated the first sealant material, methyl cyanoacrylate, but it was not marketed. This material, however, was prone to bacterial disintegration in the oral cavity over time [16]. Later on, Bowen invented a viscous resin, called bisphenol-a-glycidyl dimethacrylate, and this has become known as BIS-GMA [17]. This class was found to be resistant to degradation and successfully produced a bond with etched enamel. Buonocore made further advances and published his first paper about pit and fissure sealant, describing his successful use of BIS-GMA resin with the use of ultraviolet light in 1970 [18].

3. Pit and Fissure Sealant Materials

Sealants are classified into three sealant materials (Figure 1). The predominant types of sealant materials in the market at present are resin-based sealants and glass ionomer cement-based sealants [19].

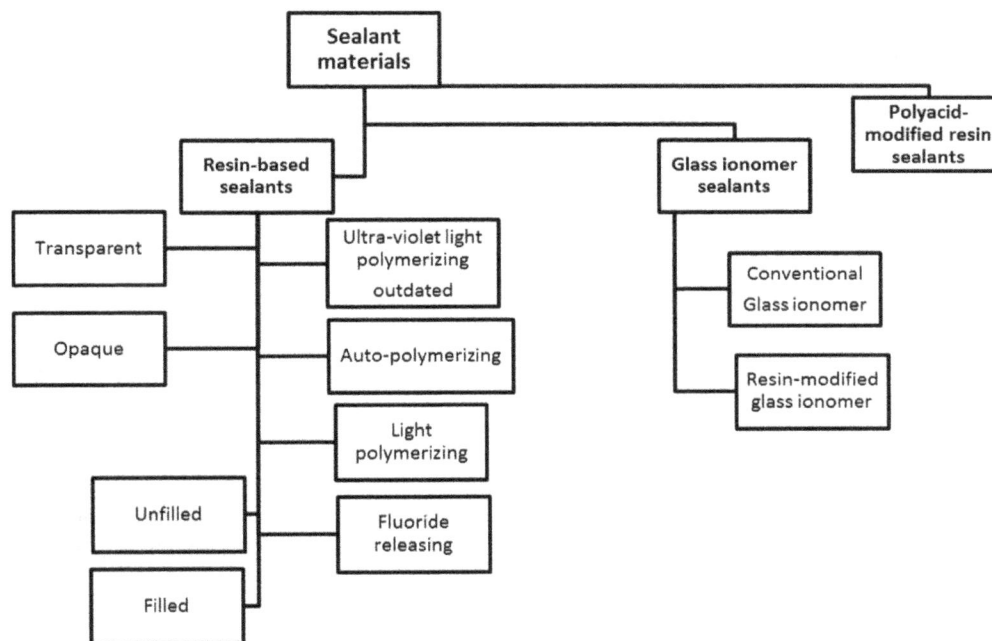

Figure 1. Classification of sealant materials.

3.1. Resin-Based Sealant Materials (RBSs)

Resin-based sealants (RBS) are classified into four generations, determined by the method of polymerization. The first generation of RBS was polymerized by the action of ultraviolet rays on the initiators in the material that initiate polymerization; this type, however, is no longer used [20]. Nuva-Seal® (LD. Caulk Co.: Milford, DE, USA) was the sealant first introduced to the market and is an example of a resin-based sealant polymerized by an ultraviolet light source. The second generation was the auto-polymerizing resin-based sealants (ARBS) or chemically-cured sealants; tertiary amine (the activator) is added to one component and mixed with another component. The reaction between these two components produces free radicals that initiate the polymerization of the resin sealant material [20]. Such autopolymerizing resin-based sealants have now largely been replaced by the third generation, which comprises visible light-polymerizing resin-based sealants (LRBS). In this type of sealant, the visible light activates photoinitiators that are present in the sealant material and are sensitive to visible light in the wavelength region of around 470 nm (blue region) [21]. On comparing this visible light polymerizing to its previous generation, the autopolymerizing resin-based sealant, LRBS, sets in a shorter time, namely, 10–20 s, compared to the 1 to 2 min setting time of ARBS. The working time is longer and the material does not set until exposure to the polymerizing light. Through the elimination of the mixing step, fewer air bubbles are incorporated with the sealant application [22]. The fourth generation is the fluoride-releasing resin-based sealants (FRBS). Fluoride resin-based sealant is the product resulting from adding fluoride-releasing particles to LRBS in an attempt to inhibit caries. According to the literature, however, FRBS cannot be considered as a fluoride reservoir providing a long-term release of fluoride, and, as such, this kind of sealant provides no additional clinical benefit to LRBS [23–25].

RBS can also be classified according to their viscosity (filled and unfilled). The addition of filler particles to fissure sealant material seems to have only a small effect on clinical outcomes. Although filled sealants have a higher wear resistance, their ability to penetrate into fissures is low. The filled sealants usually require occlusal adjustments, which lengthen the procedure unnecessarily. The unfilled resin sealants on the other hand have a lower viscosity and provide greater penetration into fissures and better retention [23,26].

Sealant materials can also be classified according to their translucency (opaque and transparent) [23]. Opaque material can be white or tooth-colored, and transparent sealants can be clear, pink, or amber. White opaque fissure sealantsare easier to see during application and to detect clinically at recall examinations, compared to tooth-colored, opaque, or clear sealants [20]. A study has shown that the identification error was only 1% for the opaque resin sealant, compared to 23% for clear resin sealant [27]. However, the choice of the sealant material is usually a matter of personal preference.

Advances in the technology of resin sealant materials include the incorporation of a color change property. The change of this color property is either in the curing phase, such as Clinpro (3M ESPE, Saint Paul, MN, USA), or in the phase after polymerization, such as Helioseal Clear (Ivoclar Vivadent, Schaan, Liechtenstein). The advantage of this technology has not yet been fully proven but it may indeed offer the advantage of the better recognition of sealed surfaces [20,23]. It therefore seems that the most suitable choice of resin-based sealant would be the light polymerizing, unfilled, opaque sealant.

3.2. Glass Ionomer Sealant Materials

Conventional glass ionomer (GI) material has also been used as pit and fissure sealants. It bonds chemically to enamel and dentin through an acid-base reaction between an aqueous-based polyacrylic acid solution and fluoroaluminosilicate glass powder [28]. GI sealants can be classified into low viscosity and high viscosity types. It is important to recognize that most of the studies on GI sealants used old-generation, low-viscosity GI, such as Fuji III GI sealant that has poor physical properties. It has now been replaced with a later generation, such as Fuji Triage (VII) (GC, Tokyo, Japan), that has better physical properties and is designed to release a higher amount of fluoride [29]. High viscosity glass ionomer cement (HVGIC), such as Ketac Molar Easymix (3M ESPE, Seefeld, Germany) and Fuji IX (GC, Tokyo, Japan), has been used in studies following atraumatic restorative treatment approach (ART). The ART concept consists of two components, namely, ART sealant and ART restoration. ART sealant is the preventive component that includes the application of HVGIC on vulnerable pits and fissures using the finger-press technique [30].

When resin is incorporated with glass ionomer, it is called a resin-modified glass ionomer (RMGI). It has also been used as a pit and fissure sealant material. The setting reaction of this type of sealant is initiated by the photoactivation of the resin component, followed by the acid-based reaction for the ionomer component. Its resin component has improved its physical characteristics, compared to conventional GI [22]. In fact, when compared to conventional GI, RMGI has less sensitivity to water and a longer working-time [28].

In general, the main advantage of a glass ionomer cement-based sealant is the continuous fluoride release and the fluoride recharging ability. Its preventive effect may even last after the visible loss of the sealant material as some parts of the sealant may remain deep in the fissures. It is moisture-friendly and easier to place and is not vulnerable to moisture, compared to the hydrophobic resin-based sealants [22]. It can be used as a transitional sealant when resin-based sealants cannot be used due to difficult moisture control in, for example, partially erupted permanent teeth, especially when the operculum is covering the distal part of the occlusal surface [31]. GI sealant can also be useful in deeply fissured, primary molars that are difficult to isolate due to a child's pre-cooperative behavior [20]. It is considered a provisional sealant and has to be replaced with a resin-based sealant when better isolation is possible [32].

3.3. Polyacid-Modified Resin Based Sealants

Polyacid-modified, resin-based composite material, which is also referred to as compomer, has been used as a fissure sealant. It combines the advantageous properties of a visible light polymerized resin-based sealant with the fluoride releasing property of the GI sealant. A polyacid-modified resin-based sealant has a better adhesion property to enamel and dentin and is also less water-soluble, compared to GI sealant material [33], and less technique-sensitive, compared to resin-based sealants.

4. Different Sealant Materials and Caries Prevention

4.1. Sealant vs. No Sealant

The role of fissure sealants in caries prevention is well established in the literature. There is also a moderate quality of evidence that sealants reduce the incidence of caries by 76% on sound occlusal surfaces, compared to the non-use of sealants during the two to three year follow-up period [28].

A recent update of a Cochrane review evaluated the caries preventive effect of sealants in children and adolescents, compared with a no sealant control group. Thirty eight trials with a total of 7924 participants, aged between 5 and 16 years old, were included. Fifteen trials compared resin-based sealants when applied to the first permanent molars with no sealant and showed a moderate quality of evidence that resin sealants reduced caries increment by between 11 percent and 51 percent in a two year follow-up period. If caries increment was 40 percent in control teeth surfaces, the application of sealant reduced the caries increment to 6.25 percent. At longer follow-up periods of 48 to 54 months, the caries preventive effect of sealants was retained but the quality of evidence was low [34]. This is in agreement with the results of the previously published review [35].

When comparing the caries preventive effect of glass-ionomer based sealants with the use of no sealant, no conclusion could be drawn on whether GI sealant prevented caries, compared to no sealant, at a two year follow-up, due to the very low quality of evidence [34,36].

4.2. Sealant vs. Fluoride Varnish

Several published studies compared pit and fissure sealants' effectiveness to that of fluoride varnish in caries prevention on occlusal surfaces. A recent update of a Cochrane review concluded that there is only a low quality of evidence that pit and fissure sealants have a superior outcome, when compared to fluoride varnish application, in the prevention of occlusal caries. This conclusion is similar to that found in the previous review in 2010 [37]. Two out of three studies included in the last updated review showed a significantly better performance of sealants, compared to fluoride varnish, while the third study reported that the benefits of sealant were not statistically significant, compared to fluoride varnish. Two of the included studies were assessed as having a high overall risk of bias and the third as having an unclear overall risk of bias [38]. The recent evidence-based guidelines of the American Dental Association (ADA), in collaboration with the American Academy of Pediatric Dentistry (AAPD), recommend the use of sealants in preference to no sealant or fluoride varnish, although the quality of evidence for this recommendation was found to be low [5,28]. In fact, this runs counter to the results from a recent randomized clinical trial that compared the clinical effectiveness for caries prevention of fluoride varnish and fissure sealants at a three year follow-up among a 6 to 7 years old population. After three years of follow-up, 17.5% of the fluoride varnish group and 19.6% of the fissure sealant group developed caries in their dentin. The difference between the two groups was not statistically significant [39].

4.3. Resin Based Sealant vs. Glass Ionomer Sealant

The caries preventive effect of resin-based sealants was compared to GI-based sealants in a recent update of a systematic review. Six trials were included in the meta-analysis and they found no statistical significant difference in the caries preventive effect when comparing RBS with GI-based sealants at 24, 36, and 48-month follow-up periods. At the 60-month follow-up, there was a border-line significance in favour of GI-based sealants. However, all the included trials were judged to be at a high risk of bias [40]. The outcome was therefore in agreement with the previously published review [41]. However, the recent update was more concerned with studies about HVGIC rather than low viscosity GIC sealants.

A meta-analysis investigated the survival rates of atraumatic restorative treatment (ART) sealants and restorations using high viscosity glass ionomers (HVGIC). It was concluded that ART sealants have a high caries preventive effect (97%) after three years of application and a survival rate of 72%. This would make them effective alternatives to resin-based sealants [42].

Another recent clinical trial compared the effectiveness of caries prevention between GI sealants and RBS after 48 months and found four carious lesions in the GI group and 12 in the RBS group, but the difference was not statistically significant. The GI sealant was therefore shown to be an effective measure in caries prevention, although it had a significantly lower retention rate compared to RBS [43]. A possible reason behind the caries preventive effect of of GIC, despite it not being as retentive as RBS, is that GI remains in the deepest areas of the fissures, even though it is not clinically evident [44]. When HVGIC is used as part of the ART sealant technique, as described earlier, the sealant may penertrate even deeper into the fissures, compared to the conventional sealant application technique [40]. The anti-caries effect is also related to the fluoride release property of the cement [45]. Nevertheless,in a recent update, the American Dental Association recommendations, in collaboration with the American Academy of Pediatric Dentistry, could not draw any conclusion as to which of the two sealant materials was better due to the very low quality of the evidence available. Table 2 summarizes their findings from comparing the different sealant materials (Table 2) [5,28].

Table 2. Summary of evidence-based findings when comparing different sealant materials.

Sealant Materials	Summary of Findings	Level of Significance	Quality of Evidence
GI vs. RBS	**Sound occlusal surface:** GI reduces caries incidence by 37%	Non-significant	Very low
	Non-cavitated occlusal carious lesion: GI increases incidence of caries by 53%	Non-significant	
	Risk of retention loss: GI has a 5× greater risk of loss	Significant	
GI vs. RMGI	**Sound occlusal surface:** GI increases caries incidence by 41%	Non-significant	Very low
	Risk of retention loss: GI has a 3× greater risk of loss	Significant	
RMGI vs. Polyacid-modified resin sealant	**Sound occlusal surface:** RMGI reduces caries incidence by 56%	Non-significant	Very low
	Risk of retention loss: RMGI has an increased risk of loss of 17%	Non-significant	
Polyacid-modified resin sealant vs. RBS	**Sound occlusal surface:** Poly-acid modified resin sealant increases caries incidence by 1%	Non-significant	Very low
	Risk of retention loss: Poly-acid modified resin sealant has a decreased risk of loss of 13%	Non-significant	

In partially erupted teeth, GI-based sealants may give better results in caries prevention effectiveness, compared to resin-based fissure sealants. A clinical trial compared the retention, marginal staining, and caries prevention properties of GI-based sealants and RBS, when placed on partially erupted, permanent molars. Thirty-nine molar pairs were included in the trial. Both types of sealants had no significant difference in their retention rates; however, the marginal staining was significantly higher for RBS. The GI-sealant group had no caries, while the RBS group had two carious molars and some others showed signs of demineralization. It was concluded that GI might be the better material for sealing partially erupted molars, as well as when salivary contamination is expected [31].

5. Sealant Retention of Different Materials

Previously, when investigating the effectiveness of sealants in preventing caries, half-mouth study designs were used, in which sealed teeth were compared with unsealed teeth as controls. Once the protective role of pit and fissure sealants was established in the 1980s, this type of study design became unethical. In other words, it was no longer acceptable to leave teeth with no sealant as a control after the efficiency of sealant in preventing caries had been proven. Since then, the retention rate has become the true determinant and a valid surrogate endpoint for sealant effectiveness in preventing caries [24,46]. The retention rate in most studies is classified into "intact sealant", "partial loss", and "complete loss" [47]. However, Mickenautsch and Yengopal in their recent systematic review do not support the use of sealant retention as a valid predictor for caries manifestation [48,49].

A systematic review evaluated the retention rate of the different materials of resin-based sealants (RBSs) placed on permanent molars. There was no significant difference between the complete retention of LRBS and ARBS. No statistically significant difference was observed when comparing LRBS with FRBS either at eight or 12 months. However, at the 48-month follow-up, the results indicated a significantly better retention for LRBS compared with FRBS. The overall decrease in the complete retention rate was observed over time in all types of sealant materials [24].

A recent meta-analysis investigated the clinical retention rates of pit and fissure sealants with regard to different types of materials at different observation-times. The resin-based sealants showed the best retention rates: the five-year retention rates for light-polymerizing, autopolymerizing, and fluoride-releasing resin-based sealants were 83.8%, 64.7%, and 69.9%, respectively. The GI-based fissure sealants, on the other hand, had a 5.2% retention rate at the five-year observation-time. Polyacid modified resin sealants also showed low retention rates [46]. However, studies that used HVGIC [50,51] or Fuji Triage [52] have shown improved retention rate results for GI sealants that are comparable to resin-based sealants.

When comparing filled and unfilled resin-based sealant retention rates, a study evaluated the retention of resin-based filled sealant Helioseal F (Ivoclar Vivadent, Schaan, Liechtenstein) and resin-based unfilled sealant Clinpro (3M ESPE, Saint Paul, MN, USA). They concluded that unfilled resin-based sealants showed slightly higher retention rates at the 12-month follow-up compared to those for filled resin-based sealants. Complete retention was 53.57% for filled RBS and 64.39% for unfilled RBS, but the difference was not statistically significant. Sealants without fillers appear to have better penetration into fissures than sealants incorporating filler particles, due to their lower viscosity [26].

The recent update of the American Dental Association's recommendations, in collaboration with the American Academy of Pediatric Dentistry, reported that the GI sealant retention loss is five times greater compared to RBS and three times greater compared to RMGI sealant. The difference here is statistically significant, but the quality of evidence was assessed as being very low (Table 2) [5,28].

6. Techniques for the Placement of Resin-Based Sealants

6.1. Tooth-Cleaning, Enamel Preparation, and Tooth Surface Treatment Prior to Sealant Placement

Most of the manufacturers' instructions for the use of fissure sealants recommend careful cleaning of the pits and fissures before acid etching. A study reported that there is in fact no difference in sealant retention between toothbrush and handpiece prophylaxis at two to five year follow-ups [53].

Some manufacturers' instructions state that the use of fluoride before sealant placement is contraindicated as it decreases enamel solubility in acid and thus inhibits proper etching of the enamel. However, Warren et al. compared the sealant retention of two sealant materials before and after fluoride treatment over an 18-month period. They reported a significantly greater retention on fluoridated teeth when LRBS was used and no significant difference in retention when ARBS was used. This suggested that sealant retention may not be impaired by fluoride application immediately prior to sealant placement [54]. Similarly, another study reported that the use of fluoride-containing prophylaxis paste or any fluoride treatment before sealant application does not adversely affect the sealant's bonding to enamel [55]. One more study also evaluated sealant retention when treating the enamel with a topical fluoride gel before acid etching clinically and in-vitro. It was found that there was no statistically significant difference between the retention rate of the sealant applied after tooth surface treatment with topical fluoride and the control group that did not receive any fluoride treatment prior to the sealant application [56]. Furthermore, many studies have investigated different methods of mechanical preparation of the fissures, such as air abrasion, eliminating fissures with a dental bur, and sandblasting, prior to the sealant placement . Interestingly, it was found that fissure eradication is not necessary. Enameloplasty, using any of the above-mentioned techniques, removes the enamel layer overlying the dentin at the bottom of the fissure, making the tooth more susceptible to caries if the sealant is lost [20,57]. There is conflicting and limited evidence regarding the benefits of using a bur for fissure cleaning or for the purpose of increasing retention, prior to sealant placement [32,58].

6.2. Isolation

Adequate moisture isolation during resin sealant placement is the most critical step in sealant application. If the etched enamel gets exposed to salivary proteins for as little as 0.5 s, it can be contaminated [36]. If this occurs, re-etching is required. The use of a rubber dam is the ideal way to achieve optimum moisture control. The use of cotton rolls and a saliva ejector is also a valid option [59]. The use of moisture control systems, such as the Isolite® system (Innerlite Incorporation, Santa Barbara, CA, USA) provides less time for the procedure and offers comparable sealant retention rates to cotton roll isolation or the use of a rubber dam [60].

A systematic review has suggested that four-handed delivery, compared to two-handed delivery, increases sealant retention by 9% when other factors, such as the surface cleaning method, were controlled [61]. The use of the four-handed technique facilitates sealant placement and is also associated with improved retention [32].

6.3. Acid Etching and Rinsing

The phosphoric acid concentration that was originally used for etching by Buonocore in 1955 was 85%, but it was then reduced in his early clinical studies to 50% [18]. Nowadays, 35% and 37% are the commonly used concentrations. Acid-etching times have also been reduced from 60 s down to 20 s [62].

Early recommendations for primary teeth enamel etching time were double the accepted time for permanent enamel, namely, 120 s for primary enamel and 60 s for permanent enamel. The early in vitro studies showed that 120 s are necessary for an adequate etching pattern in primary teeth enamel to eliminate the identification of prismless enamel. This finding was found not to be clinically significant for sealant retention, as demonstrated by Simonsen et al. in 1978. His study included 56 children between the ages of 3–8 years with 373 deciduous first and second molars that were sealed and examined six months post-application; 178 teeth were etched for 60 s and 195 teeth were etched for 120 s. The retention rate for the 60 s etched teeth was 100%, and for the 120 s etched teeth, it was 99% [8,23]. Moreover, the shorter etching time decreases the chance of saliva contamination, particularly in pre-cooperative children.

An in-vitro study evaluated the etching depth and bonding strength of 130 exfoliated primary teeth after the following four different etching times: 15, 30, 60, and 120 s. Despite the greater increase in depth after 120 s etching time, the mean bond strengths obtained for the four etching times were not significantly different [63]. Another study showed that the length of etching time has little effect on sealant retention. No significant difference in fissure sealants' retention on primary or permanent molars was found after a one-year follow-up with different etching times of 15, 30, 45, and 60 s [64].

A rinsing time of 30 s and drying the tooth for 15 s should be sufficient to remove all acid etchant residues and achieve the characteristic chalky white enamel frosty appearance [20,22].

6.4. Bonding Agents

The idea of using a bonding agent under the sealant came from Feigal et al. in 1993 when they used hydrophilic bonding materials to aid the bond strength when the sealant is applied in a moist environment [65].

There have already been eight generations of bonding agents [66–68], the latest and eighth one being introduced in 2010. It is characterized by the incorporation of nano-fillers into the adhesive composition to improve the mechanical properties of the adhesive system. However, the most recent type in adhesive dentistry is called the universal adhesive or the multi-mode adhesive. It was first introduced in 2011. This kind of adhesive system can be used as an etch and rinse adhesive, a self-etch adhesive or to do self-etch on dentin and etch-and-rinse on enamel; this particular technique is called selective enamel etching. Its composition differs from the other adhesive systems that allow chemical and micromechanical bonding [67]. All the various adhesive types are summarized in Table 3. Several studies evaluated the use of a bonding agent before sealant application. A randomized controlled trial compared fourth generation (three-step-etch-and-rinse) and fifth generation (two-step-etch-and-rinse) adhesives when used under sealants. They found that the two-step adhesives reduced the risk of sealant loss by half (Hazard ratio = 0.53) when applied on occlusal surfaces. On the other hand, the three-step adhesives had a detrimental effect on the sealant retention rate, which can be explained by the composition of the adhesive, as it is water-based, and water has a deleterious effect on sealant bonding. The two-step adhesive is acetone- or ethanol-based, which may be more effective in bonding to etched enamel [69].

With regard to self-etch adhesives, a recent clinical trial evaluated the sealant retention rate and caries preventive efficacy over a three-year period. They compared three adhesive generations, namely, fourth generation (three-step-etch-and-rinse), fifth generation (two-step-etch-and-rinse), and sixth generation (one-step, two-component-self-etch) with the conventional technique, which is etching with no adhesive application as a control. There was a significant difference between the retention rates of sealants combined with the various adhesive systems used ($p < 0.05$). The highest retention rates of sealants on the first permanent molars at a 36-month recall were combined with the fourth and fifth generation adhesive systems and were 80.01% and 74.27%, respectively. In contrast, the lowest retention rates were combined with the sixth generation adhesive system (42.84%) and with the conventional acid-etch technique (62.86%). They also found that the fissure caries incidence rate in first permanent molars that had been sealed after using the sixth generation adhesive system was 34.28%, which was significantly higher than when other adhesive systems had been used [70]. This was in agreement with a previously published study that reported a significantly better retention rate with the etch-and-rinse adhesive system (fifth generation) compared to the self-etch adhesive system (sixth generation) at a 12-month follow-up [71]. Another study, on the other hand, evaluated the retention rate of fissure sealants in primary molars using a sixth generation (one-step, two-component-self-etch) adhesive compared to the conventional phosphoric acid-etching technique with no bonding agent application. They found no statistically significant difference in sealant retention in the two groups after a one-year follow-up period [72].

Table 3. Historical development of dentin bonding agents.

Generation	Steps	Description	Examples
First Generation mid-1950s and early 1960s	2-steps	Etching enamel only and adhesive application	Cervident (S.S. White, Lakewood, NJ, USA) No longer used
Second Generation Late 1970s	2-steps	Etching enamel only followed by adhesive application, slightly improved bond strength due to modifications in the coupling agent	Clearfil™ Bond system F (Kuraray, Tokyo, Japan) Scotchbond™ (3M ESPE, Saint Paul, MN, USA) Bondlite (Kerr, Orange, CA, USA) No longer used
Third Generation 1980s	3-steps	Partial removal of smear layer acid etching, primer, then unfilled adhesive resin application	Scotchbond™ 2 (3M ESPE, Saint Paul, MN, USA) Clearfil™ New Bond (Kuraray, Tokyo, Japan)
Fourth Generation 1990s	3-step etch-and-rinse adhesive	Complete removal of the smear layer and the formation of a hybrid layer Total etch technique (etching enamel and dentin, rinsing, primer, adhesive)	Scotchbond™ Multi-Purpose (3M ESPE, Saint Paul, MN, USA) All-Bond 2® (BISCO, Schaumburg, IL, USA)
Fifth Generation mid 1990s	2-step etch-and-rinse adhesive	Separate etching step, rinsing enamel and dentin, followed by application of combined primer-adhesive solution	OptiBond® Solo (Kerr, Orange, CA, USA) Adper™ Single Bond (3M ESPE, Saint Paul, MN, USA) Prime&Bond® (DENTSPLY, York, PA, USA)
Sixth Generation late 1990s and early 2000s	2-step self-etching adhesive	Alter the smear layer forming a thin hybrid layer It is composed of an acidic primer (etchant + primer in one bottle) followed by bonding resin—no rinsing step	Clearfil™ SE Bond (Kuraray, Tokyo, Japan) OptiBond® Solo Plus Self-Etch (Kerr, Orange, CA, USA)
	1-step 2 component self-etching adhesive	It combines etchant, primer and adhesive in one step but requires pre-mixing before application	Adper™ Prompt™ L-Pop™ (3M ESPE, Saint Paul, MN, USA) Xeno® III (DENTSPLY, York, PA, USA)
Seventh Generation 2002	1-step self-etching adhesive	It combines etchant, primer and adhesive in a single bottle	Clearfil™ S³ Bond (Kuraray, Tokyo, Japan) G-Bond™ (GC America, Alsip, IL, USA) iBond® (Heraeus Kulzer, Hanau, Germany)
Eighth Generation 2010	1-step self-etching adhesive	Acidic hydrophilic adhesive in a single bottle	Futurabond DC (Voco, Cuxhaven, Germany) Nanobonding agent
Multimode or Universal 2011	Self-etching adhesive or etch and rinse adhesive or selective enamel etching	Phosphoric acid pre-etching in total or selective etching	Scotchbond™ Universal (3M ESPE, Saint Paul, MN, USA) Futurabond U (Voco, Cuxhaven, Germany)

A recent systematic review compared the retention rate of sealants, combined with self-etch adhesive systems(sixth or seventh generation), with that of etch-and-rinse adhesive systems (fourth and fifth generations). Five studies were involved: three studies showed that etch-and-rinse adhesive systems had significantly better retention than self-etch adhesive systems. The other two included studies showed no significant difference between the two adhesive systems. Feigal and Quelhas in 2003, for example, reported similar retention rates of 61% at 24 months. However, the sample in this study was small (18 molars only) [73]. The systematic review concluded that the retention of occlusal fissure sealants is higher when applied with the etch-and-rinse adhesive system than with the self-etch adhesive system [74].

Finally, a recent systematic review by Bagherian et al. evaluated the fissure sealant retention rate with or without the use of an adhesive system and also compared the retention rate of sealants when using etch-and-rinse adhesive systems (fourth or fifth generations) versus the rate achieved when self-etching adhesive systems (sixth or seventh generations) were used. They found that the adhesive system has a positive effect on the retention of the fissure sealant. The adhesive components may increase the penetration into enamel porosities and thus increase bond strength. It was also found that etch-and-rinse adhesive systems are superior to self-etch adhesive systems in terms of sealant retention [75]. However, in a recent, randomized controlled trial, Khare et al. evaluated the integrity of fissure sealants by comparing the use of fifth, seventh, or Universal bonding systems with a no bonding protocol at 3-, 6- and 12-month follow-ups. At the 12-month follow-up, fifth generation bonding and universal bonding protocols performed better than seventh generation or no-bonding protocols, but the difference between the groups was not statistically significant [76].

In summary, the above-mentioned studies indicated that the use of adhesive systems prior to fissure sealant application had a positive effect on increasing penetration and improving the retention rate. It also appears that the use of bonding-agents that involve a separate acid-etching step (fourth and fifth generations) provides better sealant retention than self-etching adhesives (sixth and seventh generations). Etch- and-rinse adhesive systems produce better penetration of the enamel surface than self-etch adhesive systems, and this may result in a better bond strength.

An evidence-based 2008 report from the American Dental Association and the American Academy of Pediatric Dentistry supports the use of adhesive systems before sealant application for better sealant retention [32,58].

6.5. Sealant Evaluation After Placement

After curing the sealant and before the removal of the isolation material, the operator should examine the sealant for any voids, bubbles, or deficient material. Sealant retention should also be checked using the explorer in attempt to remove the sealant. If the sealant is dislodged, the fissures should be re-checked for any remaining food debris that may have caused the debonding of the sealant material. The tooth should be re-etched and a new sealant material should be applied. The operator should also be cautious enough to remove excess sealant material over the distal margin that may create a ledge [44].

7. Sealing Primary Teeth

On the basis of caries risk assessment, primary teeth can be judged to be at risk due to fissure anatomy or patient caries risk factors, and would therefore benefit from sealant application [55]. Therefore, pit and fissure sealants are indicated in primary teeth, if such teeth have deep retentive or stained pits and fissures with signs of decalcification or if the child has caries or restorations in the contralateral primary molar or any other primary teeth [44]. Sealing should be considered particularly for children and young people with medical, physical, or intellectual impairment [59].

Pit-and-fissure sealants were found to be retained on primary molars at a rate of 74 to 96.3% at one year and 70.6–76.5% at 2.8 years [58]. However, the focus of most sealant studies is the occlusal surfaces of permanent molars and there is still insufficient evidence to support the use of fissure sealants in primary molars [32]. Rathnam and Madan maintain that it is difficult to conduct clinical studies on primary teeth due to several confounding factors, such as age, cooperation, and the behavior of the child when presented within an unfamiliar set-up, such as in the dental clinic [77]. To simplify the clinical procedure and make fissure sealant application more acceptable to young children, a shorter etching time may be used to decrease the chance of saliva contamination. As mentioned earlier, several studies showed that the length of etching time has a minimal effect on sealant retention [64]. Another measure that can be used with young children in an attempt to shorten the procedure time is to use self-etching bonding agents as an alternative to the conventional acid etching technique. Several studies have shown an insignificantly lower sealant retention rate in primary teeth when self-etching bonding agents have been used, compared to conventional acid etching [72,78]. Moreover, studies have shown that using a GI sealant may be a good interim option when salivary contamination is expected because it has a higher toleration to moisture compared to resin-based sealants [31]. However, studies on the use of GI sealants in primary teeth are very limited [79] and considerably more research is therefore needed in this area [42].

8. Cost-Effectiveness of Dental Sealants

A cost-effectiveness analysis can be used to analyze the cost in relation to the outcome. In the case of sealants, we must ask how many carious lesions are prevented when dental sealants are applied [80]. Dental sealants do seem to be a cost-effective intervention; sealing permanent molars reduces the total cost by preventing the need for more expensive and invasive restorative treatment. Sealants are considered to be more cost-effective if they are used with children at a high risk of caries and with teeth surfaces susceptible to caries. It is therefore recommended that sealants should be used selectively, based on the child's caries risk and the anatomy of the fissures [5,32,81,82]. Developing methods for targeting children at a high caries risk is therefore important to ensure the cost-effective use of sealants [82]. Perception of the susceptibility of pits and fissures to caries varies from practitioner to practitioner, when simple terms such as "deep occlusal anatomy"are used. Practitioners should be aware of the teeth and teeth surfaces that are most susceptible to caries and include them in treatment planning for sealants. For example, deep, narrow, I-shaped fissures are relatively more caries-susceptible, compared to shallow, wide, V-shaped fissures [22]. Newly erupted permanent first molars should also be seen as susceptible teeth, prior to full eruption. Dentists should think about how to protect such teeth from getting carious and whether to seal at an early or late stage of eruption. Buccal pits and lingual grooves are also considered caries-susceptible areas that are difficult to seal [83]. Sealant application is part of caries management protocol for high caries risk patients [84]. It is therefore important to evaluate to what extent other preventive approaches are used, such as professional topical fluoride application, regular daily toothbrushing with fluoridated toothpaste, the use of fluoride supplements, and diet counseling [59,84]. Caries risk is assessed using indicators such as low socio-economic status, previous caries experience, sugar consumption between meals, the presence of active white spot lesions, and low salivary flow [84].

A study showed that risk-based sealing improves clinical outcomes and saves money over never sealing. It should also be mentioned that sealing permanent molars in all patients further improves the outcome, adding only a small incremental cost relative to risk-based sealing [85]. A recent Cochrane review concluded that sealants have proved to be effective in preventing caries in high caries risk children [35]. Another study concluded that sealing primary molars reduces restorations and extractions, but is more expensive than not sealing [81]. It is therefore recommended that, to be more cost-effective, sealants be used only in children at a caries risk of develping caries [32].

9. Sealing Non-Cavitated Carious Lesions

Non-cavitated carious lesions refer to initial caries lesion development without any cavitation. They are defined by a change in color, surface structure, and glossiness due to demineralization before macroscopic breakdown occurs. Re-establishing the balance between remineralization and demineralization may stop the progress of caries leaving a clear clinical sign of past disease [1].

Due to the difficulty in diagnosing non-cavitated occlusal caries, dentists may have been inadvertently sealing caries over the years [36]. Many studies suggest that caries progression is slowed or arrested under sealants [86]. Blocking the bacterial nutritional supply may be the explanation for the arrest of caries progression observed under sealants [87]. A meta-analysis examined the caries progression under sealed permanent teeth. Six studies were included in the analysis, representing 840 teeth. Four of them sealed non-cavitated lesions and the other two used sealant over restorations. The median annual percentage of progression of non-cavitated caries lesions was 2.6% for sealed teeth and 12.6% for not-sealed teeth. This suggests that sealing non-cavitated lesions is effective in reducing progression [86]. Another randomized, controlled trial evaluated the progression of non-cavitated dentinal lesions under sealants. They included 30 molars in the sealant group (experimental group) and 30 molars in the no-sealant group (control group). The results showed a remarkable difference between the two groups; at the eight month-recall, 25 out of 26 molars (96.1%) in the control group showed caries progression. At the 12-month-recall, three out of 26 molars (11.5%) in the experimental group were present with caries progression. These molars were observed to have partial or complete sealant loss. The partial and total loss of sealant thus limited the effectiveness in arresting caries lesions [88]. Moreover, a recent critical appraisal provided evidence from clinical trials about sealing incipient occlusal caries lesions and concluded that caries lesions do not progress under well-sealed surfaces. However, the clinical success of sealing non-cavitated lesions is dependent on the complete retention of the sealants [89].

Sealing non-cavitated carious lesions seems to also have an effect on bacterial count. A systematic review that included six studies reported that sealing was associated with at least a 10-fold decrease in bacterial counts. About 47% percent of sealed teeth had viable bacteria, compared to 89% of unsealed lesions. They concluded that sealants were effective in reducing bacterial counts in carious lesions, but a limited number of organisms neverthless persisted [87]. Another recent systematic review supported sealing non-cavitated dentinal lesions and concluded that resin-based sealants are able to arrest the caries progression of non-cavitated dentinal lesions, while GI sealants showed low retention rates and are not able to arrest caries progression [90].

Dentists, on the other hand, have not yet adopted these findings in their clinical decision-making. A questionnaire was mailed to a randomly selected sample of 2400 dentists, of whom 771 responded. When there was no radiographic evidence of caries extending to dentin, only 38.2% of the dentists claimed that they would seal the tooth's occlusal surface, and 23% chose the option of opening the fissure [91].

The available evidence and the recommendations from the ADA Council, as well as the AAPD guidelines, support sealing occlusal non-cavitated early carious lesions in children and young adults. However, sealants are most effective if they are regularly monitored and repaired [28,32,58].

10. Follow-Up (Recall-and-Repair)

The average sealant loss from permanent molars is between five to ten percent per year [83]. Regular sealant maintenance is therefore essential to maximize efficiency, maintain marginal integrity, and provide the protection given by optimal sealant coverage [32,92]. A study evaluated more than 8000 sealants over a period of ten years; its authors reported a sealant success rate of 85 percent after eight to ten years, due to the incorporation of an annual recall and repair program. Complete sealant retention without any need for resealing was 41 percent at ten years [93]. In another study where only a single sealant application was performed, 69 percent of the group with sealed surfaces were sound, whereas 17 percent of the group without sealants were sound. However, only 28 percent were completely retained after 15 years in the group with sealants [94]. Full retention of sealants can be checked visually, tactilely, and radiographically.

There were concerns about partially lost sealant in that it may leave sharp margins that trap food and eventually lead to caries [83]. An interesting systematic review aimed to evaluate if the risk of developing caries in previously sealed teeth with fully or partially lost sealant surpasses the risk in teeth that have never been sealed. Seven studies were included and the participants were aged between 5- and 14-year-old. It was found that the risk of caries development in previously sealed teeth after a four-year follow-up is less than or equal to that for never-sealed teeth. In other words, teeth with partial or complete sealant loss are not at a higher risk of developing caries compared to never-sealed teeth, and the relative risk (RR) ranged between 0.693 and 1.083 [95]. This does not suggest that operators should be less careful with the application technique of sealants or in the evaluation and maintainenace after placement. This suggests, however, that a child should not be forbidden to get the benefits of a sealant even if recall cannot be ensured [32,95].

11. Esterogenicity

Bisphenol-A (BPA) is the precursor chemical component of bisphenol-a dimethacrylate (Bis-DMA) and bisphenol-a glycidyl dimethacrylate (Bis-GMA), which are the most common monomers used in resin composite restorations and resin-based sealants. It is known for its estrogenic property with potential reproductive and developmental human toxicity [96,97]. BPA is not present in monomers as a raw material but as BPA derivatives that can sometimes be hydrolyzed and found in saliva [34].

It has been reported in a systematic review that high levels of BPA were found in saliva samples that had been collected immediately or one hour after resin-based sealant placement. High levels of BPA were also detected in urine samples [98]. However, a report by the American Dental Association and the American Academy of Pediatric Dentistry did not support the occurrence of adverse effects after sealant placement and described the BPA effect as a small transient effect [5,28].

Some studies have reported techniques, such as the immediate cleaning of the sealed surface, or the removal of the oxygen inhibition layer of the unreacted monomer, which is present on the outer layer of the sealant surface to reduce the amount of unreacted monomer. This can be done using a pumice or a rotating rubber cup [98], to reduce the potential BPA exposure.

12. Conclusions

Pit and fissure sealant is an effective means of preventing pit and fissure caries in primary and permanent teeth. Dentists should therefore be encouraged to apply pit and fissure sealants in combination with other preventive measures in patients at a high risk of caries. Selection of sealant material is dependent on the patient's age, child's behavior, and the time of teeth eruption. Teeth that present with early non-cavitated carious lesions would also benefit from sealant application to prevent any caries progression. Sealant placement is a sensitive procedure that should be performed in a moisture-controlled environment. Maintenance is essential and the reapplication of sealants, when required, is important to maximize the effectiveness of the treatment.

Author Contributions: Literature search and studies selection were conducted by Reem Naaman, Azza A. El-Housseiny and Najlaa Alamoudi. Reem Naaman: provided the research idea and wrote the manuscript. Azza A. El-Housseiny: Participated in the design and made manuscript revisions. Najlaa Alamoudi: Made contributions to manuscript revisions. All authors have read and approved the final manuscript.

Conflicts of Interest: The authors declare no conflict of interest.

Abbreviations

AAPD	American Academy of Pediatric Dentistry
ADA	American Dental Association
ARBS	autopolymerizing resin based sealants
BIS GMA	bisphenol-a-glycidyl dimethacrylate
BPA	bisphenol-A

FRBS	fluoride releasing resin based sealants
FS	fissure sealant
GI	glass ionomer
LRBS	light polymerizing resin based sealants
NHANES	National health and nutrition examination survey
RBS	resin based sealants
RMGI	resin modified glass ionomer
SE	self-etch adhesives
SES	socioeconomic status
TE	total-etch concept
USA	United States of America
UV	ultraviolet

References

1. Young, D.A.; Novy, B.B.; Zeller, G.G.; Hale, R.; Hart, T.C.; Truelove, E.L. The American Dental Association Caries Classification System for clinical practice: A report of the American Dental Association Council on Scientific Affairs. *J. Am. Dent. Assoc.* **2015**, *146*, 79–86. [CrossRef] [PubMed]

2. Dye, B.A.; Tan, S.; Smith, V.; Lewis, B.G.; Barker, L.K.; Thornton-Evans, G.; Eke, P.I.; Beltran-Aguilar, E.D.; Horowitz, A.M.; Li, C.H. Trends in oral health status: United States, 1988–1994 and 1999–2004. *Vital Health Stat.* **2007**, *11*, 1–92.

3. Dye, B.A.; Thornton-Evans, G.; Li, X.; Iafolla, T.J. Dental caries and sealant prevalence in children and adolescents in the United States, 2011–2012. *NCHS Data Br.* **2015**, *191*, 1–8.

4. Macek, M.D.; Beltran-Aguilar, E.D.; Lockwood, S.A.; Malvitz, D.M. Updated comparison of the caries susceptibility of various morphological types of permanent teeth. *J. Public Health Dent.* **2003**, *63*, 174–182. [CrossRef] [PubMed]

5. Wright, J.T.; Crall, J.J.; Fontana, M.; Gillette, E.J.; Novy, B.B.; Dhar, V.; Donly, K.; Hewlett, E.R.; Quinonez, R.B.; Chaffin, J.; et al. Evidence-based clinical practice guideline for the use of pit-and-fissure sealants: A report of the American Dental Association and the American Academy of Pediatric Dentistry. *J. Am. Dent. Assoc.* **2016**, *147*, 672–682. [CrossRef] [PubMed]

6. Beltran-Aguilar, E.D.; Barker, L.K.; Canto, M.T.; Dye, B.A.; Gooch, B.F.; Griffin, S.O.; Hyman, J.; Jaramillo, F.; Kingman, A.; Nowjack-Raymer, R.; et al. Surveillance for dental caries, dental sealants, tooth retention, edentulism, and enamel fluorosis: United States, 1988–1994 and 1999–2002. *MMWR Surveil. Summ.* **2005**, *54*, 1–43.

7. Kitchens, D.H. The economics of pit and fissure sealants in preventive dentistry: A review. *J. Contemp. Dent. Pract.* **2005**, *6*, 95–103. [PubMed]

8. Simonsen, R.J. Pit and Fissure Sealants. In *Clinical Applications of the Acid Etch Technique*, 1st ed.; Quintessence Publishing: Hanover Park, IL, USA, 1978.

9. Veiga, N.J.; Pereira, C.M.; Ferreira, P.C.; Correia, I.J. Prevalence of dental caries and fissure sealants in a Portuguese sample of adolescents. *PLoS ONE* **2015**, *10*. [CrossRef] [PubMed]

10. Oulis, C.J.; Berdouses, E.D.; Mamai-Homata, E.; Polychronopoulou, A. Prevalence of sealants in relation to dental caries on the permanent molars of 12 and 15-year-old Greek adolescents. A national pathfinder survey. *BMC Public Health* **2011**, *11*. [CrossRef] [PubMed]

11. Al Agili, D.E.; Niazy, H.A.; Pass, M.A. Prevalence and socioeconomic determinants of dental sealant use among schoolchildren in Saudi Arabia. *East. Mediterr. Health J.* **2012**, *18*, 1209–1216. [CrossRef] [PubMed]

12. Bodecker, C. Eradication of enamel fissures. *Dent. Items Int.* **1929**, *51*, 859–866.

13. Klein, H.; Knutson, J.W. XIII. Effect of Ammoniacal Silver Nitrate on Caries in the First Permanent Molar. *J. Am. Dent. Assoc.* **1942**, *29*, 1420–1426. [CrossRef]

14. Hyatt, T.P. Prophylactic odontotomy: The cutting into the tooth for the prevention of disease. *J. Am. Dent. Assoc. Dent. Cosm.* **1923**, *65*, 234–241. [CrossRef]

15. Buonocore, M.G. A simple method of increasing the adhesion of acrylic filling materials to enamel surfaces. *J. Dent. Res.* **1955**, *34*, 849–853. [CrossRef] [PubMed]

16. Cueto, E.I. *Adhesive Sealing of Pits and Fissures for Caries Prevention*; Dentistry and Dental Research, University of Rochester: Rochester, NY, USA, 1965.

17. Bowen, R.L. Method of Preparing a Monomer Having Phenoxy and Methacrylate Groups Linked by Hydroxy Glyceryl Groups. US Patent 3,179,623 A, 20 April 1965.

18. Buonocore, M. Adhesive sealing of pits and fissures for caries prevention, with use of ultraviolet light. *J. Am. Dent. Assoc.* **1970**, *80*, 324–330. [CrossRef] [PubMed]

19. Anusavice, K.J.; Shen, C.; Rawls, H.R. *Phillips' Science of Dental Materials*; Elsevier Health Sciences: Amsterdam, The Netherlands, 2013.

20. Dean, J.A. *McDonald and Avery's Dentistry for the Child and Adolescent*, 10th ed.; Elsevier Health Sciences: Amsterdam, The Netherlands, 2016.

21. Santini, A.; Gallegos, I.T.; Felix, C.M. Photoinitiators in dentistry: A review. *Prim. Dent. J.* **2013**, *2*, 30–33. [CrossRef] [PubMed]

22. Pinkham, J.R.; Casamassimo, P.S.; Fields, H.W., Jr.; McTigue, D.J.; Nowak, A. *Pediatric Dentistry: Infancy through Adolescence*, 4th ed.; Elsevier Health Sciences: Amsterdam, The Netherlands, 2005.

23. Simonsen, R.J. Pit and fissure sealant: Review of the literature. *Pediatr. Dent.* **2002**, *24*, 393–414. [CrossRef] [PubMed]

24. Muller-Bolla, M.; Lupi-Pégurier, L.; Tardieu, C.; Velly, A.M.; Antomarchi, C. Retention of resin-based pit and fissure sealants: A systematic review. *Community Dent. Oral Epidemiol.* **2006**, *34*, 321–336. [CrossRef] [PubMed]

25. Wright, J.T.; Retief, D.H. Laboratory evaluation of eight pit and fissure sealants. *Pediatr. Dent.* **1984**, *6*, 36–40. [PubMed]

26. Reddy, V.R.; Chowdhary, N.; Mukunda, K.; Kiran, N.; Kavyarani, B.; Pradeep, M. Retention of resin-based filled and unfilled pit and fissure sealants: A comparative clinical study. *Contemp. Clin. Dent.* **2015**, *6*, S18–S23. [CrossRef] [PubMed]

27. Rock, W.P.; Potts, A.J.; Marchment, M.D.; Clayton-Smith, A.J.; Galuszka, M.A. The visibility of clear and opaque fissure sealants. *Br. Dent. J.* **1989**, *167*, 395–396. [CrossRef] [PubMed]

28. American Academy of Pediatric Dentistry. Evidence-based Clinical Practice Guideline for the Use of Pit-and-Fissure Sealants. *Pediatr. Dent.* **2016**, *38*, 263–279.

29. Limeback, H. *Comprehensive Preventive Dentistry*, 1st ed.; John Wiley & Sons: Hoboken, NJ, USA, 2012.

30. Frencken, J.E. Atraumatic restorative treatment and minimal intervention dentistry. *Br. Dent. J.* **2017**, *223*, 183–189. [CrossRef] [PubMed]

31. Antonson, S.A.; Antonson, D.E.; Brener, S.; Crutchfield, J.; Larumbe, J.; Michaud, C.; Yazici, A.R.; Hardigan, P.C.; Alempour, S.; Evans, D. Twenty-four month clinical evaluation of fissure sealants on partially erupted permanent first molars: Glass ionomer versus resin-based sealant. *J. Am. Dent. Assoc.* **2012**, *143*, 115–122. [CrossRef] [PubMed]

32. American Academy of Pediatric Dentistry. Guideline on Restorative Dentistry. *Pediatr. Dent.* **2016**, *38*, 250–262.

33. Puppin-Rontani, R.M.; Baglioni-Gouvea, M.E.; deGoes, M.F.; Garcia-Godoy, F. Compomer as a pit and fissure sealant: Effectiveness and retention after 24 months. *J. Dent. Child.* **2006**, *73*, 31–36.

34. Ahovuo-Saloranta, A.; Forss, H.; Walsh, T.; Nordblad, A.; Makela, M.; Worthington, H.V. Pit and fissure sealants for preventing dental decay in permanent teeth. *Cochrane Database Syst. Rev.* **2017**. [CrossRef] [PubMed]

35. Ahovuo-Saloranta, A.; Hiiri, A.; Nordblad, A.; Mäkelä, M.; Worthington, H.V. Sealants for preventing dental decay in the permanent teeth—A review. *Cochrane Database Syst. Rev.* **2013**. [CrossRef]

36. Deery, C. Strong evidence for the effectiveness of resin based sealants. *Evid. Based Dent.* **2013**, *14*, 69–70. [CrossRef] [PubMed]

37. Hiiri, A.; Ahovuo-Saloranta, A.; Nordblad, A.; Mäkelä, M. Pit and fissure sealants versus fluoride varnishes for preventing dental decay in children and adolescents. *Cochrane Database Syst. Rev.* **2010**. [CrossRef]

38. Ahovuo-Saloranta, A.; Forss, H.; Hiiri, A.; Nordblad, A.; Makela, M. Pit and fissure sealants versus fluoride varnishes for preventing dental decay in the permanent teeth of children and adolescents. *Cochrane Database Syst. Rev.* **2016**. [CrossRef]

39. Chestnutt, I.G.; Playle, R.; Hutchings, S.; Morgan-Trimmer, S.; Fitzsimmons, D.; Aawar, N.; Angel, L.; Derrick, S.; Drew, C.; Hoddell, C.; et al. Fissure Seal or Fluoride Varnish? A Randomized Trial of Relative Effectiveness. *J. Dent. Res.* **2017**, *96*, 754–761. [CrossRef] [PubMed]

40. Mickenautsch, S.; Yengopal, V. Caries-Preventive Effect of High-Viscosity Glass Ionomer and Resin-Based Fissure Sealants on Permanent Teeth: A Systematic Review of Clinical Trials. *PLoS ONE* **2016**, *11*. [CrossRef] [PubMed]

41. Mickenautsch, S.; Yengopal, V. Caries-preventive effect of glass ionomer and resin-based fissure sealants on permanent teeth: An update of systematic review evidence. *BMC Res. Notes* **2011**, *4*. [CrossRef] [PubMed]

42. De Amorim, R.G.; Leal, S.C.; Frencken, J.E. Survival of atraumatic restorative treatment (ART) sealants and restorations: A meta-analysis. *Clin. Oral Investig.* **2012**, *16*, 429–441. [CrossRef] [PubMed]

43. Haznedaroglu, E.; Guner, S.; Duman, C.; Mentes, A. A 48-month randomized controlled trial of caries prevention effect of a one-time application of glass ionomer sealant versus resin sealant. *Dent. Mater. J.* **2016**, *35*, 532–538. [CrossRef] [PubMed]

44. Casamassimo, P.S.; Henry, W.; Fields, J.; McTigue, D.J.; Nowak, A. *Pediatric Dentistry Infancy through Adolescence*, 5th ed.; Elsevier: Amsterdam, The Netherlands, 2013.

45. Sidhu, S.K.; Nicholson, J.W. A Review of Glass-Ionomer Cements for Clinical Dentistry. *J. Funct. Biomater.* **2016**, *7*. [CrossRef] [PubMed]

46. Kühnisch, J.; Mansmann, U.; Heinrich-Weltzien, R.; Hickel, R. Longevity of materials for pit and fissure sealing—Results from a meta-analysis. *Dent. Mater.* **2012**, *28*, 298–303. [CrossRef] [PubMed]

47. Simonsen, R.J. From prevention to therapy: Minimal intervention with sealants and resin restorative materials. *J. Dent.* **2011**, *39*, S27–S33. [CrossRef] [PubMed]

48. Mickenautsch, S.; Yengopal, V. Retention loss of resin based fissure sealants—A valid predictor for clinical outcome? *Open Dent. J.* **2013**, *7*, 102–108. [CrossRef] [PubMed]

49. Mickenautsch, S.; Yengopal, V. Validity of sealant retention as surrogate for caries prevention—A systematic review. *PLoS ONE* **2013**, *8*. [CrossRef] [PubMed]

50. Beiruti, N.; Frencken, J.E.; van't Hof, M.A.; Taifour, D.; van Palenstein Helderman, W.H. Caries-preventive effect of a one-time application of composite resin and glass ionomer sealants after 5 years. *Caries Res.* **2006**, *40*, 52–59. [CrossRef] [PubMed]

51. Chen, X.; Du, M.; Fan, M.; Mulder, J.; Huysmans, M.C.; Frencken, J.E. Effectiveness of two new types of sealants: Retention after 2 years. *Clin. Oral Investig.* **2012**, *16*, 1443–1450. [CrossRef] [PubMed]

52. Al-Jobair, A.; Al-Hammad, N.; Alsadhan, S.; Salama, F. Retention and caries-preventive effect of glass ionomer and resin-based sealants: An 18-month-randomized clinical trial. *Dent. Mater. J.* **2017**, *36*, 654–661. [CrossRef] [PubMed]

53. Kolavic Gray, S.; Griffin, S.O.; Malvitz, D.M.; Gooch, B.F. A comparison of the effects of toothbrushing and handpiece prophylaxis on retention of sealants. *J. Am. Dent. Assoc.* **2009**, *140*, 38–46. [CrossRef] [PubMed]

54. Warren, D.P.; Infante, N.B.; Rice, H.C.; Turner, S.D.; Chan, J.T. Effect of topical fluoride on retention of pit and fissure sealants. *J. Dent. Hyg.* **2001**, *75*, 21–24. [PubMed]

55. Feigal, R.J. The use of pit and fissure sealants. *Pediatr. Dent.* **2002**, *24*, 415–422. [PubMed]

56. El-Housseiny, A.; Sharaf, A. Evaluation of fissure sealant applied to topical fluoride treated teeth. *J. Clin. Pediatr. Dent.* **2005**, *29*, 215–219. [CrossRef] [PubMed]

57. Dhar, V.; Chen, H. Evaluation of resin based and glass ionomer based sealants placed with or without tooth preparation-a two year clinical trial. *Pediatr. Dent.* **2012**, *34*, 46–50. [PubMed]

58. Beauchamp, J.; Caufield, P.W.; Crall, J.J.; Donly, K.; Feigal, R.; Gooch, B.; Ismail, A.; Kohn, W.; Siegal, M.; Simonsen, R. Evidence-based clinical recommendations for the use of pit-and-fissure sealants: A report of the American Dental Association Council on Scientific Affairs. *J. Am. Dent. Assoc.* **2008**, *139*, 257–268. [CrossRef] [PubMed]

59. Welbury, R.; Raadal, M.; Lygidakis, N. EAPD guidelines for the use of pit and fissure sealants. *Eur. J. Paediatr. Dent.* **2004**, *5*, 179–184. [PubMed]

60. Alhareky, M.S.; Mermelstein, D.; Finkelman, M.; Alhumaid, J.; Loo, C. Efficiency and Patient Satisfaction with the Isolite System Versus Rubber Dam for Sealant Placement in Pediatric Patients. *Pediatr. Dent.* **2014**, *36*, 400–404. [PubMed]

61. Griffin, S.O.; Jones, K.; Gray, S.K.; Malvitz, D.M.; Gooch, B.F. Exploring four-handed delivery and retention of resin-based sealants. *J. Am. Dent. Assoc.* **2008**, *139*, 281–289. [CrossRef] [PubMed]

62. Zero, D.T. How the introduction of the acid-etch technique revolutionized dental practice. *J. Am. Dent. Assoc.* **2013**, *144*, 990–994. [CrossRef] [PubMed]

63. Redford, D.A.; Clarkson, B.; Jensen, M. The effect of different etching times on the sealant bond strength, etch depth, and pattern in primary teeth. *Pediatr. Dent.* **1986**, *8*, 11–15.

64. Duggal, M.S.; Tahmassebi, J.F.; Toumba, K.; Mavromati, C. The effect of different etching times on the retention of fissure sealants in second primary and first permanent molars. *Int. J. Paediatr. Dent.* **1997**, *7*, 81–86. [CrossRef] [PubMed]

65. Feigal, R.J.; Hitt, J.; Splieth, C. Retaining sealant on salivary contaminated enamel. *J. Am. Dent. Assoc.* **1993**, *124*, 88–97. [CrossRef] [PubMed]

66. Ozer, F.; Blatz, M.B. Self-etch and etch-and-rinse adhesive systems in clinical dentistry. *Compend. Contin. Educ. Dent.* **2013**, *34*, 12–14. [PubMed]

67. Sofan, E.; Sofan, A.; Palaia, G.; Tenore, G.; Romeo, U.; Migliau, G. Classification review of dental adhesive systems: From the IV generation to the universal type. *Ann. Stomatol.* **2017**, *8*, 1–17. [CrossRef]

68. Kugel, G.; Ferrari, M. The science of bonding: From first to sixth generation. *J. Am. Dent. Assoc.* **2000**, *131*, 20S–25S. [CrossRef] [PubMed]

69. Feigal, R.; Musherure, P.; Gillespie, B.; Levy-Polack, M.; Quelhas, I.; Hebling, J. Improved sealant retention with bonding agents: A clinical study of two-bottle and single-bottle systems. *J. Dent. Res.* **2000**, *79*, 1850–1856. [CrossRef] [PubMed]

70. Sakkas, C.; Khomenko, L.; Trachuk, I. A comparative study of clinical effectiveness of fissure sealing with and without bonding systems: 3-year results. *Eur. Arch. Paediatr. Dent.* **2013**, *14*, 73–81. [CrossRef] [PubMed]

71. Burbridge, L.; Nugent, Z.; Deery, C. A randomized controlled trial of the effectiveness of a one-step conditioning agent in fissure sealant placement: 12-month results. *Eur. Arch. Paediatr. Dent.* **2007**, *8*, 49–54. [CrossRef] [PubMed]

72. Maher, M.M.; Elkashlan, H.I.; El-Housseiny, A.A. Effectiveness of a self-etching adhesive on sealant retention in primary teeth. *Pediatr. Dent.* **2013**, *35*, 351–354. [PubMed]

73. Feigal, R.; Quelhas, I. Clinical trial of a self-etching adhesive for sealant application: Success at 24 months with Prompt L-Pop. *Am. J. Dent.* **2003**, *16*, 249–251. [PubMed]

74. Botton, G.; Morgental, C.S.; Scherer, M.M.; Lenzi, T.L.; Montagner, A.F.; Rocha, R.D.O. Are self-etch adhesive systems effective in the retention of occlusal sealants? A systematic review and meta-analysis. *Int. J. Paediatr. Dent.* **2015**, *26*, 402–411. [CrossRef] [PubMed]

75. Bagherian, A.; Sarraf Shirazi, A.; Sadeghi, R. Adhesive systems under fissure sealants: Yes or no?: A systematic review and meta-analysis. *J. Am. Dent. Assoc.* **2016**, *147*, 446–456. [CrossRef] [PubMed]

76. Khare, M.; Suprabha, B.S.; Shenoy, R.; Rao, A. Evaluation of pit-and-fissure sealants placed with four different bonding protocols: A randomized clinical trial. *Int. J. Paediatr. Dent.* **2016**, *27*, 444–453. [CrossRef] [PubMed]

77. Rathnam, A.; Nidhi, M.; Shigli, A.L.; Indushekar, K.R. Comparative evaluation of slot versus dovetail design in class III composite restorations in primary anterior teeth. *Contemp. Clin. Dent.* **2010**, *1*, 6–9. [CrossRef] [PubMed]

78. Peutzfeldt, A.; Nielsen, L.A. Bond strength of a sealant to primary and permanent enamel: Phosphoric acid versus self-etching adhesive. *Pediatr. Dent.* **2004**, *26*, 240–244. [PubMed]

79. Chadwick, B.L.; Treasure, E.T.; Playle, R.A. A randomised controlled trial to determine the effectiveness of glass ionomer sealants in pre-school children. *Caries Res.* **2005**, *39*, 34–40. [CrossRef] [PubMed]

80. Deery, C. The economic evaluation of pit and fissure sealants. *Int. J. Paediatr. Dent.* **1999**, *9*, 235–241. [CrossRef] [PubMed]

81. Chi, D.L.; van der Goes, D.N.; Ney, J.P. Cost-effectiveness of pit-and-fissure sealants on primary molars in Medicaid-enrolled children. *Am. J. Public Health* **2014**, *104*, 555–561. [CrossRef] [PubMed]

82. Weintraub, J.A. Pit and fissure sealants in high-caries-risk individuals. *J. Dent. Educ.* **2001**, *65*, 1084–1090. [PubMed]

83. Feigal, R.J. Sealants and preventive restorations: Review of effectiveness and clinical changes for improvement. *Pediatr. Dent.* **1998**, *20*, 85–92. [PubMed]

84. American Academy of Pediatric Dentistry. Guideline on caries-risk assessment and management for infants, children, and adolescents. *Pediatr. Dent.* **2014**, *36*, 127–134.

85. Quinonez, R.B.; Downs, S.M.; Shugars, D.; Christensen, J.; Vann, W.F., Jr. Assessing cost-effectiveness of sealant placement in children. *J. Public Health Dent.* **2005**, *65*, 82–89. [CrossRef] [PubMed]

86. Griffin, S.O.; Oong, E.; Kohn, W.; Vidakovic, B.; Gooch, B.F.; Bader, J.; Clarkson, J.; Fontana, M.R.; Meyer, D.M.; Rozier, R.G.; et al. The effectiveness of sealants in managing caries lesions. *J. Dent. Res.* **2008**, *87*, 169–174. [CrossRef] [PubMed]

87. Oong, E.M.; Griffin, S.O.; Kohn, W.G.; Gooch, B.F.; Caufield, P.W. The effect of dental sealants on bacteria levels in caries lesions: A review of the evidence. *J. Am. Dent. Assoc.* **2008**, *139*, 271–278. [CrossRef] [PubMed]

88. Borges, B.C.; de Souza Borges, J.; Braz, R.; Montes, M.A.; de Assuncao Pinheiro, I.V. Arrest of non-cavitated dentinal occlusal caries by sealing pits and fissures: A 36-month, randomised controlled clinical trial. *Int. Dent. J.* **2012**, *62*, 251–255. [CrossRef] [PubMed]

89. Zandona, A.F.; Swift, E.J. Evidence for Sealing versus Restoration of Early Caries Lesions. *J. Esthet. Restor. Dent.* **2015**, *27*, 55–58. [CrossRef] [PubMed]

90. De Assuncao, I.V.; da Costa Gde, F.; Borges, B.C. Systematic review of noninvasive treatments to arrest dentin non-cavitated caries lesions. *World J. Clin. Cases* **2014**, *2*, 137–141. [CrossRef] [PubMed]

91. Tellez, M.; Gray, S.L.; Gray, S.; Lim, S.; Ismail, A.I. Sealants and dental caries: Dentists' perspectives on evidence-based recommendations. *J. Am. Dent. Assoc.* **2011**, *142*, 1033–1040. [CrossRef] [PubMed]

92. Nunn, J.; Murray, J.; Smallridge, J. British Society of Paediatric Dentistry. British Society of Paediatric Dentistry: A policy document on fissure sealants in paediatric dentistry. *Int. J. Paediatr. Dent.* **2000**, *10*, 174–177. [PubMed]

93. Romcke, R.G.; Lewis, D.W.; Maze, B.D.; Vickerson, R.A. Retention and maintenance of fissure sealants over 10 years. *J. Can. Dent. Assoc.* **1990**, *56*, 235–237. [PubMed]

94. Simonsen, R.J. Retention and effectiveness of dental sealant after 15 years. *J. Am. Dent. Assoc.* **1991**, *122*, 34–42. [CrossRef] [PubMed]

95. Griffin, S.O.; Gray, S.K.; Malvitz, D.M.; Gooch, B.F. Caries risk in formerly sealed teeth. *J. Am. Dent. Assoc.* **2009**, *140*, 415–423. [CrossRef] [PubMed]

96. Eliades, T.; Eliades, G. *Plastics in Dentistry and Estrogenicity: A Guide to Safe. Practice*; Springer: Berlin, Germany, 2014.

97. Fleisch, A.F.; Sheffield, P.E.; Chinn, C.; Edelstein, B.L.; Landrigan, P.J. Bisphenol A and related compounds in dental materials. *Pediatrics* **2010**, *126*, 760–768. [CrossRef] [PubMed]

98. Kloukos, D.; Pandis, N.; Eliades, T. In vivo bisphenol-a release from dental pit and fissure sealants: A systematic review. *J. Dent.* **2013**, *41*, 659–667. [CrossRef] [PubMed]

6

Public Health Aspects of Paediatric Dental Treatment under General Anaesthetic

William Murray Thomson

Sir John Walsh Research Institute, Department of Oral Sciences, School of Dentistry, The University of Otago, Dunedin 9054, New Zealand; murray.thomson@otago.ac.nz;

Academic Editor: Barbara Cvikl

Abstract: Early childhood caries (ECC) has negative psychosocial effects on children, with chronic pain, changed eating habits, disrupted sleep and altered growth very common, and it disrupts the day-to-day lives of their families. The treatment of young children with ECC places a considerable burden on health systems, with a considerable amount having to be provided under general anaesthesia (GA), which is resource-intensive. Justifying its use requires evidence of the efficacy of treatment in improving the lives of affected children and their families. This paper discusses the available evidence and then makes some suggestions for a research agenda.

Keywords: anesthesia; dental; child; preschool; quality of life

1. Introduction

Despite improvements in dental caries rates over recent decades, early childhood caries (ECC) remains a highly prevalent, chronic disease among young children [1]. It places a considerable burden on health systems; in New Zealand, for example, dental treatment under general anaesthesia (DGA) is provided to approximately 5000 New Zealand children each year [2], with disproportionate numbers of Māori and Pacific Island children undergoing such treatment, along with those residing in deprived areas [3].

Dental caries is a multifactorial disease with causes and influences at a number of levels [4]. In fact, as with other chronic noncommunicable diseases, early childhood caries meets the criteria for designation as a "wicked" health promotion problem [5]: it is difficult to solve because of its complex, multi-level causes, and there is no single, universal solution. Preventive efforts are imperfect: relying solely on people's personal behaviour is inadequate, because to be effective, self-care—such as sustained, long-term plaque control [6] and the use of self-applied topical fluorides (such as fluoride toothpaste)—needs to be done well and be carried out over the long term. The effectiveness of clinical preventive efforts (those administered by dental practitioners) for the group at highest ECC risk remains unclear at this stage. At community level, water fluoridation is effective [7], but it does not eliminate the disease; rather, it shifts the population disease distribution, and the problem of its long "tail" and the numbers requiring DGA remain [8]. Not only is sugar intake the most important person-level risk factor for the disease [9], the marketing and consumption of sugars is increasing [10] as part of the energy-dense and nutritionally compromised industrial diet—highly processed and convenient "junk" food—which has become more and more common, especially in the groups of low socio-economic status. Such food is high in sugar (much of which comes from high-fructose corn syrup), salt and fat, and it has low nutritional value. Being cheap, readily available and requiring minimal preparation, it tends to be consumed by those on low and/or insecure incomes [11], among whom the caries burden is greatest.

There are strong socio-economic gradients in ECC occurrence, and it is likely that, as societal inequality continues to increase under the neoliberal hegemony [11], the incidence of the disease will continue to rise, leading to further increases in the numbers of children requiring dental treatment under GA. The bulk of those cases will be residing in deprived households, and so it is unlikely that there will be a fall in the numbers of children requiring DGA in the medium term.

2. The Effects of ECC on Children and Their Families

ECC has been shown to have negative psychosocial effects on children and to disrupt the day-to-day lives of their families. These effects are worsened by time spent on waiting lists for treatment.

Chronic pain, changed eating habits, disrupted sleep and altered growth are very common [12]. Among children prior to being treated under GA, chronic pain has been reported for at least two-thirds of them; eating difficulties have been experienced by 42% to 71%, and sleep disruption has affected between one-quarter and one half [13–15], although a Turkish study reported that 95% had sleeping difficulties [16]. Anyone who has children will recognise that a child with sleeping difficulties also disrupts the sleep of at least one parent. Indeed, the data show that the effects on the wider family are considerable [17]. Perhaps the greatest evidence for the impact of ECC on children and their families is the improvement in oral-health-related quality of life (OHRQoL) scale scores which is observed after the condition has been treated. This issue is further explored later in this paper.

3. Treating Children under GA

The number of children requiring dental treatment under GA has been a problem in New Zealand since the 1980s [8], but the problem is not confined to that country. The intervention rate in Australia trebled over the two decades from 1993–94 [18], and similar observations were reported from England [19].

Providing dental treatment under GA is far more expensive than conventional care, given that it requires an operating theatre, dentist, dental assistant, anaesthetist, anaesthetic technician and a recovery nurse (and room), as well as the conventional dental operating equipment. Given the expense (At around NZD$2,400 per case; [20]) and the sheer volume of cases, dental GA lists are vulnerable to the scrutiny of health service managers, whose brief includes maintaining and improving (where possible) the system's efficiency. By contrast, the clinician's main concern is treating the problem of the patient in his/her dental surgery at the time; if that can be achieved less traumatically and more efficiently by treating a case of early childhood caries under GA, that will be the option chosen. Repeated fruitless attempts at treating a young child with too much disease are traumatic for patient and clinician alike. Some years ago, a manager in New Zealand's health system suggested that the paediatric dental "logjam" in his service's theatres could be virtually eliminated by halting all treatment for the deciduous dentition; after all, went his logic, they were only baby teeth and would be replaced in time anyway. Those of us working in the dental care system reacted with predictable horror: we were aware of the benefits for child and parent alike from such treatment, but we had no data with which to demonstrate that. At best, we had some routinely collected statistics on throughput and, in some services, information on the treatment provided was able to be gleaned from claims data. Curtailing the treatment of paediatric caries cases under GA would have adverse consequences for children, households and the school dental services (who would have to struggle with treating those cases conventionally). There was an urgent need to obtain data on the wider effects of the disease and its treatment upon children and their families, and on their oral-health-related quality of life (OHRQoL).

4. Effects of Dental Treatment under GA on OHRQoL

OHRQoL has been defined as "a standard of the oral tissues which contributes to overall physical, psychological and social wellbeing by enabling individuals to eat, communicate and socialise without discomfort, embarrassment or distress and which enables them to fully participate in their chosen social roles" [21]. It seemed as if it should be relatively easy to determine the effects on children (and their families) of treatment under GA. The problem was that there was (as yet) no validated scale for use with preschool children and their parents. Early studies had used single-item approaches or batteries of items to quantify individual aspects of the improvements associated with treatment under GA [22–25], but these had not been psychometrically validated and did not allow determination of effect sizes.

What was needed was a way of placing sufferers (whether children or their families) accurately on what would effectively be a "continuum of misery" and then observing their treatment-associated movement towards the less severe end of such a continuum. Fortunately, it was not long before the means to do so was available, with the emergence of the Parental-Caregivers Perceptions Questionnaire (P-CPQ), the first OHRQoL scale developed for use with very young children [26]. A separate Family Impact Scale (FIS) was developed for use alongside it. The higher the scale score, the more severe the impact. The scales are intended for use with younger children and their families. The 33-item P-CPQ has four subscales (oral symptoms, functional limitation, emotional well-being and social well-being), and the 14-item FIS has three (parental emotions, parental/family activity, and family conflict).

Short-form versions have been developed more recently in order to lessen the respondent burden. This process has resulted in two closely related sets of measures: the 13-item Early Childhood Oral Health Impact Scale (ECOHIS) [27]; and the short-form P-CPQ (with 8- and 16-item versions available) and 8-item FIS [28]. Both measures arose from the pioneering work of Jokovic and Locker, but differ in how they were developed [29]. In short, the ECOHIS was developed using an epidemiological sample, and the short-form P-CPQ and FIS measures arose from secondary analysis of data from two New Zealand studies of OHRQoL changes in ECC-affected children undergoing dental treatment under GA. Unsurprisingly, perhaps, a direct comparison of the properties and responsiveness of the measures found that the ECOHIS was less suitable for investigating DGA-treatment-associated changes in OHRQoL in young children, but the findings suggested that it might be more suitable for epidemiological use [29].

Such scales have been used extensively in observing treatment-associated changes in OHRQoL (Table 1). The design used in those studies has usually been a pre-/post-intervention one, with the same children assessed before treatment and again some time after it. Ethical and practical challenges have meant that only one [30] used a concurrent control group which did not receive treatment. The children in that control group were eventually treated, however. To date, 10 such studies have been published [13–16,30–35], with patient numbers at baseline ranging from 31 to 311, and follow-up rates ranging from 64% to 100% (with the latter seen in half of the studies). Of the five studies with less-than-perfect follow-up rates, three included attrition analyses, and none reported any statistically significant (or otherwise important) differences between those assessed at follow-up and those who were lost.

Table 1. Overview of studies of changes in child oral-health-related quality of life (OHRQoL) scale scores following dental treatment under GA.

Study	Country	Number at Baseline	Number at Follow-Up	Scale Used
Malden et al. [13]	New Zealand	202	130 (64%)	P-CPQ and FIS (full scales) [a]
Klaasen et al. [31]	The Netherlands	31	31 (100%)	P-CPQ and FIS (full scales) [b]
Klaasen et al. [30]	The Netherlands	144	104 (72%)	ECOHIS
Lee et al. [32]	Hong Kong	32	32 (100%)	ECOHIS
Gaynor et al. [14]	New Zealand	157	144 (92%)	P-CPQ and FIS (full scales) [a]
Baghdadi et al. [33]	Saudi Arabia	67	67 (100%)	P-CPQ and FIS (short-form version)
Jankauskiene et al. [15]	Lithuania	140	122 (87%)	ECOHIS
Cantekin et al. [16]	Turkey	311	311 (100%)	ECOHIS
Almaz [34]	Turkey	120	98 (82%)	ECOHIS
Ridell et al. [35]	Sweden	75	75 (100%)	P-CPQ and FIS (full scales)

[a] Data were subsequently reanalysed by Thomson et al. [28] using the short-form versions. [b] Scale data were not reported appropriately in this study.

Examining before- and after-treatment scores on OHRQoL scales can be done in two main ways. The first involves comparing mean scale (and subscale) scores before and after treatment, with the computation of effect sizes. The effect size is a unitless measure of change which is calculated by dividing the mean change score (the difference between the baseline and follow-up score) by the standard deviation of the baseline scores, in order to give a dimensionless measure of effect. Effect size statistics of less than 0.2 indicate a "small" clinically meaningful magnitude of change, 0.2 to 0.7 a "moderate" change, and more than 0.7 a "large" change [13]. Effect sizes reported to date are presented in Table 2. Most are moderate or large, and there is little difference between the different scales which were used.

Table 2. Treatment-associated effect sizes detected, by scale.

Study	Scale Which Was Used			
	P-CPQ	FIS	ECOHIS-Child	ECOHIS-Family
Malden et al. [13]	0.9	0.8	—	—
Klaasen et al. [30] [a]	—	—	0.9	—
Lee et al. [32]	—	—	0.6	0.8
Gaynor et al. [14]	0.9	0.5	—	—
Baghdadi et al. [33]	1.6	1.5	—	—
Jankauskiene et al. [15]	—	—	1.6	2.4
Cantekin et al. [16]	—	—	0.9	1.3
Almaz [34]	—	—	1.0	1.2
Ridell et al. [35]	0.7	0.7	—	—
Mean effect size detected	1.0	0.9	1.0	1.4
Thomson et al. [29] [b]	1.2	0.9	0.9	0.6

[a] Effect sizes were unable to be calculated from the study data of Klaasen et al. [b] This was a secondary analysis of pooled data from the Malden et al and Gaynor et al studies; it calculated short-form scores for the P-CPQ and FIS, allowing direct comparison with ECOHIS scale scores in the same cohort.

The second approach is to determine the prevalence of one or more impacts (say, "fairly often" or "very often") at baseline and follow-up, and then to report the treatment-associated fall in prevalence. The latter does not use the full range of observed scores (and their variance) in the sample, but it has the distinct advantage of being easier to explain to lay people (including the all-important policy-makers and health service managers who control the resources for dental care). Data on DGA-associated changes in impact prevalence have not yet been reported in the literature.

Data on changes in the prevalence of impacts do indeed make interesting reading. In the Lithuanian sample [15], the prevalence of any impact determined by the ECOHIS-Child and ECOHIS-Family fell from 98.4% and 95.9% (respectively) at baseline to 73.8% and 46.7% (respectively) at follow-up [36]. Reanalysis of the data from the Wellington (New Zealand) sample [13] showed that the prevalence of any impact determined by the P-CPQ fell from 96.3% to 67.5% (for one or more impacts reported "Sometimes", "Often" or "Every day or almost every day"), and from 68.8% to 26.3% (for one or more impacts reported "Often" or "Every day or almost every day"). For the Auckland (New Zealand) sample [14], the prevalence of any impact determined by the P-CPQ fell from 95.5% to 75.5% (for one or more impacts reported "Sometimes", "Often" or "Every day or almost every day"), and from 60.0% to 29.1% (for one or more impacts reported "Often" or "Every day or almost every day"). In other words, impact prevalence fell from about two-thirds to just over one-quarter of the children treated. Where the FIS was concerned, impact prevalence in the Wellington and Auckland samples fell from 82.5% and 67.3% to 33.8% and 44.5% (respectively) for one or more impacts reported "Sometimes", "Often" or "Every day or almost every day". For one or more impacts reported "Often" or "Every day or almost every day", those proportions fell from 50.0% and 35.5% to 12.5% and 10.9% (respectively). As previously mentioned, falls in impact prevalence are likely to be a more effective "sell" to managers and policy-makers. Overall, the international data indicate that treating severe ECC cases under GA has benefits for both child and family.

5. Qualitative Investigations

Recent years have seen qualitative studies of the DGA experience appearing in the literature. These both complement and extend the quantitative reports. The first to appear was a study [37] in which Vancouver parents' experiences of their child's DGA were explored through interviews conducted at a postoperative follow-up appointment. The study's aim was to shed light on the reasons for the DGA event not invariably being a spur to subsequent caries-promoting practices and behaviours in the affected household. Interestingly, one of the main themes to emerge was the role of the stresses of daily life in creating and sustaining barriers to caring for the child's teeth. This raises the interesting possibility that children from more resilient and better-functioning families might not only have less disease but the effects of that disease on the family when it does occur might also be less disruptive. Guilt, stress and anxiety all featured in parental responses, as did affirmation of the positive benefits of the child having had the disease treated.

In contrast to the parent-focused Canadian work, two recent reports by researchers at the University of Sheffield described their novel approaches to investigating the DGA experience from the child's viewpoint. Video diaries were used alongside semi-structured interviews to obtain new insights into the process; these were not entirely negative, with greater attention and positive feedback from family members going some way to offsetting the more predictable anxiety, pre-operative hunger and discomfort [38]. The second report highlighted the need for greater involvement of the children in both the decision-making and the actual DGA process [39].

6. A Research Agenda—What Else Do We Need to Know?

There are a number of areas where more research is required (summarised in Table 3), and those can be considered under the three domains of the instrument, the care provided, and the household context (Table 3). Each will be discussed briefly.

Table 3. Areas requiring more research in the dental treatment under general anaesthesia (DGA) field.

Domain	Issues for investigation
The instruments	ECOHIS vs P-CPQ/FIS
	Test-retest reliability
	Reference period
	Response shift, sustainability of effects
	Regression to the mean
The care provided	Restorative/rehabilitative *versus* exodontic
	Longer-term orthodontic and other effects
The context	Roles of family function, parental personality
	The nature and extent of any cross-cultural differences

Concerning the instrument used, the first decision is which one to use. Of the studies to date, exactly half have used the ECOHIS and half have used the P-CPQ/FIS, and there were similar findings in terms of responsiveness and the effect sizes which were observed (although the ECOHIS-Family did show a substantially smaller effect size). A recent study directly compared the performance of the two measures in a secondary analysis of data from two pre-post-DGA studies conducted in New Zealand [29]. It found that, overall, the ECOHIS-Child and the P-CPQ scales are very similar in their internal consistency reliability, cross-sectional construct validity and responsiveness, at least for determining changes in OHRQoL associated with treatment for ECC. By contrast, the ECOHIS-Family and the FIS-8 differ in some important ways, despite being similar in their responsiveness. The former's face validity is the most important weakness; of the three family impact domains (parental emotions, parental/family activity and family conflict) one is not sampled at all, and another is represented by a single item. In particular, the omission of the disrupted sleep item is particularly curious, given the high prevalence and impact of disrupted sleep for the parents of a child with ECC [29]. Accordingly, the P-CPQ and FIS scales are likely to be more suitable for use in DGA outcomes research.

Test-retest reliability remains an issue in this work. To date, there have been no investigations of this. Ethical concerns are likely to be the reason for this: requiring parents who are already undergoing a stressful time (as highlighted by the Canadian study [37]) would have been an undue imposition on them. Moreover, it would probably have affected follow-up rates.

Other technical issues are those of (a) regression to the mean; (b) response shift; and (c) the sustainability of effects. Regression to the mean is always an issue with any examination of change scores, whereby some of the observed change arises from a phenomenon whereby those with more extreme baseline scores tend to have less extreme scores at follow-up, regardless of any real change in the characteristic being measured [40]. The Wellington study [13] examined this issue and adjusted the change scores by the mean change score for children for whom OHRQoL since the operation was judged (by parents using the global measure) to be "the same". To do this, the mean baseline scores were corrected by that amount and then the effect sizes were recalculated. This did attenuate the effect sizes somewhat, but they were still substantial and clinically important, meaning that the OHRQoL of children undergoing DGA does improve measurably. Response shift is a phenomenon whereby individuals' internal standards, values and view of their quality of life change as they adapt to their new situation [41]. To date, the nature, timing and extent of any response shift in respect of DGA and OHRQoL remain unclear, but it is likely to be detectable. This then raises the issue of the sustainability of the effects of DGA on OHRQoL: how long do they last, given the likelihood of response shift recalibrating informants' perspectives? To date, this has not been reported, although Jankauskiene and co-workers are currently investigating it [36].

The nature of the treatment rendered under DGA is another important aspect. The two alternative approaches to treatment provision in such situations are: (1) the restorative/rehabilitative one (where every effort is made to restore diseased teeth, and extraction is undertaken only as a last resort); and (2) the exodontic one (where affected teeth are usually extracted and little or no effort is expended on saving teeth). It might be expected that the two would differ in terms of their effects on child and family OHRQoL, but that has not yet been reported in the literature. Similarly, their respective longer-term effects on the occlusion remain unknown because of a lack of good-quality longitudinal data.

Parents' reports of their child's OHRQoL and its effects on the family are likely to be influenced by characteristics such as personality and family functioning. Personality is known to influence people's self-reported oral health, with those scoring higher on negative emotionality (or neuroticism) likely to report more negative impacts, other factors being equal [42]. What remains currently unclear is the influence of family functioning on the changes in OHRQoL: that is, whether the effects of the child's condition on the family differ according to how well (or conversely how badly) the family (household) operates from day to day anyway. Domains of interest include problem-solving, communication, roles, affective responsiveness and involvement, and behaviour control, all of which can be captured in an instrument such as the McMaster Family Assessment Device [43]. All could be considered to have some effect on responses to the ECOHIS-Family or the FIS. To date, that has not been investigated, but it is likely that those from families which are more dysfunctional or chaotic will report less favourable outcomes from the DGA experience. It is surely only a matter of time before an expansion of knowledge in this area. There are also likely to be cross-cultural differences in ECC impact and in the responsiveness of the measures used; to date, these have not been explored. However, it is worth noting that the P-CPQ, FIS and ECOHIS were all developed from a common item pool which was generated from a wide variety of cultures, and so this may not be as important a consideration as might be expected.

Acknowledgments: I thank Birute Jankauskiene for willingly undertaking further analyses with her data at my request. I am grateful to my NZ co-researchers in this field (Penny Malden, Wanda Gaynor, Heather Anderson, Geoff Hunt, Associate Professor Lyndie Foster Page and Professor Bernadette Drummond), all of whom have made important contributions to it. The seminal work of Professor David Locker and Aleksandra Jokovic is acknowledged with affection and respect.

References

1. Ministry of Health. *Our Oral Health. Key Findings of the 2009 New Zealand Oral Health Survey*; Ministry of Health: Wellington, New Zealand, 2010.
2. Lingard, G.L.; Drummond, B.K.; Esson, I.A.; Marshall, D.W.; Durward, C.S.; Wright, F.A.C. The provision of dental treatment for children under general anaesthesia. *N. Z. Dent. J.* **2008**, *104*, 10–18. [PubMed]
3. Whyman, R.A.; Mahoney, E.K.; Stanley, J.; Morrison, D. *Admissions to New Zealand Public Hospitals for Dental Care. A 20 Years Review*; Ministry of Health: Wellington, New Zealand, 2012.
4. Fisher-Owens, S.A.; Gansky, S.A.; Platt, L.J.; Weintraub, J.A.; Soobader, M.J.; Bramlett, M.D.; Newacheck, P.W. Influences on children's oral health: A conceptual model. *Pediatrics* **2007**, *120*, e510–e520. [CrossRef] [PubMed]
5. Signal, L.N.; Walton, M.D.; Ni Mhurchu, C.; Maddison, R.; Bowers, S.G.; Carter, K.N.; Gorton, D.; Heta, C.; Lanumata, T.S.; McKerchar, C.W.; *et al.* Tackling "wicked" health promotion problems: A New Zealand case study. *Health Promot. Int.* **2012**, *28*, 84–94. [CrossRef] [PubMed]
6. Broadbent, J.M.; Thomson, W.M.; Boyens, J.V.; Poulton, R. Dental plaque and oral health during the first 30 years of life. *J. Am. Dent. Assoc.* **2011**, *142*, 415–426. [CrossRef] [PubMed]
7. Griffin, S.O.; Regnier, E.; Griffin, P.M.; Huntley, V. Effectiveness of fluoride in preventing caries in adults. *J. Dent. Res.* **2007**, *86*, 410–415. [CrossRef] [PubMed]
8. Kamel, M.S.; Thomson, W.M.; Drummond, B.K. Fluoridation and dental caries severity in young children treated under general anaesthesia: An analysis of treatment records in a 10-year case series. *Community Dent. Health* **2013**, *30*, 15–18. [PubMed]
9. Sheiham, A. Dietary effects on dental diseases. *Public Health Nutr.* **2001**, *4*, 569–591. [CrossRef] [PubMed]
10. Moynihan, P.J.; Kelly, S.A.M. Effect on caries of restricting sugars intake: Systematic review to inform WHO guidelines. *J. Dent. Res.* **2014**, *93*, 8–18. [CrossRef] [PubMed]
11. Otero, G.; Pechlaner, G.; Liberman, G.; Gurcan, E. The neoliberal diet and inequality in the United States. *Soc. Sci. Med.* **2015**, *142*, 47–55. [CrossRef] [PubMed]
12. Davidson, L.E.; Drummond, B.K.; Williams, S.M.; Boyd, D.H.; Meldrum, A.M. Comprehensive dental care under general anaesthesia from 1997–1999 for children under age 6 years. *N. Z. Dent. J.* **2002**, *98*, 75–78.
13. Malden, P.E.; Thomson, W.M.; Jokovic, A.; Locker, D. Changes in parent-assessed oral-health-related quality of life among young children following dental treatment under general anaesthetic. *Community Dent. Oral Epidemiol.* **2008**, *36*, 108–117. [CrossRef] [PubMed]
14. Gaynor, W.N.; Thomson, W.M. Changes in young children's OHRQoL after dental treatment under general anaesthesia. *Int. J. Paediatr. Dent.* **2012**, *22*, 258–264. [CrossRef] [PubMed]
15. Jankauskiene, B.; Virtanen, J.I.; Kubilius, R.; Narbutaite, J. Oral health-related quality of life after dental general anaesthesia treatment among children: A follow-up study. *BMC Oral Health* **2014**, *14*, 81. [CrossRef] [PubMed]
16. Cantekin, K.; Yildirim, M.D.; Cantekin, I. Assessing change in quality of life and dental anxiety in young children following dental rehabilitation under general anesthesia. *Pediatr. Dent.* **2014**, *36*, 12E–17E. [PubMed]
17. Jankauskiene, B.; Narbutaite, J. Changes in oral health-related quality of life among children following dental treatment under general anaesthesia. A systematic review. *Stomatologija* **2010**, *12*, 60–64. [PubMed]
18. Jamieson, L.M.; Roberts-Thomson, K. Dental general anaesthetic trends among Australian children. *BMC Oral Health* **2006**, *6*. [CrossRef] [PubMed]
19. Moles, D.R.; Ashley, P. Hospital admissions for dental care in children: England 1997–2006. *Br. Dent. J.* **2009**, *206*. [CrossRef] [PubMed]
20. Whyman, R.A.; Hawke's Bay District Health Board, Napier, New Zealand. Personal communication, 10 May 2016.
21. Locker, D. Does dental care improve the oral health of older adults? *Community Dent. Health* **2001**, *18*, 7–15. [PubMed]
22. Acs, G.; Pretzer, S.; Foley, M.; Ng, M.W. Perceived outcomes and parental satisfaction following dental rehabilitation under general anesthesia. *Pediatr. Dent.* **2001**, *23*, 419–423. [PubMed]
23. Thomas, C.W.; Primosch, R.E. Changes in increemental weight and well-being of children with rampant caries following complete dental rehabilitation. *Pediatr. Dent.* **2002**, *24*, 109–113. [PubMed]

24. White, H.; Lee, J.Y.; Vann, W.F., Jr. Parental evaluation of quality of life measures following pediatric dental treatment using general anesthesia. *Anesthesia Prog.* **2003**, *50*, 105–110.

25. Anderson, H.K.; Drummond, B.K.; Thomson, W.M. Changes in aspects of children's oral-health-related quality of life following dental treatment under general anaesthesia. *Int. J. Paediatr. Dent.* **2004**, *14*, 317–325. [CrossRef] [PubMed]

26. Jokovic, A.; Locker, D.; Stephens, M.; Kenny, D.; Tompson, B.; Guyatt, G. Measuring parental perceptions of child oral health-related quality of life. *J. Public Health Dent.* **2003**, *63*, 67–72. [CrossRef] [PubMed]

27. Pahel, B.T.; Rozier, R.G.; Slade, G.D. Parental perceptions of children's oral health: The Early Childhood Oral Health Impact Scale (ECOHIS). *Health Qual. Life Outcomes* **2007**, *5*. [CrossRef] [PubMed]

28. Thomson, W.M.; Foster Page, L.A.; Gaynor, W.N.; Malden, P.E. Short-form versions of the Parental-Caregivers Perceptions Questionnaire (P-CPQ) and the Family Impact Scale (FIS). *Community Dent. Oral Epidemiol.* **2013**, *41*, 441–450. [PubMed]

29. Thomson, W.M.; Foster Page, L.A.; Malden, P.M.; Gaynor, W.N.; Nordin, N. Comparison of the ECOHIS and short-form P-CPQ and FIS scales. *Health Qual. Life Outcomes* **2014**, *12*. [CrossRef] [PubMed]

30. Klaassen, M.A.; Veerkamp, J.S.; Hoogstraten, J. Young children's Oral Health-Related Quality of Life and dental fear after treatment under general anaesthesia: A randomized controlled trial. *Eur. J. Oral Sci.* **2009**, *117*, 273–278. [CrossRef] [PubMed]

31. Klaasen, M.A.; Veerkamp, J.S.; Hoogstraten, J. Dental treatment under general anaesthesia: the short-term change in young children's oral-health-related quality of life. *Eur. Arch. Paediatr. Dent.* **2008**, *9*, 130–137. [CrossRef]

32. Lee, G.H.; McGrath, C.; Yiu, C.K.; King, N.M. Sensitivity and responsiveness of the Chinese ECOHIS to dental treatment under general anaesthesia. *Community Dent. Oral Epidemiol.* **2011**, *39*, 372–377. [CrossRef] [PubMed]

33. Baghdadi, Z.D. Effects of dental rehabilitation under general anesthesia on children's oral health-related quality of life using proxy short versions of OHRQoL instruments. *Sci. World J.* **2014**, *2014*. [CrossRef] [PubMed]

34. Almaz, E.M.; Sonmez, S.; Oba, A.A.; Alp, S. Assessing changes in oral health-related quality of life following dental rehabilitation under general anesthesia. *J. Clin. Pediatr. Dent.* **2014**, *38*, 263–267. [PubMed]

35. Ridell, K.; Borgstrom, M.; Lager, E.; Magnusson, G.; Brogardh-Roth, S.; Matsson, L. Oral health-related quality-of-life in Swedish children before and after dental treatment under general anaesthesia. *Acta Odontol. Scand.* **2015**, *73*, 1–7. [CrossRef] [PubMed]

36. Jankauskiene, B. Lithuanian University of Health Sciences, Kaunas, Lithuania. Personal communication, April 2016.

37. Amin, M.; Harrison, R.L.; Weinstein, P. A qualitative look at parents' experience of their child's dental general anaesthesia. *Int. J. Paediatr. Dent.* **2006**, *16*, 309–319. [CrossRef] [PubMed]

38. Rodd, H.; Hall, M.; Deery, C.; Gilchrist, F.; Gibson, B.; Marshman, Z. Video diaries to capture children's participation in the dental GA pathway. *Eur. Arch. Paediatr. Dent.* **2013**, *14*, 325–330. [CrossRef] [PubMed]

39. Rodd, H.; Hall, M.; Deery, C.; Gilchrist, F.; Gibson, B.; Marshman, Z. "I felt weird and wobbly". Child-reported impacts associated with a dental general anaesthetic. *Br. Dent. J.* **2014**, *216*. [CrossRef] [PubMed]

40. Barnett, A.G.; van der Pols, J.C.; Dobson, A.J. Regresson to the mean: what it is and how to deal with it. *Int. J. Epidemiol.* **2005**, *34*, 215–220. [CrossRef] [PubMed]

41. Sprangers, M.A.; Schwartz, C.E. Integrating response shift into health-related quality of life research: A theoretical model. *Soc. Sci. Med.* **1999**, *48*, 1507–1515. [CrossRef]

42. Thomson, W.M.; Caspi, A.; Poulton, R.; Moffitt, T.E.; Broadbent, J.M. Personality and oral health. *Eur. J. Oral Sci.* **2011**, *119*, 366–372. [CrossRef] [PubMed]

43. Boterhaven de Haan, K.L.; Hafekost, J.; Lawrence, D.; Sawyer, M.G.; Zubrick, S.R. Reliability and validity of a short version of the general functioning subscale of the McMaster Family Assessment device. *Fam. Process* **2015**, *54*, 116–123. [CrossRef] [PubMed]

Green Tea Polyphenol Epigallocatechin-3-Gallate-Stearate Inhibits the Growth of *Streptococcus mutans*: A Promising New Approach in Caries Prevention

Amy Lynn Melok [1], **Lee H. Lee** [1], **Siti Ayuni Mohamed Yussof** [1,2] **and Tinchun Chu** [2,*] **ID**

[1] Department of Biology, Montclair State University, Montclair, NJ 07043, USA; meloka1@mail.montclair.edu (A.L.M.); leel@montclair.edu (L.H.L.); mohamedyusss@montclair.edu (S.A.M.Y.)

[2] Department of Biological Sciences, Seton Hall University, South Orange, NJ 07079, USA

* Correspondence: Tin-Chun.Chu@shu.edu;

Abstract: *Streptococcus mutans* (*S. mutans*) is the main etiological bacteria present in the oral cavity that leads to dental caries. All of the *S. mutans* in the oral cavity form biofilms that adhere to the surfaces of teeth. Dental caries are infections facilitated by the development of biofilm. An esterified derivative of epigallocatechin-3-gallate (EGCG), epigallocatechin-3-gallate-stearate (EGCG-S), was used in this study to assess its ability to inhibit the growth and biofilm formation of *S. mutans*. The effect of EGCG-S on bacterial growth was evaluated with colony forming units (CFU) and log reduction; biofilm formation was qualitatively determined by Congo red assay, and quantitatively determined by crystal violet assay, fluorescence-based LIVE/DEAD assays to study the cell viability, and scanning electron microscopy (SEM) was used to evaluate the morphological changes. The results indicated that EGCG-S was able to completely inhibit growth and biofilm formation at concentrations of 250 µg/mL. Its effectiveness was also compared with a commonly prescribed mouthwash in the United States, chlorhexidine gluconate. EGCG-S was shown to be equally effective in reducing *S. mutans* growth as chlorhexidine gluconate. In conclusion, EGCG-S is potentially an anticariogenic agent by reducing bacterial presence in the oral cavity.

Keywords: epigallocatechin-3-gallate-stearate; *Streptococcus mutans*; biofilm; colony forming assay

---

1. Introduction

Dental caries, or tooth decay, is a multifactorial disease that affects a large percentage of today's society [1,2]. Of the thousands of resident bacteria present in the oral cavity, they maintain a relatively neutral pH of around 6.8 [3]. Problems arise when this pH drops to a more acidic value, which promotes the demineralization of the enamel resulting in dental caries.

While it is obvious that dental caries are extremely problematic in underdeveloped and underprivileged areas, this disease is also seen extensively among privileged societies [4,5]. Dental caries pathogenesis involves several steps including the formation of a biofilm. A biofilm is defined as a community of bacteria that attach to a surface. While dental plaque is moderately specialized, it still shares the main properties of all biofilms. Biofilm formation is a three-stage process: docking, locking, and maturation [6,7]. *S. mutans* often gets the most attention in dental related studies because it has been previously shown to favor attachment to tooth enamel [8,9].

A popular drink around the world, tea is made from the infusion of dried *Camellia sinensis* leaves. Eastern cultures, such as China and Japan, are known to use tea medicinally based on its many health benefits. Previous studies have established that *Camellia sinensis*, especially the non-fermented type commonly known as green tea, has numerous medicinal advantages. These preceding studies have recognized green tea to have anti-inflammatory, antiviral, antifungal, antioxidant, protein-denaturing, anti-mutagenic, anti-diabetic, anticarcinogenic, and antibacterial characteristics [10–19]. The remedial effects of green tea are thought to be a result of the polyphenolic catechins present in green tea. The most active catechin, epigallocatechin-3-gallate (EGCG), makes up most of the content of the catechins at 59% [20]. However, several studies indicated that EGCG is unstable and less bioavailable [21–24]. A modified lipophilic derivative of EGCG called epigallocatechin-3-gallate-stearate (EGCG-S) has been synthesized with better stability and improved bioavailability [24]. Because these green tea components are known to have antibacterial activity, it has been shown that these bioactive components are also anticariogenic. Dental research has been completed in vivo in both animal and human participants demonstrating that green tea reduces carious incidents [15,25]. Previous literature reported that green tea extracts have short-term anti-plaque capabilities [26].

In order to determine EGCG-S's effect on *S. mutans*, both qualitative and quantitative analyses were performed to observe its effect on growth inhibition and biofilm reduction. Furthermore, EGCG-S was compared with chlorhexidine gluconate, a common prescription for dental infections.

2. Materials and Methods

2.1. Culturing and Maintenance of Bacterial Cultures

Streptococcus mutans (*S. mutans*) Clarke was purchased from ATCC (ATCC® 25175™) and maintained at 37 °C aerobically with consistent shaking at 250 rpm. All cultures were maintained in nutrient agar (Difco™, Detroit, MI, USA) or nutrient broth (Difco™, Detroit, MI, USA). Fresh overnight cultures were used for each experiment. The purity of the culture was checked periodically.

2.2. Preparation of EGCG-S

EGCG-S was purchased from Camellix LLC, Augusta, GA, USA. EGCG-S was prepared using ethanol. Stock concentrations (5 mg/mL or 2.5 mg/mL) were prepared and diluted to the required concentrations needed for each experiment. The media containing ethanol were used as negative controls according to the EGCG-S concentration.

2.3. Colony Forming Unit (CFU) Assay

Each culture was treated with 0, 100, 200 and 250 μg/mL of EGCG-S respectively and was incubated at 37 °C for 1 h. These samples were serial diluted (from 10^{-2} to 10^{-8}) and 100 μL of each dilution was spread onto nutrient agar plates aseptically and incubated overnight at 37 °C. All experiments were carried out in triplicates. Colony forming units (CFU) were recorded and the percentage of inhibition was calculated as follows:

$$\% \text{ of Inhibition} = [(\text{CFUcontrol} - \text{CFUtreated})/\text{CFUcontrol}] \times 100 \tag{1}$$

2.4. Viability Assay

The LIVE/DEAD® BacLight™ Bacterial Viability Kit (Thermo Fisher, Catalog number: L7007) was used according to the manufacture recommendation. Molecular probes used in this kit include SYTO 9, green fluorescent dye stains intact cell membrane, and propidium iodide (PI), red fluorescence dye for damaged cell membrane. All samples were viewed under a fluorescent microscope (ZEISS Axio Scope A1).

2.5. Congo Red Assay

Congo red (Sigma-Aldrich C6767) agar was prepared according to the procedure outlined by Schwartz [27]. Positive, negative controls and EGCG-S (50, 100, 200 and 250 μg/mL) treated cultures were placed onto the respective wells and the plates were observed every day over a 4-day period. Black precipitation on the red agar indicates positive results for biofilm formation. All assays were done in triplicates.

2.6. Crystal Violet Assay

The cultures were treated with 100, 200, and 250 µg/mL of EGCG-S respectively and allowed to incubate at 37 °C for 4 days. The plates were aspirated, washed with 1X PBS and stained with 0.1% crystal violet for 30 min. The crystal violet was then aspirated, washed, and the plates were inverted until completely dry. One milliliter of 30% acetic acid was added into each well. OD readings were taken at 595 nm [28]. All experiments were done in triplicates with mean and standard deviation calculated. These readings were then used to determine the percentage of biofilm inhibition.

$$\% \text{ of Inhibition} = [(OD_{control} - OD_{treated})/OD_{control}] \times 100 \tag{2}$$

2.7. Scanning Electron Microscopy (SEM)

A sterile coverslip was placed at the bottom of each well in 6-well plates. Overnight cultures with or without EGCG-S 250 µg/mL were pipetted into the well and allowed to incubate at 37 °C for 4 days. Samples were prepared according to the procedure reported previously [29]. Finally, the samples were mounted onto a stub and coated with a thin layer of metal film using the Denton IV Sputter Coater before microscopic observation.

2.8. Time Course Study

This study is to determine different treatment times of EGCG-S and chlorhexidine gluconate on *S. mutans*. The times selected for this study were 5 s, 30 s, 1 min, and 5 min. One mL of overnight culture was centrifuged and the pellet was then suspended in either EGCG-S (250 µg/mL), or chlorhexidine gluconate (0.1%). At each time point, serial dilutions were made, 100 µL of the sample was retrieved and plated onto nutrient agar plates. Cultures suspended in nutrient agar were used as controls. All plates were incubated at 37 °C overnight and CFUs were determined.

2.9. Statistical Analysis

All assays were performed in triplicates and the data analyzed using one-way Analysis of Variance (ANOVA) with Dunnett's Post Hoc Test using SPSS Version 20.0 (IBM Corp. Armonk, NY, USA).

3. Results

3.1. The Effect of EGCG-S on S. mutans

The effect of different concentrations EGCG-S on the growth of *S. mutans* was monitored using a colony forming unit (CFU) assay. No inhibition of *S. mutans* in all negative controls were observed. Log reduction was calculated from the results obtained from the CFU assay (Table 1). Compared with control, log reduction was 1.19 ± 0.02 when cells were treated with 100 µg/mL EGCG-S; 2.04 ± 0.02 at 200 µg/mL EGCG-S; and 2.65 ± 0.01 at 250 µg/mL EGCG-S.

Table 1. Colony forming units (CFU) (cells/mL) and log reduction of epigallocatechin-3-gallate-stearate (EGCG-S) treated samples.

EGCG-S Concentration (µg/mL)	CFU (cells/mL)	Log Reduction
0	$1.01 \times 10^{12} \pm 9.24 \times 10^{10}$	0
100	$6.57 \times 10^{10} \pm 3.20 \times 10^{9}$	1.19 ± 0.02
200	$9.20 \times 10^{9} \pm 4.00 \times 10^{8}$	2.04 ± 0.02
250	$2.30 \times 10^{9} \pm 2.65 \times 10^{8}$	2.65 ± 0.01

Fluorescent microscopy was used to evaluate cell viability with BacLight™ Bacterial Viability Kit. Cell viability was assessed before and after treatment with 250 μg/mL EGCG-S as shown in Figure 1. The control group was shown to have a high population density and fluoresced the green color (Figure 1A), indicating that most of the population was alive and viable. After treatment with 250 μg/mL EGCG-S, nearly the entire population fluoresced red indicating that most cells were not viable post-treatment (Figure 1B).

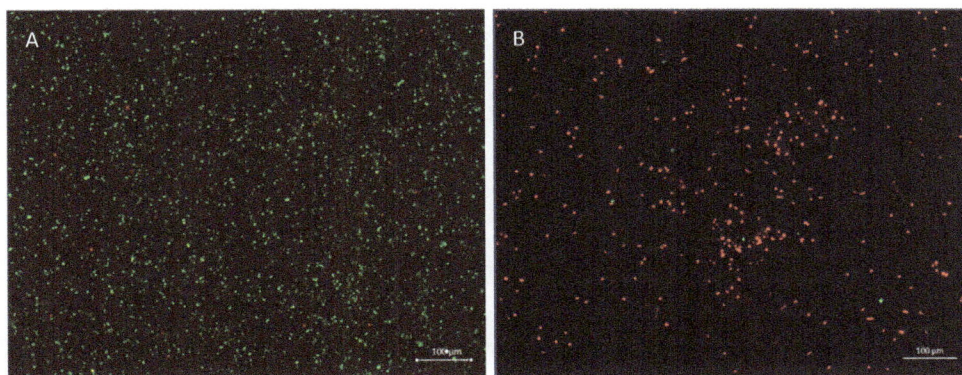

Figure 1. Cell viability assay. (**A**) Control (untreated *S. mutans*). Cells fluorescent green are viable cells. (**B**) *S. mutans* treated with EGCG-S 250 μg/mL for 1 h (430X). Cells fluorescent red indicated dead cells.

3.2. The Effect of EGCG-S on Biofilm of S. mutans

EGCG-S at 250 μg/mL was able to inhibit the growth of cells. In this study, Congo red agar was used to qualitatively examine the effects of EGCG-S on biofilm formation. The results of Congo red analysis are shown in Figure 2. Results with a black color on agar, as shown, are Positive Control; Negative Control, with a red color, represents no biofilm formation. It demonstrated that for samples treated with 50 μg/mL and 100 μg/mL of EGCG-S for 2 and 4 h treatment, the biofilm was significantly reduced but not completely inhibited, as it appeared as partially black. When treated with 200 μg/mL the biofilm was nearly completely inhibited at 2 h treatment and completely inhibited at 4 h treatment. With the concentration of 250 μg/mL at 2 h and 4 h, biofilm formation was completely inhibited. These results indicated that EGCG-S could completely inhibit biofilm formation of *S. mutans* at 200 μg/mL for 4 h and 250 μg/mL for 2 to 4 h. Lower concentrations were not able to completely inhibit the formation of biofilm.

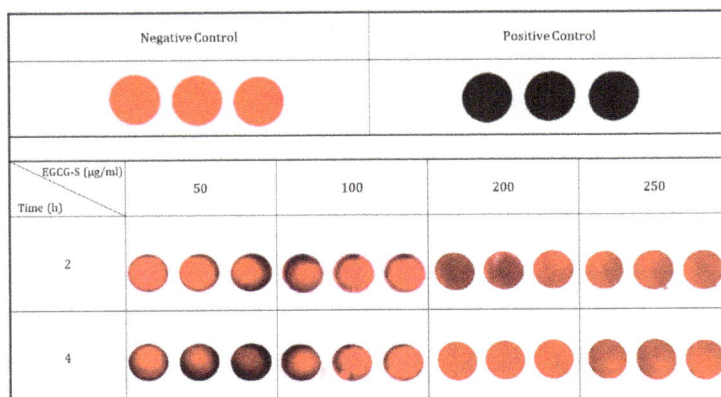

Figure 2. Congo red biofilm assay. Negative controls are represented by a red color and signify no biofilm growth. Positive controls are represented by a dark color and signify that biofilm growth has occurred. At concentrations of 200 and 250 μg/mL biofilm formation was inhibited completely.

In order to quantitatively study the effect of EGCG-S on biofilm formation, the crystal violet assay was carried out. The results exhibited that 100, 200, and 250 µg/mL of EGCG-S were able to inhibit biofilm formation by $82.49 \pm 8.50\%$, $92.75 \pm 2.9\%$, and $100 \pm 4.7\%$, respectively, as shown in Figure 3. The concentration of 250 µg/mL EGCG-S was able to completely inhibit biofilm formation from occurring, which further supported the results from Congo red analysis. Although no biofilm dark precipitation was observed at a concentration of 200 µg/mL (92.75%), the complete inhibition was determined to be 250 µg/mL.

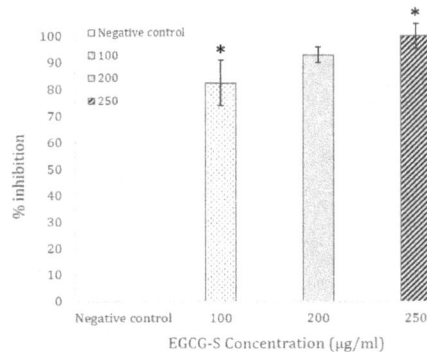

Figure 3. The percentage of inhibition of EGCG-S treated samples vs. control from the Crystal Violet Assay. EGCG-S demonstrates an excellent inhibitory effect by having 100% inhibition at the concentration of 250 µg/mL. Results were shown with mean and standard deviation ($n = 3$). Data analysis indicated significant difference between 100 and 250 µg/mL EGCG-S (with asterisks).

Scanning electron microscopy (SEM) images were taken before and after treatment with 250 µg/mL EGCG-S. The control of untreated cells confirmed the morphology of *S. mutans* (Figure 4A) and after 4 days, biofilm was observed (Figure 4B). After 4 days of 250 µg/mL EGCG-S treatment, the morphology of the cells was altered suggested the integrity of the cells was damaged. There is no biofilm observed as shown in Figure 4C.

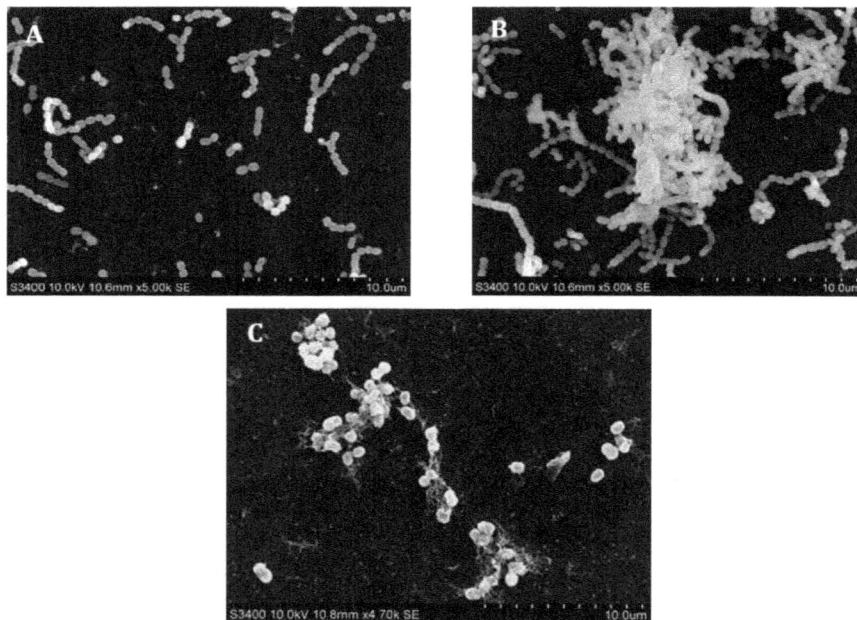

Figure 4. Scanning electron microscopy (SEM) of *S. mutans*. (**A**) Control *S. mutans* cells; (**B**) Untreated *S. mutans* cells were grown for 4 days; (**C**) *S. mutans* cells treated with 250 µg/mL EGCG-S for 4 days.

3.3. Time Course Study of S. mutans treated with 250 μg/mL EGCG-S and Chlorhexidine Gluconate

For evaluating if EGCG-S can be a potential organic mouthwash, the short term time course study was carried out for 0 to 5 min to determine the minimum time needed to inhibit *S. mutans*. In this study, 0 s, 15 s, 30 s, 1 min, and 5 min were used, CFU was determined and the percentage of viability was calculated. Untreated bacteria were used as the control. A parallel study using 0.1% chlorhexidine gluconate was also carried out to compare their effects. The results are shown in Figure 5 and clearly indicated that by 1 min, both EGCG-S and chlorhexidine gluconate were able to completely inhibit the growth of the cells.

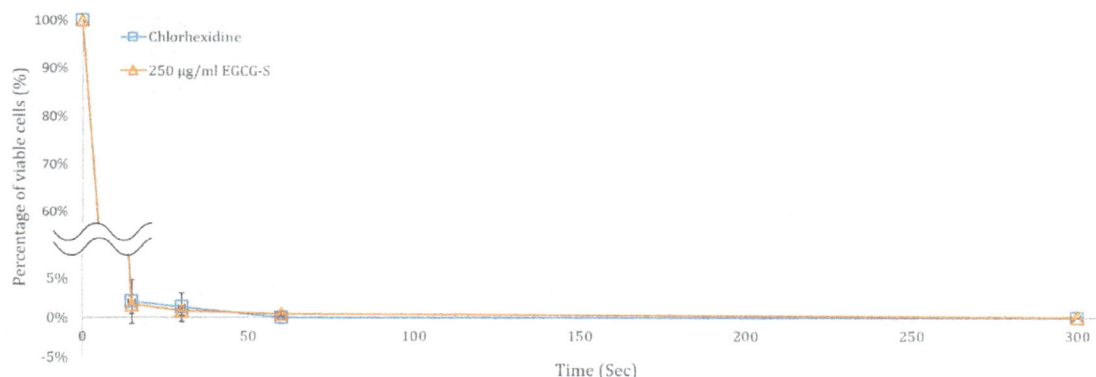

Figure 5. Time course study of 250 μg/mL EGCG-S and 0.1% chlorhexidine gluconate on the growth of *S. mutans*.

4. Discussion

This is the first study investigating EGCG-S as a potential anticariogentic agent. In this study, it suggested that EGCG-S can inhibit the growth of *S. mutans*. The Congo red assay provided preliminary information for the exposure time and concentrations necessary for EGCG-S on their effect on biofilm formation and indicate the presence/absence of biofilm. The Crystal Violet (CV) assay showed that 250 μg/mL EGCG-S was able to completely inhibit biofilm formation. Both experiments confirmed that EGCG-S was able to reduce bacterial growth and biofilm formation in a dose-dependent manner.

While the mechanism of EGCG-S is not yet fully understood, both the fluorescence microscopy and scanning electron microscopy results displayed a possible association to cell surface integrity. This suggested the possible mechanisms of EGCG-S may be similar to one of the mechanisms of EGCG that have been reported previously to damage the cell membrane [30–36], or cell wall [37–39] or interfere with polysaccharides interaction [6]. Molecular research should be carried out to further elucidate the mechanism of EGCG-S on *S. mutans* and other biofilm forming bacteria.

It is common for patients with infections of the oral cavity to be prescribed with 0.1% chlorhexidine gluconate. This comparative study was conducted over a period of 5 min and EGCG-S was effective in reducing bacterial growth at 1 min similar to the prescribed mouth wash chlorhexidine gluconate.

Author Contributions: Conceptualization, L.H.L. and T.C.; Methodology, L.H.L. and T.C.; Validation, L.H.L. and T.C.; Formal Analysis, T.C., A.L.M. and L.H.L.; Investigation, A.L.M. and S.A.M.Y.; Resources, L.H.L. and T.C.; Data Curation, A.L.M., L.H.L., S.A.M.Y. and T.C.; Writing—Original Draft Preparation, A.L.M., L.H.L. and T.C.; Writing—Review & Editing, T.C. and L.H.L.; Visualization, T.C., L.H.L. and T.C.; Supervision, LH.L. and T.C.; Project Administration, L.H.L. and T.C.; Funding Acquisition, L.H.L. and T.C.

Acknowledgments: The authors thank Laying Wu at MMRL for her generous time and assistance on SEM imaging. This work was supported by Montclair State University (MSU) Faculty Scholarship Program (FSP) to L.H.L.; S.A.M.Y. is supported by Seton Hall University (SHU) Graduate Teaching Assistantship in the Department of Biological Sciences; SHU Biological Sciences Department Annual Research Fund and William and Doreen Wong Foundation to T.C.

References

1. Aas, J.A.; Paster, B.J.; Stokes, L.N.; Olsen, I.; Dewhirst, F.E. Defining the normal bacterial flora of the oral cavity. *J. Clin. Microbiol.* **2005**, *43*, 5721–5732. [CrossRef] [PubMed]

2. Gao, X.; Jiang, S.; Koh, D.; Hsu, C.-Y.S. Salivary biomarkers for dental caries. *Periodontology 2000* **2016**, *70*, 128–141. [CrossRef] [PubMed]

3. Aframian, D.J.; Davidowitz, T.; Benoliel, R. The distribution of oral mucosal pH values in healthy saliva secretors. *Oral Dis.* **2006**, *12*, 420–423. [CrossRef] [PubMed]

4. Downer, M.C.; Drugan, C.S.; Blinkhorn, A.S. Dental caries experience of British children in an international context. *Community Dent. Health* **2005**, *22*, 86–93. [PubMed]

5. Marsh, P.D. Dental plaque as a microbial biofilm. *Caries Res.* **2004**, *38*, 204–211. [CrossRef] [PubMed]

6. Blanco, A.R.; Sudano-Roccaro, A.; Spoto, G.C.; Nostro, A.; Rusciano, D. Epigallocatechin gallate inhibits biofilm formation by ocular staphylococcal isolates. *Antimicrob. Agents Chemother.* **2005**, *49*, 4339–4343. [CrossRef] [PubMed]

7. Dunne, W.M. Bacterial adhesion: Seen any good biofilms lately? *Clin. Microbiol. Rev.* **2002**, *15*, 155–166. [CrossRef] [PubMed]

8. Duchin, S.; van Houte, J. Colonization of teeth in humans by Streptococcus mutans as related to its concentration in saliva and host age. *Infect. Immun.* **1978**, *20*, 120–125. [PubMed]

9. Kolenbrander, P.E.; Jakubovics, N.S.; Chalmers, N.I.; Palmer, R.J. Human Oral multispecies biofilms: Bacterial communities in health and disease. In *The Biofilm Mode of Life: Mechanisms and Adaptations*; Kjelleberg, S., Givskov, M., Eds.; Horizon Scientific Press: Poole, UK, 2007; pp. 175–190.

10. Chu, T.-C.; Adams, S.D.; Lee, L.H. Tea polyphenolic compounds against herpes simplex viruses. In *Cancer-Causing Viruses and Their Inhibitors*; Gupta, S.P., Ed.; CRC Press, Taylor & Francis Group: Boca Raton, FL, USA, 2014.

11. de Oliveira, A.; Adams, S.D.; Lee, L.H.; Murray, S.R.; Hsu, S.D.; Hammond, J.R.; Dickinson, D.; Chen, P.; Chu, T.C. Inhibition of herpes simplex virus type 1 with the modified green tea polyphenol palmitoyl-epigallocatechin gallate. *Food Chem. Toxicol.* **2013**, *52*, 207–215. [CrossRef] [PubMed]

12. de Oliveira, A.; Prince, D.; Lo, C.Y.; Lee, L.H.; Chu, T.C. Antiviral activity of theaflavin digallate against herpes simplex virus type 1. *Antivir. Res.* **2015**, *118*, 56–67. [CrossRef] [PubMed]

13. Elvinlewis, M.; Steelman, R. The anticariogenic effects of tea drinking among Dallas schoolchildren. *J. Dent. Res.* **1986**, *65*, 198.

14. Haghjoo, B.; Lee, L.H.; Habiba, U.; Tahir, H.; Olabi, M.; Chu, T.-C. The synergistic effects of green tea polyphenols and antibiotics against potential pathogens. *Adv. Biosci. Biotechnol.* **2013**, *4*, 959. [CrossRef]

15. Hamilton-Miller, J.M. Anti-cariogenic properties of tea (Camellia sinensis). *J. Med. Microbiol.* **2001**, *50*, 299–302. [CrossRef] [PubMed]

16. Otake, S.; Makimura, M.; Kuroki, T.; Nishihara, Y.; Hirasawa, M. Anticaries effects of polyphenolic compounds from Japanese green tea. *Caries Res.* **1991**, *25*, 438–443. [CrossRef] [PubMed]

17. Sakanaka, S.; Kim, M.; Taniguchi, M.; Yamamoto, T. Antibacterial substances in Japanese green tea extract against Streptococcus mutans, a cariogenic bacterium. *Agric. Biol. Chem.* **1989**, *53*, 2307–2311. [CrossRef]

18. Xu, X.; Zhou, X.D.; Wu, C.D. Tea catechin epigallocatechin gallate inhibits Streptococcus mutans biofilm formation by suppressing gtf genes. *Arch. Oral Biol.* **2012**, *57*, 678–683. [CrossRef] [PubMed]

19. Zhao, M.; Zheng, R.; Jiang, J.; Dickinson, D.; Fu, B.; Chu, T.-C.; Lee, L.H.; Pearl, H.; Hsu, S. Topical lipophilic epigallocatechin-3-gallate on herpes labialis: A phase II clinical trial of AverTeaX formula. *Oral Surg. Oral Med. Oral Pathol. Oral Radiol.* **2015**, *120*, 717–724. [CrossRef] [PubMed]

20. Taylor, P.W.; Hamilton-Miller, J.M.; Stapleton, P.D. Antimicrobial properties of green tea catechins. *Food Sci. Technol. Bull.* **2005**, *2*, 71. [CrossRef] [PubMed]

21. Hong, J.; Lu, H.; Meng, X.; Ryu, J.-H.; Hara, Y.; Yang, C.S. Stability, cellular uptake, biotransformation, and efflux of tea polyphenol (−)-epigallocatechin-3-gallate in HT-29 human colon adenocarcinoma cells. *Cancer Res.* **2002**, *62*, 7241–7246. [PubMed]

22. Su, Y.L.; Leung, L.K.; Huang, Y.; Chen, Z.-Y. Stability of tea theaflavins and catechins. *Food Chem.* **2003**, *83*, 189–195.

23. Venkateswara, B.; Sirisha, K.; Chava, V.K. Green tea extract for periodontal health. *J. Indian Soc. Periodontol.* **2011**, *15*, 18. [CrossRef] [PubMed]

24. Chen, P.; Dickinson, D.; Hsu, S.D. Lipid-soluble green tea polyphenols: Stabilized for effective formulation. In *Handbook of Green Tea and Health Research*; McKinley, H., Jamieson, M., Eds.; Nova Science: New York, NY, USA, 2009; pp. 45–61.

25. Xu, X.; Zhou, X.D.; Wu, C.D. The tea catechin epigallocatechin gallate suppresses cariogenic virulence factors of Streptococcus mutans. *Antimicrob. Agents Chemother.* **2011**, *55*, 1229–1236. [CrossRef] [PubMed]

26. You, S.Q. Study on feasibility of Chinese green tea polyphenols (CTP) for preventing dental caries. *Zhonghua Kou Qiang Yi Xue Za Zhi* **1993**, *28*, 197–199, 254. [PubMed]

27. Schwartz, K.; Syed, A.K.; Stephenson, R.E.; Rickard, A.H.; Boles, B.R. Functional amyloids composed of phenol soluble modulins stabilize Staphylococcus aureus biofilms. *PLoS Pathog.* **2012**, *8*, e1002744. [CrossRef] [PubMed]

28. Nowak, J.; Cruz, C.D.; Palmer, J.; Fletcher, G.C.; Flint, S. Biofilm formation of the *L. monocytogenes* strain 15G01 is influenced by changes in environmental conditions. *J. Microbiol. Methods* **2015**, *119*, 189–195. [PubMed]

29. Newby, J.R.; Lee, L.H.; Perez, J.L.; Tao, X.; Chu, T. Characterization of zinc stress response in Cyanobacterium *Synechococcus* sp. IU 625. *Aquat. Toxicol.* **2017**, *186*, 159–170. [CrossRef] [PubMed]

30. Anita, P.; Sivasamy, S.; Madan Kumar, P.D.; Balan, I.N.; Ethiraj, S. In vitro antibacterial activity of Camellia sinensis extract against cariogenic microorganisms. *J. Basic Clin. Pharm.* **2015**, *6*, 35–39. [CrossRef] [PubMed]

31. Caturla, N.; Vera-Samper, E.; Villalain, J.; Mateo, C.R.; Micol, V. The relationship between the antioxidant and the antibacterial properties of galloylated catechins and the structure of phospholipid model membranes. *Free Radic. Biol. Med.* **2003**, *34*, 648–662. [CrossRef]

32. Gordon, N.C.; Wareham, D.W. Antimicrobial activity of the green tea polyphenol (−)-epigallocatechin-3-gallate (EGCG) against clinical isolates of Stenotrophomonas maltophilia. *Int. J. Antimicrob. Agents* **2010**, *36*, 129–131. [CrossRef] [PubMed]

33. Hamilton-Miller, J.M. Antimicrobial properties of tea (*Camellia sinensis* L.). *Antimicrob. Agents Chemother.* **1995**, *39*, 2375–2377. [CrossRef] [PubMed]

34. Ikigai, H.; Nakae, T.; Hara, Y.; Shimamura, T. Bactericidal catechins damage the lipid bilayer. *Biochim. Biophys. Acta* **1993**, *1147*, 132–136. [CrossRef]

35. Tamba, Y.; Ohba, S.; Kubota, M.; Yoshioka, H.; Yamazaki, M. Single GUV method reveals interaction of tea catechin (−)-epigallocatechin gallate with lipid membranes. *Biophys. J.* **2007**, *92*, 3178–3194. [CrossRef] [PubMed]

36. Yanagawa, Y.; Yamamoto, Y.; Hara, Y.; Shimamura, T. A combination effect of epigallocatechin gallate, a major compound of green tea catechins, with antibiotics on Helicobacter pylori growth in vitro. *Curr. Microbiol.* **2003**, *47*, 244–249. [PubMed]

37. Koech, K.R.; Wachira, F.N.; Ngure, R.M.; Wanyoko, J.K.; Bii, C.C.; Karori, S.M.; Kerio, L.C. Antioxidant, antimicrobial and synergistic activities of tea polyphenols. *Afr. Crop Sci. J.* **2014**, *22*, 837–846. [CrossRef]

38. Osterburg, A.; Gardner, J.; Hyon, S.H.; Neely, A.; Babcock, G. Highly antibiotic-resistant Acinetobacter baumannii clinical isolates are killed by the green tea polyphenol (−)-epigallocatechin-3-gallate (EGCG). *Clin. Microbiol. Infect.* **2009**, *15*, 341–346. [CrossRef] [PubMed]

39. Zhao, W.H.; Hu, Z.Q.; Okubo, S.; Hara, Y.; Shimamura, T. Mechanism of synergy between epigallocatechin gallate and beta-lactams against methicillin-resistant Staphylococcus aureus. *Antimicrob. Agents Chemother.* **2001**, *45*, 1737–1742. [CrossRef] [PubMed]

8

Probiotics: A Promising Role in Dental Health

Sari A. Mahasneh [1] and Adel M. Mahasneh [2,*]

[1] School of Dental Medicine, The University of Manchester, Manchester, M13 9PL, UK;
    sari-mahasneh@hotmail.com
[2] Department of Biological Sciences, The University of Jordan, Amman 11942, Jordan
*   Correspondence: amahasneh@ju.edu.jo;

Abstract: Probiotics have a role in maintaining oral health through interaction with oral microbiome, thus contributing to healthy microbial equilibrium. The nature and composition of any individual microbiome impacts the general health, being a major contributor to oral health. The emergence of drug resistance and the side effects of available antimicrobials have restricted their use in an array of prophylactic options. Indeed, some new strategies to prevent oral diseases are based on manipulating oral microbiota, which is provided by probiotics. Currently, no sufficient substantial evidence exists to support the use of probiotics to prevent, treat or manage oral cavity diseases. At present, probiotic use did not cause adverse effects or increased risks of caries or periodontal diseases. This implicates no strong evidence against treatment using probiotics. In this review, we try to explore the use of probiotics in prevention, treatment and management of some oral cavity diseases and the possibilities of developing designer probiotics for the next generation of oral and throat complimentary healthcare.

Keywords: probiotics; *Lactobacillus*; dental healthcare; periodontitis; caries; halitosis

1. Introduction

It is well recognized that the human microbiome including bacteria, fungi, and viruses is ten times the number of cells of our body [1,2]. For obvious reasons, great attention in healthcare focused on the gut microbiota until recently, when microbial populations of other body regions, especially of the oral cavity, became of concern [3,4].

In the oral cavity, a diverse population has been estimated to include more than 700–1000 bacterial species spread on the tongue, teeth, gum, inner cheeks, palate and tonsils. Streptococci form about 20% of these bacteria, in addition to viruses, fungi and some archaea. It is generally accepted that oral health is affected by residing bacteria as well as the individual's age, health, nutritional status and lifestyle [5].

With the slow progress of isolating new antibiotics coupled with the increase of emerging resistant pathogenic bacteria, it has become imperative to try and enhance the use of living therapeutics. Probiotics form the cornerstone of such biotherapy. According to World Health Organization, the definition of probiotics refers to "live microorganisms which when administered in adequate amounts, confer benefits to the health of the host". Probiotic effect on human health has been substantiated for many years [6]. Research results have confirmed the positive activity of probiotic lactic acid bacteria in prevention and treatment of antibiotic associated diarrhea rota virus infections and many gastrointestinal diseases [7]. It is also known that probiotic bacteria including lactobacilli and bifidobacteria are good colonizers of the gastrointestinal tract, vagina and oral cavity of humans [8], which broaden the prospective role of biotherapy. On the other hand, recent studies suggested a role of periodontopathic bacteria in enhancing systemic diseases including diabetes, respiratory and cardiovascular cases [9]. Probiotic preparations are increasingly used to confer good health substantiated with successful randomized clinical trials. Table 1 presents results of some randomized clinical trials on the use of probiotics in clinical applications. Table 1 shows the little attention given to the use of probiotics for a healthy oral cavity. However, in the last decade, more research has been carried out in this direction and it was extended to the oral cavity where probiotics are expected to play an important therapeutic and/or preventive role in the development of oral diseases.

Table 1. Totally or partially proven probiotic activity and mode of action on oral pathogens.

Probiotic	Activity	References
S. salivarius K12	Antagonism	[10]
L. reuteri	Coaggregation	[11]
S. salivarius K12, M18	Interaction withepithelium	[12]
L. acidophilus LA-5	Modulation of biofilm	[13]
L. casei LC-11	Reduction of cariogenic biofilm potential	[13]
L. paracasei	Caries management	[14,15]
Lactobacilli sp	Periodontal control	[16]
Bifidobacterium sp	Gingivitis management	[16]
L. rhamnosus GG	Modulation of immune response	[17]
Bifidobacterium *Animalis subsp. lacis*	Improved resistance to oral infections	[16,18]

2. Foreseen and Research Targeted Activities of Probiotics

The envisaged role of probiotic bacteria on human health is associated with remarks of Metchnikoff, a Nobel Prize winner, at the turn of the 20th century on longevity of peasants relying on fermented dairy products as a major diet component. It is now well established that some probiotic bacteria, mainly *Lactobacillus* and *Bifidobacterium* confer health benefits. This is substantiated through continued research and randomized clinical trials [5,19,20]. Probiotics benefits tend to be widened with the development of more accurate research methods to better understand microbe–host interactions [21]. Such interactions include, but are not limited to, modulation of the immune responses [22], strengthening means of evading pathogens [23], affecting the balance of the host microbiota [24] and the metabolism of microbiota at specific locations of the host body [25,26]. All of the above observations led researchers to revisit the selection criteria of probiotics with great emphasis on the ability: (1) to harness the immune response, whether it is specific or non-specific; (2) to produce antimicrobials including bacteriocins; (3) to compete successfully for binding site; and (4) to survive during oro-gastro intestinal passage, thus resisting host defense mechanisms with assured safety to the users. Considering the accumulating literature about the proven benefits of probiotics and their inhibitory effects on the growth of pathogenic microorganisms [27–29], researchers have extended their interest to include the oral cavity where probiotics may exhibit some therapeutic or preventive outcome on the incidence and progression of oral diseases. Consequently, regarding the oral environment, some studies on oral probiotic bacteria role on prevention and control of dental caries have been promising [30–32]. Indeed, it is recognized that most new strategies to deal with oral cavity diseases are based on manipulating microbial activities through use of beneficial probiotics inhibitory activities against pathogens including cariogenic and gingivitis causing microbiota [21,26,27]. In this review, we present information on the expected beneficial role of probiotic microorganisms in the oral cavity in the context of the wider scope of the new era of biotherapeutics or biotherapy.

3. Possible Roles of Probiotics in the Oral Cavity

Accumulating research results point to the following activities of probiotics in the human oral cavity:

(1)   Antagonism with pathogens;
(2)   Aggregation with oral bacteria; and
(3)   Interaction with oral epithelium.

In Cases 1 and 2, it is expected that, through such processes, modulation of the oral–biofilm composition will take place [33–36]. This would result in reducing the pathogenicity and cariogenic potential of biofilm microorganisms [33,37–39] as well as reducing the potential pathogens burden in oral biofilm [39–41]. The final outcome will definitely present a clear path for caries, gingivitis and periodontal management [42–46].

As for interaction with oral epithelium, research results point out the ability of the probiotic bacteria to strengthen the epithelial barrier function [16,47–49], in addition to modulating the innate and adaptive immune responses [50–52]. Figure 1 summarizes the probable combined effects of probiotics on oral health.

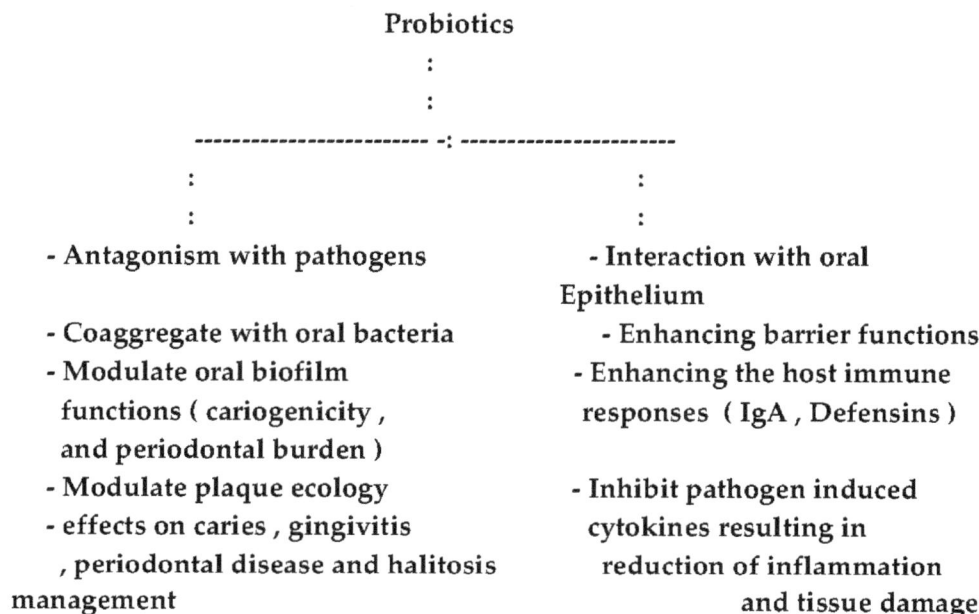

Probiotics

```
                                :
                                :
        ------------------------ -: ------------------------
             :                                    :
             :                                    :
```

- Antagonism with pathogens   - Interaction with oral
                                        Epithelium
- Coaggregate with oral bacteria   - Enhancing barrier functions
- Modulate oral biofilm   - Enhancing the host immune
  functions (cariogenicity ,   responses (IgA , Defensins)
  and periodontal burden)
- Modulate plaque ecology   - Inhibit pathogen induced
- effects on caries , gingivitis   cytokines resulting in
  , periodontal disease and halitosis   reduction of inflammation
management   and tissue damage

Figure 1. The envisaged probiotic roles in the oral cavity.

4. Oral Microbiota Characteristics

The oral microbiota develops emergent characteristics that cannot be observed from studies of single species [43,44,46,48]. This microbiota, in regards to its structure and function, is highly organized and is considered similar to multicellular organism by some researchers [44]. Usually, it is recognized in a healthy setting that the numerous interactions would contribute to resilience and stability of an ecosystem against perturbations. Consequently, if certain pathogenesis parameters that vary among patients exceed threshold, competitiveness among bacteria will be altered leading to caries and periodontal diseases [48]. Understanding of these situations will without doubt lead to strategies of better oral health control and management [45].

The tremendous nutritional and physical interactions that develop among and within the species during infection are greatly affected by an array of host factors eliciting inflammatory responses. Many studies indicated a great biomass yield when more than one species are grown in co-culture [53]. This has been explained by species responding to the presence of each other through changes in the rate of certain gene expression. Other studies highlighted the interaction role of close physical associations to biofilm formation [54].

5. The Oral Cavity and Indigenous Probiotics

Considering all of the above, the question of the presence of probiotic bacteria within the indigenous oral microbiota has been partially answered. Recent studies mention no less than 1000 bacterial species residing or transient within the oral cavity [49,55]. These bacteria in the cavity are either planktonic or integrated into an oral biofilm of diverse oral surfaces or niches. In this context, research results recorded major physiological differences between bacteria of the planktonic state and those in biofilms [43,56,57]. Keigser et al. [55] reported the presence of more than 1000 species in the oral cavity in both planktonic and biofilm statuses. Saliva also contributed to the microbial diversity through its composition and easy flow and flow effect upon continuous detachment of bacterial cells from biofilm surfaces. The question of presence of probiotics indigenously in the mouth is still unclear; however, since *Lactobacillus* and *Bifidobacterium* form the majority of probiotics in general, it could be said that some lactobacilli in the mouth would exhibit beneficial effects [58]. Although information regarding indigenous probiotics in the oral cavity is very scarce [59], Koll-Klais et al. [60] reported that healthy oral cavity was populated with *Lactobacillus gasseri* and *Lactbacillus fermentum*, whereas periodontitis patients were free of these two species but populated with *Lactobacillus plantarum*. Ample clinical studies presented results indicating the positive effects of the regular probiotic yoghurt consumption on reducing the numbers of cariogenic streptococci in the oral cavity [61–64] in both saliva and dental plaque. Further studies on periodontal diseases (gingivitis and periodontitis) presented to researchers the definite ability of certain probiotic lactobacilli to antagonize the pathogenic bacteria active in periodontitis such as *Porphyromonas gingivitis* and *Aggregatibacter* species [60,65]. The trend of these positive reports about the roe of probiotics in managing periodontal disease is of utmost significance if we couple this to the complexity of the etiology of periodontitis which is believed to be biofilm induced infection [66]. However, Bartold and Van Dyke [67] associated periodontal disease in general with imbalances with the host local microbiome pertaining to increased numbers of pathogens and reduced proportions of health associated bacteria [68]. Finally, since the aim of managing the oral cavity infections lies in reducing the pathogenic burden by antibiotics or other means, this effect is not a permanent process due to recolonization in due course [4], and there are problems associated with emerging resistant bacteria, considering probiotics and beneficial bacteria with their prospective disease preventive capabilities provides a reasonable option for safer oral health.

6. Halitosis and Probiotics

Halitosis (malodor) is primarily caused by anaerobic bacteria associated with periodontal diseases [69]. It has several causes stemming from imbalance of the oral cavity microbiota such as metabolic disorders, use of certain types of foods and some respiratory infections [64]. Cultivable oral cavity bacteria associated with halitosis include mainly *Porphyromonas gingivitis*, *Treponema denticola* and *Treponema forsythia* [70–72]. It is caused by the production of volatile sulfur compounds due to degradation of S-containing amino acids by these bacteria and others. The reduction of pathogenic bacterial counts involved in halitosis or its replacement through colonization with probiotic strains would elucidate treatment, management and control of halitosis [20,73,74]. Studies carried out on periodontitis and halitosis patients showed a high degree of heterogeneity of probiotic strains used, dosages, method and vehicle of administration, and treatment duration. Probiotic strain co-aggregating ability to dental pathogens may pave the way for wider application routes for reduction of halitosis symptoms through improving co-aggregation and/or colonization of selected probiotics to volatile sulfur compounds producing oral pathogens [4,74,75]. The complex oral microbiota is considered the major hurdle challenging researchers on prevention, treatment, management and control of dental diseases including halitosis. In future studies, it is necessary to obtain substantial data from blind and randomized large groups of patients with emphasis on strain efficacy, dose effects and most successful delivery vehicles.

7. Oral Fungal Infections

Interactions between bacteria and fungi in the oral cavity environment are dynamic and usually drive the structure and behavior of the oral cavity community resulting in pathogenesis of the oral diseases [76–79]. Vest et al. [76] studying the oral fungal communities reported diverse numbers of fungal genera including *Candida, Saccharomyces, Pencillium, Cladosporium, Malasseezia* and *Fusarium* with varying densities. However, species of *Candida* were dominant and they are known to be commensals in the oral cavity and present in about 25%–75% of the microbiota of healthy individuals [80]. These species are opportunistic pathogens and may under suitable conditions infect the oral mucosa causing infectious candidiasis [11]. The majority cases of candidiasis are associated with *Candida albican* isolates [77]. Other *Candida* species such as *C. krusei, C. tropicalis, C. glabrata, C. parapsilosis,* and *C. dubliniensis* were incriminated and isolated from oral cavity infections [78–81]. The oral cavity is among the most diverse microbiomes of the human body where different niches occur in the plaque, saliva and epithelial mucosa, thus eliciting dysbiosis by fungi and bacteria [82,83]. These dysbiotic infections could affect mucosal surfaces of the oral cavity and esophagus, and may become systemic [11]. Under certain stress conditions of debilitated patients, candidiasis would be life threatening and cause "diseases of the diseased" [84,85]. Considering the slow down in antifungals development [21] coupled with little number of new antibiotics available as well as the increased rate of emerging resistant fungal and bacterial strains [86,87], it has become very inviting to researchers and health professionals to extend the probable adoption of probiotics as an option in oral cavity care where probiotics may exert therapeutic or preventive effects on common oral diseases. Nevertheless, in vitro studies have several limitations and they never exactly mimic the microbiota of the oral cavity [11]. It is also recognized that probiotics activity is highly host and strain specific, even at strain level. Significant differences in growth inhibition and co-aggregation were observed, especially against *Candida* pathogenic species [11,85,88]. This reconfirms the notion that probiotics should not be put in one box and further in vitro and in vivo studies are needed to elucidate and understand the role of probiotics in prevention, treatment and management of fungal infections of the oral cavity.

8. Designer Probiotics as a Base for Living Therapeutics

Recent studies on the mode of action of probiotics that target the oral cavity, though not fully substantiated by in vivo studies [89,90], are presented in several categories: competition for nutrients; growth factors; adhesion; production of inhibitory substances such as enzymes, antimicrobials, bacteriocins, and H_2O_2; inhibition of pathogen induced production of cytokines; and immune system stimulation [91]. All of these envisioned activities vary according to host and microbial strains [92,93]. In the last six years, interesting reviews about the probable and real use of probiotics have been published [88–90,92,93]. Although the feeling of low degree of substantiation in vitro studies prevailed, nevertheless most authors agreed upon the great promise of the benefits of probiotic use in oral health. They also pointed out that enhancing the functional repertoire of probiotic microorganisms as biotherapeutic agents is an attractive and promising approach. This approach is being pushed to the frontiers of research due to the slow down in new drugs development and increasing rate of emerging resistant pathogens. Probiotics able to deliver new and novel therapeutics are hopefully emerging with site specific and well-defined efficacy, which is now known as designer probiotics. These emerging living improved therapeutics [designer probiotics] will without doubt transform existing paradigms of disease prevention, control and management. These awaited designer probiotics would, when fully developed, expand the efficiency and efficacy of probiotics by introducing new genetic circuits to develop new drug delivery systems [94–96]. As a result of pressing needs for alternative biotherapeutics and nutraceuticals, the science of probiotics has emerged in the post genomic era of medicine and biology as a hot research area in the quest for better healthcare areas including the oral cavity. In this context, the use of designer probiotics is being tested against infectious diseases and in anticancer therapy studies [97,98]. When used as dietary supplements or applied topically, designer probiotics would support normal physiology and immunity to improve health and prevent infections, oxidation stress, autoimmune responses and inflammatory diseases [99]. As for dental and periodontal health, an array of probiotics has demonstrated beneficial effects. Clinical studies have typically used surrogate endpoints such as *Streptococcus mutans* counts, salivary flow, plaque or gingival scores, and pocket depth to substantiate efficacy [92–94]. These studies provided promising outlook, however, need to be further confirmed in randomized double blind placebo studies with specific target sites in the oral cavity.

9. Concluding Remarks and Future Directions

In medical settings, it is now recognized that the increase in emerging resistant pathogens coupled to metabolic diseases are paramount public health and oral health concerns. This concern necessities the search for safe, cost-effective and inventive alternatives and/or complimentary means to the traditional uses of prophylactics and treatment. In this context, probiotics, both general and designer, would offer potential prospects. This conviction of the importance of biotherapeutics that integrate with clinical prescriptions should be inviting and given priority in medical research. The potential role of such living biotherapeutics should not overlook the notion that probiotic-mediated antagonism and functional characteristics may hinder some commensal bacteria and/or inter signals from indigenous microbiota. The effect of this prospective hindrance would be reduced through designer probiotic development, which needs concerted research efforts to fully understand and substantiate their safe use, specificity and efficacy. This becomes imminent if we know that most of the documented health benefits come from research and clinical trials on animal models. With all of this in mind, it appears that the stage is set not only for probiotics use in medicine but also expansion to include the oral cavity microbiome. A further outlook might be to have the personal oral microbiome characterized to the genus level by providing a saliva sample to be used as a biomarker to formulate a list of probiotic strains specifically targeting resident pathogenic bacteria. This, no doubt, will help in offering a strong complementary and/or alternative approach for the next generation [designer] probiotics for oral cavity and throat healthcare.

Acknowledgments: The University of Jordan is thanked for the direct and indirect support, which was given to the authors.

Author Contributions: Both authors contributed equally in executing the work and writing the manuscript.

References

1. Wade, W.G. The oral microbiome in health and disease. *Pharmacol. Res.* **2013**, *69*, 137–143. [CrossRef] [PubMed]

2. Shomark, D.K.; Allen, S.J. The microbiota and disease reviewing the links between the oral microbiome, aging and Alzheimer's disease. *J. Alzheimer's Dis.* **2015**, *43*, 725–738.

3. Scannapieco, F.A. The oral microbiome: Its role in health and in oral and systemic infections. *Clin. Microbiol. News* **2013**, *35*, 163–199. [CrossRef]

4. Gatej, S.; Gully, N.; Gibson, R.; Bartold, P.M. Probiotics and periodontitis—A literature review. *J. Int. Acad. Periodontol.* **2012**, *19*, 42–50.

5. Stamatova, I.; Meurman, J.H. Probiotics: Health benefits in the mouth. *Am. J. Dent.* **2009**, *22*, 329–338. [PubMed]

6. Kobayashi, R.; Kobayashi, T.; Sakai, F.; Hosoya, T.; Yamamoto, M.; Kurita-Ochiai, T. Oral administration of *Lactobacillus gasseri* SBT 2055 is effective in preventing *Porphyromonas gingivalis*—Accelerated periodontal disease. *Sci. Rep.* **2017**, *7*, 545–554. [CrossRef] [PubMed]

7. Vandenplas, Y.; Huys, G.; Daube, G. Probiotics: An update. *J. Pediatr.* **2015**, *91*, 6–21. [CrossRef] [PubMed]

8. Selle, K.; Klaenhammer, T.R. Genomic and phenotypic evidence for probiotic influences of Lactobacillus gasseri on human health. *FEMS Micrbiol. Rev.* **2013**, *37*, 915–935. [CrossRef] [PubMed]

9. Hajishengallis, G. Periodontitis from microbial immune subversion to systemic inflammation. *Nat. Rev. Immunol.* **2015**, *15*, 30–44. [CrossRef] [PubMed]

10. Maseda, L.; Kulik, E.M.; Hauser-Gerpach, I.; Ramseier, A.M.; Filipi, A.; Waltimo, T. Antimicrobial activity of *Streptococcus salivarius* K12 on bacteria involved in oral malodor. *Arch. Oral Biol.* **2012**, *57*, 1041–1047. [CrossRef] [PubMed]

11. Jorgensen, M.R.; Kragelund, C.; Jansen, P.; Keller, M.K.; Twetman, S. Probiotic *Lactobacillus reuteri* has antifungal effects on oral Candida species In Vitro. *Arch. Oral Biol.* **2017**, *9*, 127–135. [CrossRef] [PubMed]

12. Manning, J.; Dunne, E.; Wescombe, P.; Hale, J.; Mullholland, E.; Tagg, J. Investigation of *S. salivarius* mediated inhibition of pneumococcal adherence to pharyngeal cells. *BMC Microbiol.* **2016**, *16*, 225–234. [CrossRef] [PubMed]

13. Schwendicke, F.; Korte, F.; Drofer, C.; Kneist, S.; El-Sayed, F.; Paris, S. Inhibition of *Streptococcus mutans* growth and biofilm formation by probiotics In Vitro. *Caries Res.* **2017**, *51*, 87–95. [CrossRef] [PubMed]

14. Chang, L.C.; Huang, C.S.; Ou-Yang, L.W.; Lin, S.Y. Probiotic *Lactobacillus paracaesi* effect on cariogenic flora. *Clin. Oral Investig.* **2017**, *15*, 471–476. [CrossRef] [PubMed]

15. Schwendicke, F.; Dorfer, C.; Kneist, F.; Meyer-Lueckel, H.; Paris, S. Cariogenic effect of *Lactobacillus rhamnosus* GG in dental biofilm model. *Caries Res.* **2014**, *48*, 186–192. [CrossRef] [PubMed]

16. Gruner, D.; Paris, S.; Schwendicke, F. Probiotics for managing caries and periodontitis: Systematic review and meta-analysis. *J. Dent.* **2016**, *48*, 16–25. [CrossRef] [PubMed]

17. Fong, F.L.; Shah, N.P.; Kirjavainen, P.; El-Nezami, H. Mechanisms of action of probiotic bacteria on intestinal and systemic immunities and antigen-presenting cells. *Int. Rev. Immunol.* **2016**, *35*, 179–188. [CrossRef] [PubMed]

18. Oliveria, L.F.F.; Salvador, S.L.; Silva, P.H.F.; Furlaneto, F.A.; Figuiredo, L.; Casarin, R.; Ervolino, E.; Palioto, D.; Souza, S.; Taba, M.; et al. Benefits of *Bifidobacterium animalis* subsp. lactis Probiotic in Experimental Periodontitis. *J. Periodontl.* **2017**, *88*, 197–208. [CrossRef] [PubMed]

19. Para, D.; Martinez, J.A. Amino acid uptake from probiotic milk in lactose intolerance subjects. *Br. J. Nutr.* **2007**, *98*, 5101–5104.

20. Burton, J.P.; Chilcott, C.N.; Moore, C.J.; Speiser, G.; Tagg, J.R. A preliminary study of the effect of probiotic *Streptococcus salivarius* K12 on oral malodour parameters. *J. Appl. Microbiol.* **2006**, *100*, 754–764. [CrossRef] [PubMed]

21. Alok, A.; Singh, I.D.; Singh, S.; Kishore, M.; Jha, P.C.; Iqbal, M.A. A new era of biotherapy. *Adv. Biomed. Res.* **2017**, *6*, 31–37. [CrossRef] [PubMed]

22. Toshimitsu, T.; Ozaki, S.; Mochizuki, J.; Furuichi, K.; Asami, Y. Effects of *Lactobacillus plantarum* strain OLL 2712 culture conditions on the anti-inflammatory activities for murine immune cells and obese type 2 diabetic mice. *Appl. Environ. Microbiol.* **2017**, *83*, e03001-16. [CrossRef] [PubMed]

23. Bouchard, D.S.; Rault, L.; Berkova, N.; Le Loir, Y.; Evens, S. Inhibition of *Staphylococcus aureus* invasion into bovine mammary epithelial cells by contact with live *Lactobacillus casei*. *Appl. Environ. Microbiol.* **2013**, *79*, 877–885. [CrossRef] [PubMed]

24. Arumugam, S.; Lau, C.S.; Chamberlain, R.S. Probiotics and symbiotics decrease post-operation sepsis in elective gastrointestinal surgical patients: A meta-analysis. *J. Gastrointest. Surg.* **2016**, *20*, 1123–1131. [CrossRef] [PubMed]

25. Kumar, R.; Dhanda, S. Mechnistic insight of probiotic derived anticancer pharmaceuticals: A road forward for cancer therapeutics. *Nutr. Cancer* **2017**, *69*, 375–380. [CrossRef] [PubMed]

26. Laleman, I.; Teughels, W. Probiotics in dental practice: A review. *Quintessence Int.* **2015**, *46*, 255–264. [PubMed]

27. Collado, M.C.; Meriluoto, J.; Salminen, S. Adhesion and aggregation properties of probiotic and pathogen strains. *Eur. Food Restechnol.* **2008**, *226*, 1065–1075. [CrossRef]

28. Mahasneh, A.M.; Hamdan, S.; Mahasneh, S.A. Probiotic properties of *Lactobacillus* species isolated from local traditionally fermented products. *Jordan J. Biol. Sci.* **2015**, *8*, 81–87. [CrossRef]

29. Mahasneh, A.M.; Mahasneh, S.A. Probiotic characterization of lactic acid bacteria isolated from local fermented vegetables (Makdoos). *Int. J. Curr. Microbiol. Appl. Sci.* **2017**, *6*, 1673–1686. [CrossRef]

30. Bonifait, I.; Chandad, F.; Grenier, D. Probiotics for oral health: Myth or reality? *J. Can. Dent. Assoc.* **2009**, *75*, 585–590. [PubMed]

31. Nudelman, P.; Frazao, J.V.; Vieira, T.I.; Balth, C.F.; Andrade, M.M.; Alexandria, A.K.; Cruz, A.G.; Fonseca, A.; Maia, L.C. The performance of fermented sheep milk and ice cream sheep milk in inhibiting enamel loss. *Food Res. Int.* **2017**, *97*, 184–190. [CrossRef] [PubMed]

32. Thomas, I.V. Probiotics—The journey continues. *Int. J. Dairy Technol.* **2016**, *69*, 469–480. [CrossRef]

33. Ben Taheur, F.; Kouidhi, B.; Fdhila, K.; Elabed, H.; Ben Salama, R.; Mahduan, K.; Bakharouf, A.; Chaieb, K. Antibacterial and antibiofilm activity of probiotic bacteria against oral pathogens. *Microb. Pathog.* **2016**, *97*, 213–220. [CrossRef] [PubMed]

34. Samot, J.; Badet, C. Antibacterial activity of probiotic candidate for oral health. *Anaerobe* **2013**, *19*, 34–38. [CrossRef] [PubMed]

35. Lee, S.H.; Kim, Y.-J. A copmparative study on cariogenic biofilm model for preventing dental caries. *Arch. Microbiol.* **2014**, *196*, 601–609. [CrossRef] [PubMed]

36. Schwendicke, F.; Horb, K.; Kneist, S.; Dorfer, C.; Paris, S. Effects of heat-inactivated bifidobacterium BB12 on cariogenicity of *Streptococcus mutans* In Vitro. *Arch. Oral Biol.* **2014**, *59*, 1384–1390. [CrossRef] [PubMed]

37. Suzuki, N.; Uneda, M.; Hatano, Y.; Iwamoto, T.; Masuo, Y.; Hirofugi, T. *Enterococcus faecium* WB 2000 inhibits biofilm formation by oral cariogenic streptococci. *Int. J. Dent.* **2011**, *2011*, 834151. [CrossRef] [PubMed]

38. Bensalama, R.; Kouidhi, B.; Zmantar, T.; Chaieb, K.; Bakharouf, A. Antilisterial and biofilm activities of potential probiotic *Lactobacillus strains* isolated from *Tunisian traditional* fermented foods. *J. Food Saf.* **2013**, *33*, 8–16. [CrossRef]

39. Singh, V.P.; Malhotra, N.; Apratim, A.; Verma, M. Assessment and management of halitosis. *Dent. Update* **2015**, *42*, 346–353. [CrossRef] [PubMed]

40. Castalonga, M.; Herzberg, M. The oral microbiome and the immunobiology of periodontal disease and caries. *Immunol. Lett.* **2014**, *162*, 22–38. [CrossRef] [PubMed]

41. Anusha, R.L.; Umar, D.; Basheer, D.; Baroudi, K. The magic of magic bugs in oral cavity: Probiotics. *J. Adv. Pharm. Technol. Res.* **2015**, *6*, 43–47. [PubMed]

42. Russel, D.A.; Ross, R.P.; Fitzgerald, G.F.; Santon, C. Metabolic activities and probiotic potential of bifidobacteria. *Int. J. Food Microbiol* **2011**, *149*, 88–105. [CrossRef] [PubMed]

43. Marsh, P.D.; Zura, E. Dental biofilms: Ecological interactions inhealth disease. *J. Clin. Periodontol.* **2017**, *44*, S12–S22. [CrossRef] [PubMed]

44. Ereshefsky, M.; Pedroso, M. Rethinking evolutionary individuality. *Proc. Natl. Acad. Sci. USA* **2015**, *112*, 10126–10132. [CrossRef] [PubMed]

45. Burczynska, A.; Dziewit, L.; Decewit, L.; Decewicz, P.; Struzycka, I.; Wroblewska, M. Application of metagenomic analyses in dentistry and novel strategy enabling complex insight into microbial diversity of the oral cavity. *Pol. J. Microbiol.* **2017**, *66*, 9–15. [CrossRef]

46. Perez-Chaparro, P.J.; Concalves, C.; Figueirado, P.; Faveri, M.; Louo, E.; Tamashiro, N.; Durate, P.; Feres, M. Newly identified pathogens associated with periodontitis: A systematic review. *J. Dent. Res.* **2014**, *93*, 846–858. [CrossRef] [PubMed]

47. Roberts, F.A.; Darveau, R.P. Microbial protection and virulence in periodontal tissue as a function of polymicrobial communities: Symbiosis and dysbiosis. *Periodontology* **2015**, *69*, 18–27. [CrossRef] [PubMed]

48. Ng, H.M.; Kin, L.X.; Dashper, S.G.; Slakeski, N.; Butler, C.A.; Reynolds, E.C. Bacterial interactions in pathogenic subgingival plaque. *Microb. Pathog.* **2016**, *94*, 60–69. [CrossRef] [PubMed]

49. Mark-Welsh, J.L.; Rosseti, B.J.; Rieken, C.W.; Dewhirst, F.W.; Boristy, G.G. Biogeography of a human oral microbiome at the micro scale. *Proc. Natl. Acad. Sci. USA* **2016**, *113*, E791–E800. [CrossRef] [PubMed]

50. Hagishengallis, G. Immunomicrobial pathogenesis of periodontitis: Keystones, pathobionnts and host response. *Trends Immunol.* **2014**, *35*, 3–11. [CrossRef] [PubMed]

51. Schincaglia, G.P.; Hong, B.Y.; Rosania, A.; Barasz, J.; Thompson, A.; Soube, T.; Panagakos, F.; Burleson, J.A.; Dongari-Bagtzoglou, A.; Diaz, P. Clinical, immune, and microbiome traits of gingivitis and peri-implant mucositis. *J. Dent. Res.* **2017**, *96*, 47–55. [CrossRef] [PubMed]

52. Diaz, P.I.; Xie, Z.; Sobae, T.; Thompson, A.; Biyikoglu, B.; Rikers, A.; Ikonomou, I.; Dongari-Bagtazoslou, A. Synergistic interaction between *Candida albicans* and commensal oral streptococci in a novel In Vitro mucosal model. *Infect. Immun.* **2012**, *80*, 620–632. [CrossRef] [PubMed]

53. Tan, K.H.; Seers, C.A.; Dashper, S.G.; Mitchell, H.L.; Pyke, J.S.; Meuric, V.; Slakeski, N.; Cleal, S.M.; Chambers, J.L.; McConville, M.; et al. *Porphyromonas gingivalis* and *Treponema denticola* exhibits metabolic symbiosis. *PLoS Pathog.* **2014**, *10*, e1003955. [CrossRef] [PubMed]

54. Oukoda, T.; Kokubu, E.; Kawana, T.; Saito, A.; Okuda, K.; Ishihara, K. Synergy in biofilm formation between *Fusobacterium nucleatum* and *Prevotella species*. *Anaerobe* **2012**, *18*, 110–116. [CrossRef] [PubMed]

55. Keijser, B.J.; Zaura, E.; Huse, S.M.; Van der Vossen, J.M.; Schuren, F.H.; Montigen, R.C.; Ten Cate, J.M.; Crielaad, V.V. Pyrosequencing analysis of the oral microflora of healthy adults. *J. Dent. Res.* **2008**, *87*, 1016–1020. [CrossRef] [PubMed]

56. Rudney, J.D. Saliva and dental plaque. *Adv. Dent. Res.* **2000**, *14*, 29–39. [CrossRef] [PubMed]

57. Burne, R.A.; Quivey, R.G.; Marquis, R.E. Physiologic homeostasis and stress responses in oral biofilms. *Meth. Enzymol.* **1999**, *310*, 441–460. [PubMed]

58. Bernaedeau, M.; Venoux, J.P.; Henri-Dubernet, S.; Gueguen, M. Safety assessment of dairy microorganisms: The Lactobacillus genus. *Int. J. Food Microbiol.* **2008**, *85*, 88–94.

59. Yli-Knuuttila, H.; Snall, J.; Kari, K.; Meurman, J.H. Colonization of *Lactobacillus rhamnosus* GC in the oral cavity. *Oral Microbiol. Immunol.* **2006**, *21*, 129–131. [CrossRef] [PubMed]

60. Koll-Klais, P.; Mandar, R.; Leibur, E.; Marcotte, H.; Hammarstrom, L.; Mikelsaar, M. Oral lactobacilli in chronic periodontitis and periodontal health: Species composition and antimicrobial activity. *Oral Microbiol. Immunol.* **2005**, *20*, 354–361. [CrossRef] [PubMed]

61. Bizzini, B.; Pizzo, G.; Scapagnini, G. Probiotics and oral health. *Curr. Pharm. Des.* **2012**, *18*, 5522–5531. [CrossRef] [PubMed]

62. Scully, C.; Greenman, J. Halitosis (breath odour). *Periodontology* **2012**, *48*, 66–75. [CrossRef] [PubMed]

63. Islam, B.; Khan, S.; Khan, A. Dental caries: From infection to prevention. *Med. Sci. Monit.* **2007**, *13*, 196–205.

64. Ruiz-Martinez, R.C.; Bedani, R.; Saad, S.M. Scientific evidence for probiotics and prebiotics: An update for current prospectives and future challenges. *Br. J. Nutr.* **2015**, *114*, 1993–2015. [CrossRef] [PubMed]

65. Sookkhee, S.; Chulasiri, M.; Pradyabreud, W. Lactic acid bacteria from healthy oral cavity of Thai volunteers, inhibition of oral pathogens. *J. Appl. Microbiol.* **2001**, *90*, 172–179. [CrossRef] [PubMed]

66. Hajishengallis, G. The inflammophilic character of the periodontitis-associated microbiota. *Mol. Oral Microbiol.* **2014**, *29*, 248–257. [CrossRef] [PubMed]

67. Bartold, P.M.; Van Dyke, T.E. Periodontitis: A host mediated disruption of microbial homeostasis. Unlearning learned concept. *Periodontology* **2013**, *62*, 203–217. [CrossRef] [PubMed]

68. Wade, W. Has the use of molecular methods for the characterization of the human oral microbiome changed our understanding of the role of bacteria in the pathogenesis of periodontal disease? *J. Clin. Periodontol.* **2011**, *38*, 7–16. [CrossRef] [PubMed]

69. De Geest, S.; Laleman, I.; Teughels, W.; Dekeyser, C.; Quirynen, M. Periodental diseases as a source of halitosis: A review of the evidence and treatment approaches for dentists and dental hygienists. *Periodontology* **2016**, *71*, 213–227. [CrossRef] [PubMed]

70. De Boever, E.H.; Loesche, W.J. Assessing the contribution of anaerobic microflora of the tongue to oral malodor. *Am. Dent. Assoc.* **1995**, *126*, 1384–1393. [CrossRef]

71. Aung, E.; Ueno, M.; Zaitsu, T.; Furukawa, S.; Kawaguchi, Y. Effectiveness of three oral hygiene regimens on oral malodor reduction: A randomized clinical trial. *Trials* **2015**, *16*, 31–37. [CrossRef] [PubMed]

72. Takahashi, N. Oral microbiome metabolism: From who are they? To what are they doing? *J. Dent. Res.* **2015**, *94*, 1628–1637. [CrossRef] [PubMed]

73. Kang, M.S.; Kim, B.J.; Yang, K.H.; Oh, J.H. Effect of *Weissella cibaria* isolates on the formation of *S. mutans* biofilms. *Cries Res.* **2006**, *40*, 418–425. [CrossRef] [PubMed]

74. Kang, M.S.; Kim, B.J.; Chung, J.; Lee, H.C.; Oh, J.H. Inhibitory effect of *Weissella cibaria* isolates on the production of volatile sulfur compounds. *J. Clin. Periodontol.* **2006**, *33*, 226–232. [CrossRef] [PubMed]

75. Stingu, C.S.; Escherich, K.; Rodloff, A.C.; Jentsch, H. Periodontitis is associated with loss of colonization by *Streptococcus sanguinis*. *J. Med. Microbiol.* **2008**, *57*, 495–499. [CrossRef] [PubMed]

76. Vesty, A.; Biswas, K.; Taylor, M.W.; Gear, K.; Douglas, R.G. Evaluating the impact of DNA extraction-method on the representation of human oral bacterial and fungal communities. *PLoS ONE* **2007**, *12*, e0169877. [CrossRef] [PubMed]

77. Xu, H.; Dongari-Bagtzoglou, A. Shaping the oral microbiota: Interaction of opportunistic fungi with oral bacteria and the host. *Curr. Opin. Microbiol.* **2015**, *26*, 65–70. [CrossRef] [PubMed]

78. Krom, B.P.; Kidwai, S.; Ten Cate, J.M. Candida and other fungal species: Forgotten players of healthy oral microbiota. *J. Dent. Res.* **2017**, *93*, 445–451. [CrossRef] [PubMed]

79. Ghannoum, M.A.; Jurevic, R.J.; Mukherjee, P.K.; Cui, F.; Sikaroodi, M.; Naqavi, M. Characterization of the oral fungal microbiome (mycobiome) in healthy individuals. *PLoS Pathog.* **2010**, *6*, e1000713. [CrossRef] [PubMed]

80. Barros, P.P.; Ribeiro, F.C.; Rossoni, R.D. Influence of *Candida krusei* and *Candida glabrata* on *Candida albicans* gene expression In Vitro biofilms. *Arch. Oral Biol.* **2016**, *64*, 92–101. [CrossRef] [PubMed]

81. Sardi, J.S.; Scorzoni, I.; Bernardi, T.; Fusco-Almeida, A.M.; Mandis Giannini, M.J. Candida species: Current epidemiology, pathogenicity, biofilm formation natural antifungal products and new therapeutic options. *J. Med. Microbiol.* **2013**, *62*, 10–24. [CrossRef] [PubMed]

82. Wade, W.G. Characterization of the human oral microbiome. *J. Oral Biosci.* **2013**, *55*, 143–148. [CrossRef]

83. Darveau, R.P. Periodontitis: A poly microbial disruption of host homeostasis. *Nat. Rev. Microbiol.* **2010**, *8*, 481–490. [CrossRef] [PubMed]

84. Samaranayake, L.P. Superficial oral fungal infections. *Curr. Opin. Dent.* **1991**, *1*, 415–422. [PubMed]

85. Matsubara, V.H.; Bandara, H.M.; Marcia, P.; Mayer, A.; Samaranayake, P. Probiotics as antifungals in mucosal candidiasis. *Clin. Infect. Dis.* **2016**, *62*, 1143–1153. [PubMed]

86. Miceli, M.H.; Diaz, J.A.; Lee, S.A. Emerging opportunistic yeast infections. *Lancet Inf. Dis.* **2011**, *11*, 42–51. [CrossRef]

87. Oever, J.C.; Netea, M.G. The bacteriome-mycobiome interactions and antifungal host defense. *Eur. J. Immunol.* **2014**, *44*, 3182–3191. [CrossRef] [PubMed]

88. Matsubara, V.H.; Wang, Y.; Bandara, H.M.; Samaranayake, L.P. Probiotic lactobacilli inhibit early stages of *Candida albicans* biofilm development by reducing their growth, cell adhesion and filamentation. *Appl. Microbiol. Biotechnol.* **2016**, *100*, 6415–6426. [CrossRef] [PubMed]

89. Gungor, C.E.; Kirizioglu, Z.; Kivanc, M. Probiotics can they be used to improve oral health? *Benef. Microbes* **2015**, *6*, 647–656. [CrossRef] [PubMed]

90. Prodeep, K.; Kuttapa, M.A.; Prasna, K.P. Probiotics and oral health: An update. *SADJ* **2014**, *69*, 20–24.

91. Haukioja, A. Probiotics and oral health. *Eur. J. Dent.* **2010**, *4*, 348–355. [PubMed]

92. Wescombe, P.A.; Hale, J.D.; Heng, N.C. Developing oral probiotics from Streptococcus salivarius. *Future Microbiol.* **2012**, *7*, 1355–1371. [CrossRef] [PubMed]

93. Saha, S.; Tomaro-Duchesneau, C.; Tabrizian, M.; Prakash, S. Probiotics as oral health biotherapeutics. *Expert Opin. Biol. Ther.* **2013**, *12*, 1207–1220. [CrossRef] [PubMed]

94. Paton, A.W. Bioengineered microbes in disease therapy. *Trends Mol. Med.* **2012**, *18*, 417–425. [CrossRef] [PubMed]

95. Kumar, M. Bioengineered probiotics as a new hope for health and disease: Potential and prospects. *Future Microbiol.* **2015**, *11*, 585–600. [CrossRef] [PubMed]

96. Maxmen, A. Living therapeutics: Scientists genetically modify bacteria to deliver drugs. *Nat. Med.* **2017**, *25*, 5–7. [CrossRef] [PubMed]

97. Mansour, N.M.; Abdelaziz, S.A. Oral immunization of mice with engineered *Lactobacillus gasseri* NM713 strain expressing *Streptococcus pyogenes* M6 antigen. *Microbiol. Immunol.* **2016**, *60*, 527–532. [CrossRef] [PubMed]

98. Zhang, B. Recombinant *Lactococcus lactis* NZ 9000 secretes a bioactive kisspeptin that inhibits proliferation and migration of human colon carcinoma HT-29 cells. *Microb. Cell Fact.* **2016**, *15*, 102–107. [CrossRef] [PubMed]

99. Mahasneh, A.M.; Abbas, M.M. Probiotics: The possible alternative to disease therapy. In *Microbial Biotechnolgy: Progress and Trends*; CRC Press: Boca Raton, FL, USA, 2015; pp. 213–238.

9

Detection of Caries Around Resin-Modified Glass Ionomer and Compomer Restorations Using Four Different Modalities In Vitro

Tamara Abrams [1], Stephen Abrams [1,*] , Koneswaran Sivagurunathan [1], Veronika Moravan [2], Warren Hellen [3], Gary Elman [3], Bennett Amaechi [4] and Andreas Mandelis [5]

[1] Quantum Dental Technologies Inc., Toronto, ON M6B 1L3, Canada; tabrams@uoguelph.ca (T.A.); konesh@thecanarysystem.com (K.S.)

[2] VM Stats, Toronto, ON M5A 4R3, Canada; vmoravan@vmstats.ca

[3] Cliffcrest Dental Office, Toronto, ON M1M 1P1, Canada; wmph@rogers.com (W.H.); garyelman@sympatico.ca (G.E.)

[4] Department of Comprehensive Dentistry, University of Texas Health Science Center, San Antonio, TX 78229-3900, USA; amaechi@uthscsa.edu

[5] Center for Advanced Diffusion Wave and Photoacoustic Technologies (CADIPT), Department of Mechanical and Industrial Engineering, University of Toronto, Toronto, ON M5S 3G8, Canada; mandelis@mie.utoronto.ca

* Correspondence: dr.abrams4cell@sympatico.ca;

Abstract: The aim of this study was to evaluate the ability of visual examination (International Caries Detection and Assessment System—ICDAS II), light-emitting diodes (LED) fluorescence (SPECTRA), laser fluorescence (DIAGNODent, DD), photothermal radiometry and modulated luminescence (PTR-LUM, The Canary System, CS) to detect natural decay beneath resin-modified glass ionomer (RMGIC) and compomer restorations in vitro. Twenty-seven extracted human molars and premolars, consisting of 2 control teeth, 10 visually healthy/sound and 15 teeth with natural cavitated lesions, were selected. For the carious teeth, caries was removed leaving some carious tissue on one wall of the preparation. For the sound teeth, 3 mm deep cavity preparations were made. All cavities were restored with RMGIC or compomer restorative materials. Sixty-eight sites (4 sites on sound unrestored teeth, 21 sound sites and 43 carious sites with restorations) were selected. CS and DD triplicate measurements were done at 2, 1.5, 0.5, and 0 mm away from the margin of the restoration (MOR). SPECTRA images were taken, and two dentists provided ICDAS II scoring for the restored surfaces. The SPECTRA data and images were inconclusive due to signal interference from the restorations. Visual examinations of the restored tooth surfaces were able to identify 5 of the 15 teeth with caries. In these situations, the teeth were ranked as having ICDAS II 1 or 2 rankings, but they could not identify the location of the caries or depth of the lesion. CS and DD were able to differentiate between sound and carious tissue at the MOR, but larger variation in measurement, and poorer accuracy, was observed for DD. It was concluded that the CS has the potential to detect secondary caries around RMGIC and compomer restorations more accurately than the other modalities used in this study.

Keywords: caries; resin-modified glass ionomer; compomer; PTR-LUM; DIAGNODent; caries around restoration margins; SPECTRA; ICDAS II; caries detection

1. Introduction

One of the major reasons for the replacement of restorations is secondary caries or caries around the restoration margins [1,2]. Caries detection around restoration margins including RMGIC and compomers is a major challenge in clinical practice. Compomers and RMGIC restorations release fluoride which may have promising results in caries prevention around restoration margins [3–6]. Systematic reviews show significant decreases of new lesions around RMGIC restorations compared to amalgam [7] and composite restorations [8,9]. However, the challenge is to detect these lesions early; before caries has destroyed more tooth structure and larger, more invasive replacement restorations are required [1].

The detection of secondary caries in the early stages of the disease process is challenging [10], especially, with current detection methods which included visual examination, use of explorers or blunt probes, radiography, and or fluorescence-based devices [11]. Visual or visual-tactile examination, using explorers or probes, often in combination with bitewing radiographs, are the most commonly used technique in clinical practice for caries detection [12].

The International Caries Detection and Assessment System (ICDAS II) was introduced in 2009 to assist in visual ranking of caries [13–16]. The surface appearance of restorations with secondary caries is considered similar to primary caries lesions so the ICDAS II criteria can be used for ranking secondary caries around restorations [17,18]. Research has shown that the ICDAS II presents good reproducibility and accuracy for in vitro and in vivo detection of primary caries lesions at different points in the disease process [18–20].

Laser fluorescence (DIAGNODent 2095 (LF), KaVo, Biberach, Germany) has been used as an aid in detecting caries beneath restorations [12,21]. In 2006, a new laser fluorescence device (DIAGNODent 2190 (LFpen), KaVo) was introduced to aid in the detection of occlusal and interproximal caries. The LFpen, using a low powered 655 nm wavelength diode laser, can analyze and quantify the fluorescence emitted from bacterial porphyrins and other chromophores [22,23]. In vitro studies have demonstrated that LF can detect caries at the margins of amalgam restorations, but amalgam overhangs and stain reduce the sensitivity of this method [24–26].

The SPECTRA Caries Detection System (SPECTRA Air Techniques Melville, New York, NY, USA) also uses fluorescence technology as well. Light-emitting diodes (LED) projects 405 nm wavelength of light onto the tooth surface causing cariogenic bacteria to fluoresce red and healthy enamel to appear green [27,28]. SPECTRA software then quantifies the fluorescence on scale ranging from 0 to 5 [29]. SPECTRA also captures the fluorescence from bacterial porphyrins [28,30,31]. Studies have shown the ability of SPECTRA to detect caries on unrestored occlusal surfaces [32–35] but the detection around restoration margins or beneath sealants has been more challenging [36–38].

The Canary System (Quantum Dental Technologies, Toronto, ON, Canada) using a 660 nm <50 mW, pulsed laser, combines laser photothermal radiometry (PTR) and modulated luminescence (LUM) amplitude and phase signals to detect and assess caries [39]. Pulses of laser light focused on a tooth cause, the tooth to "glow" or luminesce (LUM) and releases heat (PTR). The system analyzes the response of the re-emitted radiation (luminescence or LUM) and the thermal behavior of the emitted infrared photons (PTR) to provide information about the status of the tooth's crystal structure [39]. The CS measures both the amplitude and phase delay of the PTR and LUM signals and then converts these signals into a measurement or Canary Number (CN). These pulses of laser light can detect caries lesions up to 5 mm below the tooth surface [39–41]. As a caries lesion increases in volume there is a corresponding change in the PTR and LUM signals [40]. The heat is confined to the region with crystalline disintegration (dental caries) increasing the PTR and decreasing the LUM signals [42]. During remineralization, the enamel prisms start to reform their structure and the thermal and luminescence properties begin to revert towards those of healthy tooth structure [43–46].

This study assessed the ability of four caries detection systems to detect secondary caries beneath the margins of RMGIC and compomer restorations. This in vitro model does simulate a clinical situation where restoration margins are intact but secondary caries is present beneath one section of the restoration.

2. Materials and Methods

2.1. Study Design

Following the approval of the Institutional Review Board (IRB Approval: HSC20080233N) of the University of Texas Health Science Center at San Antonio (UTHSCSA), freshly extracted unidentified human teeth appropriately disposed in various clinics of the UTHSCSA Faculty of Dentistry, were collected and examined. Twenty-seven extracted human molars and premolars, consisting of 12 visually sound/healthy teeth and 15 teeth with natural cavitated lesions were selected. Teeth with open caries lesions where selected, where the caries could be restored by the placement of an RMGIC or compomer restoration. Surface debris and stain was removed from the teeth, but the caries lesions were not touched. The teeth were stored in distilled water to avoid dehydration, using the protocol established in our earlier studies [39,47,48]. Before examination each tooth was removed from the vial, rinsed thoroughly with distilled water for 20 s and air-dried for five seconds.

Two healthy teeth were set aside as sound healthy samples. They were used to confirm that storage media and sample handling did not alter readings with the various modalities. These teeth were scanned at two spots on each tooth. Of the remaining 25 teeth, 10 teeth were identified as healthy/sound and 15 teeth had visible caries lesions.

A dentist selected the smooth surface to be restored on the tooth samples. A standard RMGIC/compomer preparation was done using high speed handpiece bur to remove enamel. A slow speed hand piece with round carbide bur was used to remove dentin and caries. The cavity preparation on the sound samples was at least 3 mm in depth. On the samples with caries, the carious tissue was removed from the tooth, except on one wall. On that wall, the caries and demineralized enamel was removed from the preparation margin, but caries was left at least 1 mm below the tooth surface with the caries covering at least 3 mm width of the preparation wall. All measurements, during the cavity preparation, were done with a periodontal probe (Williams Periodontal Probe PW6 Hu-Friedy, Chicago, IL, USA).

Three restorative materials were used:

- Dyract eXtra Dentsply Refill Compules Shade A2 Lot., 1608001074; Expiry August 2018 (3M ESPE St. Paul MN., USA).
- Ketac Nano 3M Shade A2 Ref. 3304A2 Lot., N733107; Expiry May 2017 (Dentsply DeTrey GmbH, Konstanz, Germany).
- Compoglass F Ivoclar Vivadent Refill: Shade 140/A2 Lot., V19970; Expiry October 2018 (Ivoclar Vivadent AG, Schaan, Liechtenstein).

When the preparations were completed, the teeth were photographed on all surfaces. Standard bonded compomer/RMGIC technique was used for the placement of the restorations. The cavity preparation was etched using 37% phosphoric acid gel (Temrex Gel Etch, Temrex Corporation. Freeport, NY, USA) for 30 s. The teeth were rinsed with water for 30 s to remove the phosphoric acid gel and then air-dried for 30 s. Bond1 Primer/Adhesive (Pentron Clinical Technologies, Orange County, CA, USA) was applied inside the cavity preparation to bond restoration. The bond was cured with a dental curing light (Demi-Ultra LED Curing Light Kerr, Orange County, CA, USA) for 20 s. The restorations were then placed in 3 mm depth increments and light cured. Any excess material on the surface was removed. After the restorations were placed the teeth were put back into distilled water for storage for 1 month.

Photographs were taken of all the tooth surfaces after placement of the restorations. On each photograph a section of the restoration was selected for examination. On samples with caries beneath restoration, a section of the carious margin was selected for examination and marked on the photographs.

On the ten healthy/sound teeth, a total of 21 areas were examined and on the fifteen teeth with caries a total of 43 areas were examined. On the 10 sound restored teeth, 21 sites (8 sites for Dyract eXtra, 7 sites for Ketac Nano and 6 sites for Compoglass F) were examined. On the 15 carious sample teeth, 43 sites (15 sites for Dyract eXtra, 15 sites for Ketac Nano and 13 sites for Compoglass F) were examined. In total there were 23 spots scanned with CN and DD on Dyract eXtra restorations, 22 spots scanned on Ketac Nano restorations, 19 spots scanned on Compoglass F restorations and 4 sites on standard teeth. In summary, 68 sites (4 sites on sound unrestored teeth, 21 sound sites with restorations; 43 carious sites) were examined with CN and DD.

A technician, not involved in restoration of the teeth, took DD and CS measurements at the MOR, 0.5 mm, 1.5 mm and 2.0 mm away from the MOR of the RMGIC and compomer margins. Three readings were taken at each position and the measurements were recorded. The means and standard deviation for each measurement taken at each position were calculated. The measurement scales for the various caries detection systems, used in the study, are shown in Figure 1.

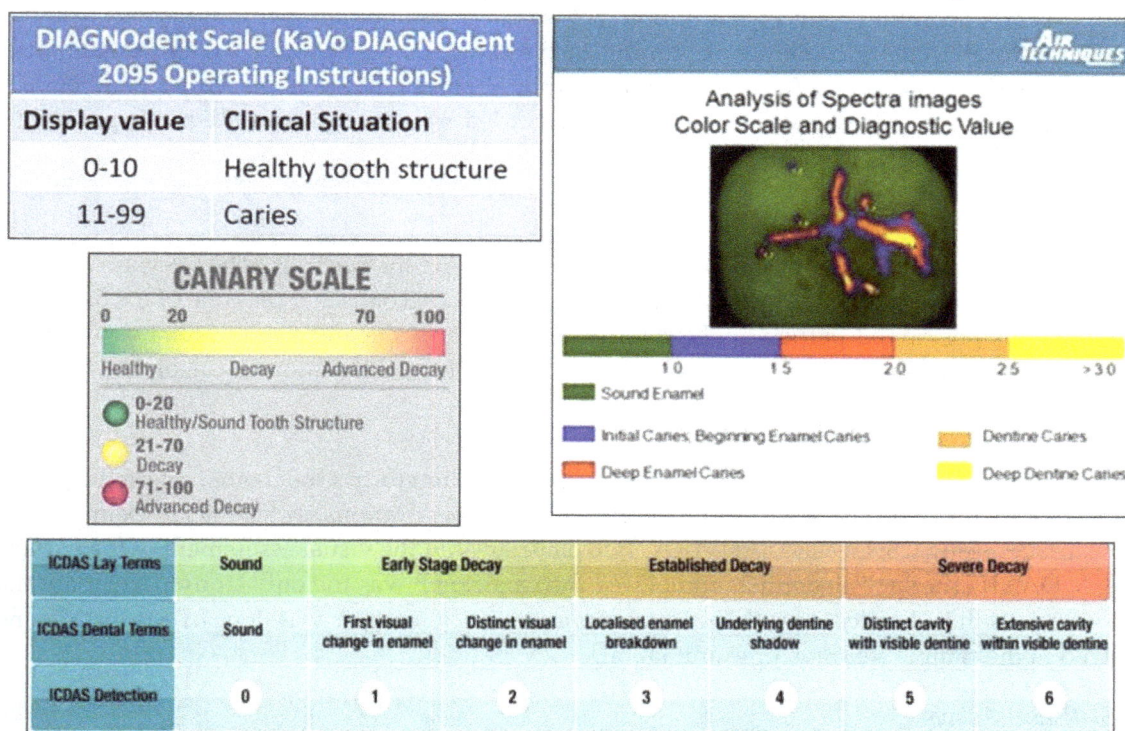

Figure 1. Caries system detection scales for devices used in this study.

2.2. ICDAS II Visual Examination

Two dentists, trained in using the ICDAS II visual scoring system [49], scored each tooth surface with a restoration independently. The ICDAS II criteria used in the study were:

0 Sound tooth surface;
1 First visual change in enamel (on a dry tooth surface);
2 Distinct visual change on enamel surface (on a moist and dry tooth surface);
3 Localized enamel breakdown due to caries with no exposed dentin or shadowing beneath the tooth surface;
4 Dark shadow beneath the tooth surface from dentin;
5 Distinct cavity with visible dentin;
6 Extensive distinct cavity with visible dentin and more than half of the surface involved.

All ICDAS examinations were conducted in a dental operatory using a dental operatory light. No visual aids such as microscopes or magnifying loupes were used. Where there was disagreement between the clinicians' scores, the tooth surfaces were re-examined by both clinicians at the same time and agreement was reached on the ICDAS score (consensus score). The clinicians' scores and consensus scores were recorded, and the consensus scores were used in this study.

2.3. SPECTRA Caries System Examination

SPECTRA recorded an image of each tooth surface being examined using SPECTRA Imaging software and stored it on a computer. A 10-mm distance spacer and the SPECTRA handpiece disposable camera covers were used (AIR TECHNIQUES, Melville, New York, NY, USA) during image acquisition.

2.4. DIAGNODent Examination

DIAGNOdent Classic (KaVo Dental model 2095, Biberach, Germany) was used following the manufacturer's operating instructions. Probe "A" was used for measurements at various distances from the restoration margin. Before examining each tooth, DD was calibrated with the calibration disc. The tooth was air-dried for five seconds and the tip of the DD was placed perpendicular to the examination site. Three measurements were recorded for each site and the mean peak value was calculated.

2.5. The Canary System Examination

The CS was used following the manufacturer's operating instructions. The CS was calibrated before each tooth was scanned. The tooth was air-dried for five seconds and the cone of the disposable plastic tip was positioned perpendicular over the examination site and a measurement was taken. Three measurements were taken at each site and recorded. The mean value was calculated.

2.6. Blinding of the Participants in This Study

Several actions were taken to blind the participants in this study. One dentist selected the tooth samples for inclusion in the study and placed the various restorations. A technician examined the tooth surfaces using CS, DD and SPECTRA. Two clinicians did the visual assessment of the surfaces using ICDAS II criteria. The dentist who placed the restoration was the only study participant that knew which teeth had caries beneath the restorations. Statistical analysis was done by a statistician not involved in the sample selection or examination.

2.7. Statistical Analysis

Since the teeth had been pre-selected as sound and carious before examination with the various systems, they were divided into these two groups for analysis. Sensitivity and specificity analysis were performed on the data collected using CS, SPECTRA, ICDAS II and DD.

Three measurements using CS and DD were conducted on each tooth spot, as per the protocol. Intra-operator repeatability analysis was done for the 3 CS and DD readings on each spot. The intraclass correlation (ICC) was used to measure intra-rater reliability of individual scans by spot scanned. The ICC was calculated using two-way random effects model, under the absolute agreement definition.

Descriptive statistics, including means, standard errors, standard deviations, and 95% confidence intervals were calculated for all measurements. The means for CS and DD were analyzed at the MOR, 0.5 mm, 1.5 mm, and 2 mm away from the restoration margin. Differences between means of restored sound and restored carious teeth were tested with two-sample t-tests, after use of Levene's test for equality of variances to determine if separate or pooled variances were called appropriate. Any testing between means involving unrestored teeth was done using Wilcoxon signed rank test because of the small sample size. All p-values were two-sided and statistical significance was determined using the traditional p-value of <0.05. The sensitivity and specificity (with 95% CI) were done for all measurements and analyzed overall and by restorative materials. The intra-operator repeatability was assessed by calculating the intraclass correlation coefficient (ICC).

All analysis was done using R software (version 3.4.3, R Core Team, Vienna, Austria) [50]. The T-test and Wilcoxon signed rank test was calculated using R software functions "t.test" and "wilcoxon.test" respectively, in R package "stats". Levene's test for equality of variances was calculated using function "LeveneTest" in R package "car". Confidence intervals for sensitivity and specificity were calculated using Wilson method, using function "binom.confint" in R package "binom" [50]. The intraclass correlation coefficient (ICC) was calculated using function "ICC" in R package "IRR" [50].

3. Results

Two clinicians using ICDAS II ranking for visual inspection of the RMGIC/compomer margins were only able to locate 5 teeth with caries beneath the restoration margins. On these 5 teeth the agreed ICDAS ranking were; 3 teeth at ICDAS 1 (2 teeth restored with Compoglass F and 1 restored with Dyract eXtra) and 2 teeth at ICDAS 2 (2 teeth restored with Ketac Nano). For healthy samples, the examiners ranked five surfaces as ICDAS 1 and the rest were ranked as ICDAS 0 or healthy. The ICDAS 1, rankings, on healthy teeth, were associated with 2 Dyract eXtra restorations, 1 Ketac Nano restoration and 1 Compoglass F restorations and one on the control tooth. All the other RMGIC or compomer margins on both carious and sound samples were ranked as ICDAS 0 (healthy). The ICDAS II, examination sensitivity and specificity were 0.35 and 0.52, respectively. Visual ranking using ICDAS II did not appear to be an accurate method for detecting caries beneath restoration margins, in this study. There appeared to be no correlation with lesion detection and restorative material in this study when using ICDAS II ranking.

The SPECTRA images of the RMGIC or compomer restoration all appeared as green. At times the color was slightly darker than the surrounding tooth structure. Near the margins of some of the restorations, there were very thin blue or red lines (see Figures 2 and 3). At times these lines were associated with the edges of the tooth surface or with stain on the surface. The majority of tooth surface examined, appeared green, indicating sound enamel, even if caries was present beneath the MOR. The compomer and RMGIC had very low reflectivity so SPECTRA was not able to accurately measure fluorescence around the MOR. This study found that the SPECTRA data and images were inconclusive due to signal interference from the restorations.

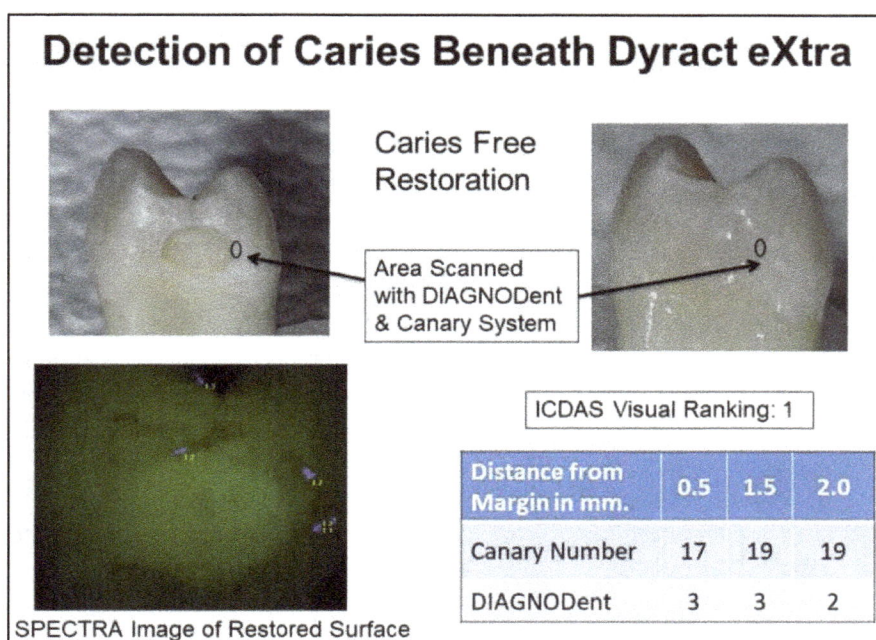

Detection of Caries Beneath Dyract eXtra

Caries Free Restoration

Area Scanned with DIAGNODent & Canary System

SPECTRA Image of Restored Surface

ICDAS Visual Ranking: 1

Distance from Margin in mm.	0.5	1.5	2.0
Canary Number	17	19	19
DIAGNODent	3	3	2

Figure 2. Examination of caries free margin of a Dyract eXtra restoration.

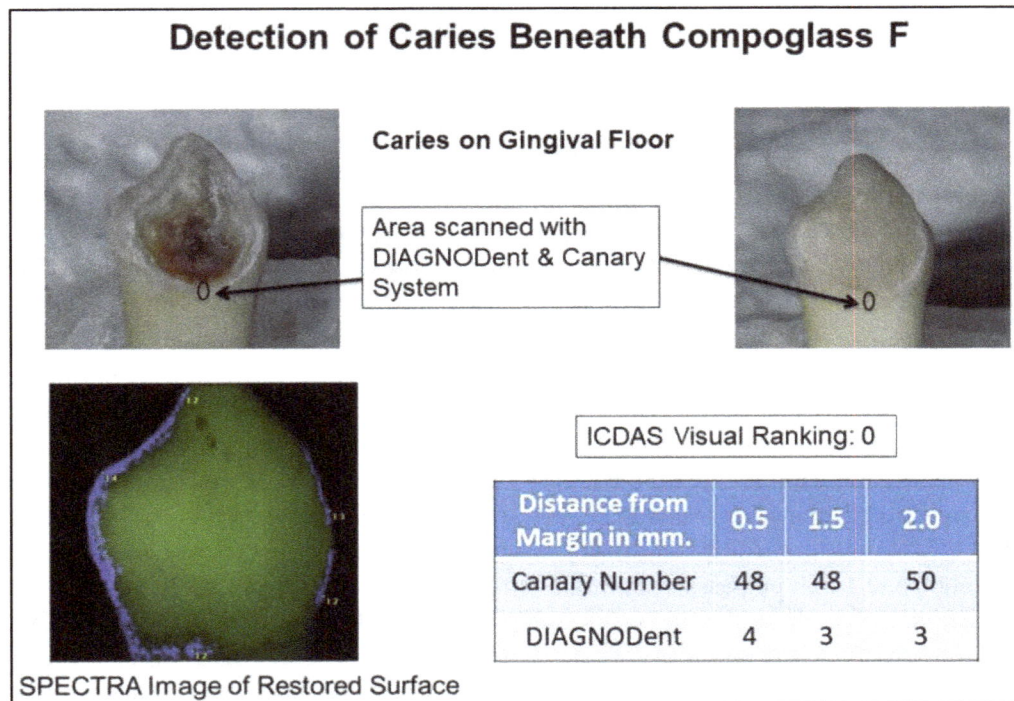

Figure 3. Detection of caries beneath Compoglass F restoration margin.

Table 1 shows the mean CN and DD readings on the compomer or RMGIC margin and at various distances from the margins of the restoration. At the MOR, the CN from teeth with caries beneath MOR were 45 ± 15.7. On healthy MOR the CN was 20.1 ± 5.7. The CN at 0.5, 1.5 and 2.0 mm away from the restoration margin on sound samples remained below 20 indicating no caries present. However, on teeth with caries beneath the restoration margin, the CN measurements at 0.5, 1.5 and 2.0 mm away from the margin gave means ranging between 45.7 and 52.2, indicating that there was caries beneath the restoration margin. The CN on caries samples did not drop significantly at 2 mm away from the restoration margin. Difference between means of sound and carious samples was statistically significant, at $p < 0.001$, at every distance from the restoration margin. Table 2 shows the sensitivity/specificity for sites at 2.0, 1.5, 0.5, 0 mm from the MOR which ranged from 0.91–1.0/0.71–0.93 for the CS.

DD gave readings of 17.2 ± 10.6 at the MOR in sound teeth. This dropped to 5 ± 3.4 at 2 mm from the restoration margin. Difference between means of sound and carious samples was not statistically significant at any distance from the margins of the restorations. On teeth with caries beneath restoration margins the DD reading was 19.5 ± 18.7 and dropped to 8.6 ± 8.81 at 2 mm away from the restoration margin. The sensitivity/specificity for sites at 2.0, 1.5, 0.5, on the margin ranged 0.19–0.7/0.14–0.93 for DD (Table 2).

From examining the data and looking at practical applications in clinical practice [38], it appeared that examining the restorations at 0.5 mm from the restoration margin provided the most accurate data for clinical assessment. Standard teeth scanned at 0.5 mm from the margin, yielded CN mean (SD) of 16.8 (2.2). This was similar to CN at 0.5 mm from margin for healthy/sound teeth 18.1 (3.3), p-value = 0.25, but differed from carious teeth 46.8 (18.7), p-value = 0.003. Using DD, standard teeth yielded 4.5 (0.6), compared to sound teeth 10 (7.3) and carious teeth 11.7 (15.4), p-values were 0.095 and 0.018. Wilcoxon signed rank test were used in all comparisons of standard teeth to sounds or carious teeth.

Table 1. Canary number and DIAGNODent readings by distance from the margin of the restoration and by material.

Distance from the Margins of the Restoration	Canary Number (21–100 Denotes Caries)			Peak DIAGNODent (11–99 Denotes Caries)		
	Sound Teeth Mean (SD)	Carious Teeth Mean (SD)	p-Value [1]	Sound Teeth Mean (SD)	Carious Teeth Mean (SD)	p-Value [1]
By Distance from Margin (All Materials)						
At margin	20.1 (5.7)	47.7 (19.9)	<0.001	17.2 (10.6)	19.5 (18.7)	0.414
0.5 mm	18.8 (3.3)	46.8 (18.7)	<0.001	10 (7.3)	11.7 (15.4)	0.396
1.5 mm	19.3 (4.7)	45 (15.7)	<0.001	7.5 (5.9)	9.4 (7.8)	0.122
2 mm	18.3 (2.6)	52.2 (19.6)	<0.001	5 (3.4)	8.6 (8.8)	0.076
Dyract eXtra						
At margin	19.9 (6.3)	32.6 (12.5)	0.014	20.5 (11.7)	21 (18.5)	0.941
0.5 mm	17.1 (2.4)	31.8 (9.4)	<0.001	5.1 (1.6)	9.6 (6.6)	0.073
1.5 mm	17.4 (1.5)	37.2 (13.4)	0.003	4.9 (1.1)	7.7 (4.1)	0.076
2 mm	18.6 (1.3)	40.3 (12.2)	0.002	4.5 (1.6)	10.8 (13.6)	0.334
Ketac Nano						
At margin	19.2 (5.8)	63.2 (14.8)	<0.001	11.7 (6.4)	23.9 (24.9)	0.211
0.5 mm	18.6 (3.7)	63.7 (13.7)	<0.001	11.5 (9.1)	18.1 (24.4)	0.496
1.5 mm	18.7 (4.1)	56.7 (16)	<0.001	8.9 (7.7)	15.1 (11.1)	0.212
2 mm	17.8 (3.9)	68.4 (22.5)	<0.001	5.8 (5.2)	10.7 (6.5)	0.127
Compoglass F						
At margin	21.4 (5.7)	47.4 (19)	0.005	19.3 (12)	12.6 (4.6)	0.238
0.5 mm	21.3 (2.7)	44.5 (16.1)	<0.001	14.8 (6.5)	6.6 (2.5)	0.028
1.5 mm	22.7 (6.7)	42.2 (11)	0.001	9.4 (6.9)	5.8 (2.2)	0.097
2 mm	18.8 (0.5)	46.8 (9.4)	<0.001	4.4 (1)	4.5 (1.3)	0.93

[1] Two-sample t-test.

Table 2. Sensitivity and specificity ICDAS II, SPECTRA, DIAGNODent and Canary System. For DIAGNODent and Canary System the sensitivity and specificity are given at various distances from the restoration margins.

Caries Detection System	Sensitivity (95% CI)	Specificity (95% CI)
ICDAS II	34.9 (22.4, 49.8)	52.4 (32.4, 71.7)
SPECTRA	34.9 (22.4, 49.8)	61.9 (40.9, 79.2)
Peak DIAGNODent at margin	69.8 (54.9, 81.4)	14.3 (5, 34.6)
Peak DIAGNODent at 0.5 mm from margin	30.2 (18.6, 45.1)	66.7 (45.4, 82.8)
Peak DIAGNODent at 1.5 mm from margin	19.5 (10.2, 34)	90.5 (71.1, 97.3)
Peak DIAGNODent at 2 mm from margin	18.8 (8.9, 35.3)	92.9 (68.5, 98.7)
Canary Number at Margin	97.7 (87.9, 99.61)	76.2 (54.9, 89.4)
Canary Number at 0.5 mm from margin	90.7 (78.4, 96.3)	81 (60, 92.3)
Canary Number at 1.5 mm from margin	95.1 (83.9, 98,7)	71.4 (50, 86.2)
Canary Number at 2 mm from margin	100 (89.3, 100)	92.9 (68.5, 98.7)

When measuring 0.5 mm away from a restoration placed on a healthy/sound tooth the DD reading was approximately 10, at the top end of the range for healthy teeth. When measuring around restorations with caries the DD measurements (Table 1) rose to around 12 indicating caries was present but not providing an indication of the size or extent of the lesion. The overall sensitivity and specificity for detection of caries around RMGIC and compomer restorations was best when using CS at 0.5 mm from the restoration margin (Table 2).

An analysis was done on the potential impact that the RMGIC or compomer material had on the ability to detect caries beneath the respective restoration margins. Table 1 shows the data for CS and DD. When scanning with CS around the 3 materials margins with caries beneath the margins, (Table 1) all had CN in the range between 30 and 68 indicating that caries was present. On restorations placed in healthy/sound teeth the CN remained below 20 indicating no caries was present. Each restoration material type showed statistically significant differences in CN means, at $p < 0.001$, between healthy restored and carious teeth. Since the scanning was done 0.5 mm from the restoration margin it is possible that the restorative material might have contributed to the size of the CN. This study did not produce standard sized lesions, so one could not assess the impact of the restorative material on CN. Even if the material did increase the CN it did not drive the number over the healthy range when scanning the margins of restorations placed in healthy/sound teeth.

In examining the DD reading around the three different materials (Table 1), the Dyract-Xtra and Ketac Nano restorations did show an increase between restorations placed in healthy and carious teeth, but the differences were not statistically significant, $p = 0.073$ and $p = 0.496$ respectively. With the Dyract eXtra restorations, beyond healthy margins measured just under 5 and the margins with caries beneath them, were just below 10. Although the readings were different on the DD scale, these measurements indicated that there were no caries on restorations placed over caries lesions. Ketac Nano restorations placed on healthy/sound teeth had DIAGNODent readings just above 10 indicating caries and the restorations placed over caries had readings around 15. Compoglass F restorations placed on healthy teeth had DD readings of 14.8 ± 6.5 and restorations placed over caries had readings of 6.6 ± 2.25. In this situation, DD was not able to accurately identify caries lesions.

The overall intra-operator repeatability [50], when using CS or DD, was high (Table 3), for both systems.

Table 3. Repeatability of DIAGNODent and Canary System measurements at 0.5 mm from the restoration margin.

Restorative Materials	Canary Number ICC [1] (95% CI)	Peak DIAGNODent ICC [1] (95% CI)
All materials	0.99 (0.99, 1.0)	0.98 (0.98, 0.99)
Dyract eXtra	0.98 (0.97, 0.99)	0.89 (0.78, 0.95)
Ketac Nano	0.99 (0.99, 1.0)	0.99 (0.98, 1.0)
Compglass F	0.99 (0.97, 0.99)	0.96 (0.92, 0.98)

[1] Intraclass Correlation Coefficient.

4. Discussion

The longevity of restorations depends upon many factors including materials used, type of restorative procedure, size and depth of the lesion, patient parameters such as caries risk, oral hygiene, operator variables and other local factors. Some of the major reasons for restoration failures are secondary caries, restoration or tooth fracture, marginal deficiencies, wear, and postoperative sensitivity [2]. The development of caries adjacent to existing restorations is a multifactorial problem that is difficult to study in vivo, due to human variability and the time required for identifiable lesion to form [51]. This in vitro model does not exactly emulate what would occur, in vivo. In clinical practice a restoration is placed into a cavity preparation that has sound, caries-free walls. This in vitro model was chosen to simulate caries on the wall of a restoration which would develop months or years after the initial placement of the restoration. The study was designed to see if various caries detection systems could detect caries beneath the visibly intact margins of RMGIC and compomer restorations.

In clinical practice, visual or visual-tactile examinations (use of an explorer or blunt probe), often combined with bitewing radiography, are still the most common techniques for examining the marginal integrity of restorations [52]. Since the study involved examining visible smooth surfaces radiographs were not included. Visual changes adjacent to restoration margins such as discoloration, staining, or dentinal shading, may be caused by a lot of clinical factors; only one of them being secondary caries [53,54]. The two dentists using ICDAS II scoring for visual assessment, could only detects caries beneath the restoration margin in a few of the samples.

Fluorescence-based caries detection devices may encounter challenges in detecting caries around RMGIC and compomer margins. Some studies have found that measuring fluorescence may not be suitable for detecting caries around restoration margins due to false positive readings [25,55–57].

The CR Clinicians Report (March 2012), found that existing restorations may cause interference in readings from these devices [58]. Fluorescence-based technologies may not give any information about lesion size, volume or depth [59,60]. Scattering of the light and fluorescence caused by stain, plaque, organic deposits and surface features such as pits and fissures may prevent deep penetration of the light below the tooth surface. In this study, SPECTRA images were not able to detect caries beneath the restoration margins in vast majority of the tooth samples (Figures 2 and 3).

DD is also a fluorescence-based device but uses a 660 nm wavelength which is not the wavelength used in SPECTRA. DIAGNOdent also does a point measurement so it was able to pick up some information from the tooth structure adjacent to the restoration margin with some interference from the restoration [61]. Overall DD was less consistently able to detect sound and carious margins. DD was not able to accurately identify sound or caries tissue beneath the margins of teeth restored with Compoglass F.

The CS can examine an area of approximately 1.5 mm in diameter and up to 5 mm below the tooth surface [42]. It provides a CN (ranging from 0–100) from an algorithm combining the PTR and LUM amplitude and phase measurements, which are directly linked to the status of the tooth's structure being examined (Figure 1) [42]. A CN of less than 20 indicates healthy tooth structure [42]. A CN greater than 70 indicates the presence of a large lesion that may justify restoration [42]. CNs falling between 20 and 70 indicate the presence of caries or cracks that may require restoration or other preventive treatments-based upon further patient evaluation including caries risk factors [38,40]. If the caries is located beneath a healthy layer of enamel, the CS measures both healthy tissue and caries around and beneath the beam. The healthy tooth overlying the caries dampens the signal, decreasing the CN but keeping it above the CN healthy range [37]. In this in vitro study, The CS was able to examine the margins of the RMGIC or compomer restoration and up to 2 mm beyond the restoration margin and in the vast majority of the tooth samples, discern if there was healthy or carious tissue present beneath the MOR.

5. Conclusions

CS and DD were able to differentiate between sound and carious tissue at the MOR more accurately than ICDAS II and SPECTRA. DD had less reliability, larger variation in measurement and poorer accuracy for detecting caries when compared to CS. When scanning at 0.5 mm from the RMGIC or compomer restoration margin DD was not able to accurately detect caries or healthy margins. Therefore, CS has the potential to detect secondary caries around RMGIC and compomer restorations more accurately than visual examination with ICDAS II, SPECTRA or DD.

Author Contributions: Conceptualization, S.A., B.A. and K.S.; Methodology, S.A., B.A. and K.S.; Investigation, T.A., S.A., W.H. and G.E.; Data Curation, V.M.; Formal Analysis, V.M. and B.A.; Validation, B.A., S.A. and K.S.; Writing-Original Draft Preparation, S.A., V.M. and K.S.; Writing-Review & Editing, B.A., S.A., V.M., A.M. and K.S.; Supervision, S.A.

Funding: Funding for this study was supported by Quantum Dental Technologies.

Conflicts of Interest: None of the authors received any compensation for work on this study and preparation of this paper. T Abrams, and K Sivagurunathan are employees of Quantum Dental Technologies, the manufacturer of The Canary System. S Abrams is President & Co-Founder of Quantum Dental Technologies and did not receive any compensation for this study. V. Moravan provided statistical analysis for this study. A. Mandelis is CTO and Co-Founder of Quantum Dental Technologies and did not receive any compensation for this study. WMP Hellen is a shareholder in Quantum Dental Technologies. GI Elman and BT Amaechi did not receive any compensation nor do they have any conflicts to disclose.

References

1. Kopperud, S.E.; Tveit, A.B.; Gaarden, T.; Sandvik, L.; Espelid, I. Longevity of posterior dental restorations and reasons for failure. *Eur. J. Oral Sci.* **2012**, *120*, 539–548. [CrossRef] [PubMed]
2. Hickel, R.; Manhart, J. Longevity of restorations in posterior teeth and reasons for failure. *J. Adhes. Dent.* **2001**, *3*, 45–64. [PubMed]

3.   Hara, A.T.; Magalhaes, C.S.; Serra, M.C.; Rodrigues, A.L., Jr. Cariostatic effect of fluoride-containing restorative systems associated with dentifrices on root dentin. *J. Dent.* **2002**, *30*, 205–212. [CrossRef]

4.   Serra, M.C.; Cury, J.A. The in vitro effect of glass-ionomer cement restoration on enamel subjected to a demineralization and remineralization model. *Quintessence Int.* **1992**, *23*, 143–147. [PubMed]

5.   Tedesco, T.K.; Bonifacio, C.C.; Calvo, A.F.; Gimenez, T.; Braga, M.M.; Raggio, D.P. Caries lesion prevention and arrestment in approximal surfaces in contact with glass ionomer cement restorations—A systematic review and meta-analysis. *Int. J. Paediatr. Dent.* **2016**, *26*, 161–172. [CrossRef] [PubMed]

6.   Raggio, D.P.; Tedesco, T.K.; Calvo, A.F.; Braga, M.M. Do glass ionomer cements prevent caries lesions in margins of restorations in primary teeth? A systematic review and meta-analysis. *J. Am. Dent. Assoc.* **2016**, *147*, 177–185. [CrossRef] [PubMed]

7.   Mickenautsch, S.; Yengopal, V. Absence of carious lesions at margins of glass-ionomer cement and amalgam restorations: An update of systematic review evidence. *BMC Res. Notes* **2011**, *4*, 58. [CrossRef] [PubMed]

8.   Yengopal, V.; Mickenautsch, S. Caries-preventive effect of resin-modified glass-ionomer cement (RM-GIC) versus composite resin: A quantitative systematic review. *Eur. Arch. Paediatr. Dent.* **2011**, *12*, 5–14. [CrossRef] [PubMed]

9.   Pendrys, D.G. Resin-modified glass-ionomer cement (RM-GIC) may provide greater caries preventive effect compared with composite resin, but high-quality studies are needed. *J. Evid.-Based Dent. Pract.* **2011**, *11*, 180–182. [CrossRef] [PubMed]

10. Kidd, E.A.; Toffenetti, F.; Mjör, I.A. Secondary Caries. *Int. Dent. J.* **1992**, *42*, 127–138. [PubMed]

11. Diniz, M.B.; Eckert, G.J.; González-Cabezas, C.; Cordeiro, R.d.C.L.; Ferreira-Zandona, A.G. Caries Detection around Restorations Using ICDAS and Optical Devices. *J. Esthet. Restor. Dent.* **2016**, *28*, 110–121. [CrossRef] [PubMed]

12. Ando, M.; González-Cabezas, C.; Isaacs, R.L.; Eckert, G.J.; Stookey, G.K. Evaluation of several techniques for the detection of secondary caries adjacent to amalgam restorations. *Caries Res.* **2004**, *38*, 350–356. [CrossRef] [PubMed]

13. Mjör, I. Clinical diagnosis of recurrent caries. *J. Am. Dent. Assoc.* **2005**, *136*, 1426–1433. [CrossRef] [PubMed]

14. FDI World Dental Federation. FDI policy statement on Classification of caries lesions of tooth surfaces and caries management systems: Adopted by the FDI General Assembly: 17 September 2011, Mexico City, Mexico. *Int. Dent. J.* **2013**, *63*, 4–5. [CrossRef] [PubMed]

15. Fisher, J.; Johnston, S.; Hewson, N.; Van Dijk, W.; Reich, E.; Eiselé, J.L.; Bourgeois, D. FDI Global Caries Initiative; implementing a paradigm shift in dental practice and the global policy context. *Int. Dent. J.* **2012**, *62*, 169–174. [CrossRef] [PubMed]

16. FDI World Dental Federation. Caries Prevention and Management Chairside Guide. 2017. Available online: http://www.fdiworlddental.org/sites/default/files/media/resources/2017-fdi_cpp-chairside_guide.pdf (accessed on 12 September 2018).

17. Ekstrand, K.; Martignon, S.; Ricketts, D.J.; Qvist, V. Detection and activity assessment of primary coronal caries lesions: A methodologic study. *Oper. Dent.* **2007**, *32*, 225–235. [CrossRef] [PubMed]

18. Rodrigues, J.A.; Hug, I.; Diniz, M.B.; Lussi, A. Performance of fluorescence methods, radiographic examination and ICDAS II on occlusal surfaces in vitro. *Caries Res.* **2008**, *42*, 297–304. [CrossRef] [PubMed]

19. Diniz, M.B.; Rodrigues, J.A.; Hug, I.; Cordeiro Rde, C.; Lussi, A. Reproducibility and accuracy of the ICDAS-II for occlusal caries detection. *Community Dent. Oral Epidemiol.* **2009**, *37*, 399–404. [CrossRef] [PubMed]

20. Jablonski-Momeni, A.; Stachniss, V.; Ricketts, D.N.; Heinzel-Gutenbrunner, M.; Pieper, K. Reproducibility and accuracy of the ICDAS-II for detection of occlusal caries in vitro. *Caries Res.* **2008**, *42*, 79–87. [CrossRef] [PubMed]

21. Bamzahim, M.; Shi, X.Q.; Angmar-Månsson, B. Secondary caries detection by DIAGNOdent and radiography: A comparative in vitro study. *Acta Odontol. Scand.* **2004**, *62*, 61–64. [CrossRef] [PubMed]

22. Lussi, A.; Hellwig, E. Performance of a new laser fluorescence device for the detection of occlusal caries in vitro. *J. Dent.* **2006**, *34*, 467–471. [CrossRef] [PubMed]

23. Spaveras, A.; Karkazi, F.; Antoniadou, M. Caries detection with laser fluorescence devices. Limitations of their use. *Stoma Educ. J.* **2017**, *4*, 46–53. [CrossRef]

24. Neuhaus, K.W.; Rodrigues, J.A.; Seemann, R.; Lussi, A. Detection of proximal secondary caries at cervical class II-amalgam restoration margins in vitro. *J. Dent.* **2012**, *40*, 493–499. [CrossRef] [PubMed]

25. Hitij, T.; Fidler, A. Effect of dental material fluorescence on DIAGNOdent readings. *Acta Odontol. Scand.* **2008**, *66*, 13–17. [CrossRef] [PubMed]

26. Nokhbatolfoghahaie, H.; Alikhasi, M.; Chiniforush, N.; Khoei, F.; Safavi, N.; Zadeh, B.Y. Evaluation of Accuracy of DIAGNOdent in Diagnosis of Primary and Secondary Caries in Comparison to Conventional Methods. *J. Lasers Med. Sci.* **2013**, *4*, 149–167.

27. Rechmann, P.; Charland, D.; Rechmann, B.M.; Featherstone, J.D. Performance of laser fluorescence devices and visual examination for the detection of occlusal caries in permanent molars. *J. Biomed. Opt.* **2012**, *17*, 036006. [CrossRef] [PubMed]

28. Achilleos, E.E.; Rahiotis, C.; Kakaboura, A.; Vougiouklakis, G. Evaluation of a new fluorescence-based device in the detection of incipient occlusal caries lesions. *Lasers Med. Sci.* **2013**, *28*, 193–201. [CrossRef] [PubMed]

29. Gutta, A.; Merdad, H.E. In vitro study of the diagnostic performance of the Spectra Caries Detection Aid. *J. Clin. Dent.* **2015**, *26*, 17–22.

30. Konigm, K.; Flelviming, G.; Hibst, R. Laser-induced autofluorescence spectroscopy of dental caries. *Cell Mol. Biol.* **1998**, *44*, 1293–1300.

31. Graye, M.; Markowitz, K.; Strickland, M.; Guzy, G.; Burke, M.; Houpt, M. In vitro evaluation of the Spectra early caries detection system. *J. Clin. Dent.* **2012**, *23*, 1–6. [PubMed]

32. Melo, M.; Pascual, A.; Camps, I.; Del Campo, A.; Ata-Ali, J. Caries diagnosis using light fluorescence devices in comparison with traditional visual and tactile evaluation: A prospective study in 152 patients. *Odontology* **2017**, *105*, 283–290. [CrossRef] [PubMed]

33. Matos, R.; Novaes, T.F.; Braga, M.M.; Siqueira, W.L.; Duarte, D.A.; Mendes, F.M. Clinical performance of two fluorescence-based methods in detecting occlusal caries lesions in primary teeth. *Caries Res.* **2011**, *45*, 294–302. [CrossRef] [PubMed]

34. Gimenez, T.; Braga, M.M.; Raggio, D.P.; Deery, C.; Ricketts, D.N.; Mendes, F.M. Fluorescence-based methods for detecting caries lesions: Systematic review, meta-analysis and sources of heterogeneity. *PLoS ONE* **2013**, *8*, e60421. [CrossRef] [PubMed]

35. Jablonski-Momeni, A.; Heinzel-Gutenbrunner, M.; Klein, S.M.C. In vivo performance of the VistaProof fluorescence-based camera for detection of occlusal lesions. *Clin. Oral Investig.* **2014**, *18*, 1757–1762. [CrossRef] [PubMed]

36. Markowitz, K.; Rosenfeld, D.; Peikes, D.; Guzy, G.; Rosivack, G. Effect of pit and fissure sealants on caries detection by a fluorescent camera system. *J. Dent.* **2013**, *41*, 590–599. [CrossRef] [PubMed]

37. Silvertown, J.D.; Wong, B.P.; Abrams, S.H.; Sivagurunathan, K.S.; Mathews, S.M.; Amaechi, B.T. Comparison of The Canary System and DIAGNOdent for the in vitro detection of caries under opaque dental sealants. *J. Investig. Clin. Dent.* **2016**. [CrossRef] [PubMed]

38. Abrams, T.E.; Abrams, S.H.; Sivagurunathan, K.; Silvertown, J.D.; Hellen, W.; Elman, G.I.; Amaechi, B.T. In Vitro Detection of Caries Around Amalgam Restorations Using Four Different Modalities. *Open Dent. J.* **2017**, *11*, 609–620. [CrossRef] [PubMed]

39. Jeon, R.J.; Phan, T.D.T.; Wu, A.; Kulkarni, G.; Abrams, S.H.; Mandelis, A. Photothermal radiometric quantitative detection of the different degrees of demineralization of dental enamel by acid etching. *J. Phys. IV Fr.* **2005**, *125*, 721–772. [CrossRef]

40. Abrams, S.H.; Sivagurunathan, K.; Silvertown, J.D.; Wong, B.; Hellen, A.; Mandelis, A.; Hellen, W.M.P.; Elman, G.I.; Mathew, S.K.; Mensinkai, P.K.; et al. Correlation with Caries Lesion Depth of The Canary System, DIAGNOdent and ICDAS II. *Open Dent. J.* **2017**, *11*, 679–689. [CrossRef] [PubMed]

41. Jeon, R.J.; Matvienko, A.; Mandelis, A.; Abrams, S.H.; Amaechi, B.T.; Kulkarni, G. Detection of interproximal demineralized lesions on human teeth in vitro using frequency-domain infrared photothermal radiometry and modulated luminescence. *J. Biomed. Opt.* **2007**, *12*, 034028. [CrossRef] [PubMed]

42. Silvertown, J.D.; Abrams, S.H.; Sivagurunathana, K.S.; Kennedy, J.; Jeon, J.; Mandelis, A.; Hellen, A.; Hellen, W.; Elman, G.; Ehrlich, R.; et al. Multi-centre clinical evaluation of photothermal radiometry and luminescence correlated with international benchmarks for caries detection. *Open Dent. J.* **2017**, *11*, 636–647. [CrossRef] [PubMed]

43. Matvienko, A.; Jeon, R.J.; Mandelis, A.; Abrams, S.H.; Amaechi, B.T. Photothermal detection of incipient dental caries: Experiment and modeling. *Proc. SPIE* **2007**, *6759*. [CrossRef]

44. Jeon, R.J.; Hellen, A.; Matvienko, A.; Mandelis, A.; Abrams, S.; Amaechi, B.T. Experimental Investigation of Demineralization and Remineralization of Human Teeth Using Infrared Photothermal Radiometry and Modulated Luminescence. *Proc. SPIE* **2008**, *6856*. [CrossRef]

45. Matvienko, A.; Mandelis, A.; Abrams, S. Robust multiparameter method of evaluating the optical and thermal properties of a layered tissue structure using photothermal radiometry. *Appl. Opt.* **2009**, *48*, 3192–3203. [CrossRef] [PubMed]

46. Silvertown, J.D.; Wong, B.P.; Sivagurunathan, K.S.; Abrams, S.H.; Kirkham, J.; Amaechi, B.T. Remineralization of natural early caries lesions in vitro by P11-4 monitored with photothermal radiometry and luminescence. *J. Investig. Clin. Dent.* **2017**. [CrossRef] [PubMed]

47. Matvienko, A.; Jeon, R.J.; Mandelis, A.; Abrams, S.H.; Amaechi, B.T. Photothermal Detection of Incipient Dental Caries: Experiment and Modeling. *Photonics East Proc. SPIE* **2007**, *6759*. [CrossRef]

48. Hellen, A.; Mandelis, A.; Finer, Y.; Amaechi, B.T. Quantitative remineralization evolution kinetics of artificially demineralized human enamel using photothermal radiometry and modulated luminescence. *J. Biophotonics* **2011**, *4*, 788–804. [CrossRef] [PubMed]

49. Pitts, N.B.; Ismail, A.I.; Martignon, S.; Ekstrand, K.; Douglas, G.A.; Longbottom, C. ICCMS Guide for Practitioners and Educators. Available online: https://www.iccms-web.com/uploads/asset/59284654c0a6f822230100.pdf (accessed on 12 September 2018).

50. R Core Team. *R: A Language and Environment for Statistical Computing*; R Core Team: Vienna, Austria, 2016.

51. Ferracane, J. Models of Caries Formation around Dental Composite Restorations. *J. Dent. Res.* **2017**, *96*, 364–371. [CrossRef] [PubMed]

52. Boston, D. Initial in vitro evaluation of DIAGNOdent for detecting secondary carious lesions associated with resin composite restorations. *Quintessence Int.* **2003**, *34*, 109–116. [PubMed]

53. Sarrett, D.C. Prediction of clinical outcomes of a restoration based on in vivo marginal quality evaluation. *J. Adhes. Dent.* **2007**, *9* (Suppl. 1), 117–120. [PubMed]

54. Lino, J.R.; Ramos-Jorge, J.; Coelho, V.S.; Ramos-Jorge, M.L.; Moyses, M.R.; Ribeiro, J.C. Association and comparison between visual inspection and bitewing radiography for the detection of recurrent dental caries under restorations. *Int. Dent. J.* **2015**, *65*, 178–181. [CrossRef] [PubMed]

55. Gostanian, H.V.; Shey, Z.; Kasinathan, C.; Caceda, J.; Janal, M.N. An in vitro evaluation of the effect of sealant characteristics on laser fluorescence for caries detection. *Pediatr. Dent.* **2006**, *28*, 445–450. [PubMed]

56. Hosoya, Y.; Matsuzaka, K.; Inoue, T. Influence of tooth-polishing pastes and sealants on DIAGNOdent values. *Quintessence Int.* **2004**, *35*, 605–611. [CrossRef]

57. Lussi, A.; Reich, E. The influence of toothpastes and prophylaxis pastes on fluorescence measurements for caries detection in vitro. *Eur. J. Oral Sci.* **2005**, *113*, 141–144. [CrossRef] [PubMed]

58. Christensen, G. New Caries Detection Systems Reliable & Accurate. *Clin. Rep.* **2012**, *5*, 1–2.

59. Liang, R.; Wong, V.; Marcus, M.; Burns, P.; McLaughlin, P. Multimodal imaging system for dental caries detection. *Proc. SPIE Lasers Dent.* **2007**, *6425*. [CrossRef]

60. Hall, A.; Girkin, J.M. A review of potential new diagnostic modalities for caries lesions. *J. Dent. Res.* **2004**, *83*, C89–C94. [CrossRef] [PubMed]

61. Bamzahim, M.; Aljehani, A.; Shi, X.-Q. Clinical performance of DIAGNOdent in the detection of secondary carious lesions. *Acta Odontol. Scand.* **2005**, *63*, 26–30. [CrossRef] [PubMed]

10

A Review of the Common Models Used in Mechanistic Studies on Demineralization-Remineralization for Cariology Research

Ollie Yiru Yu, Irene Shuping Zhao, May Lei Mei, Edward Chin-Man Lo and Chun-Hung Chu *

Faculty of Dentistry, The University of Hong Kong, Hong Kong SAR 999077, China; yuyiru@hku.hk (O.Y.Y.); irenezhao110@gmail.com (I.S.Z.); mei1123@hku.hk (M.L.M.); hrdplcm@hkucc.hku.hk (E.C.-M.L.)
* Correspondence: chchu@hku.hk;

Abstract: Mechanistic studies on demineralization-remineralization play a critical role in investigating caries pathogenicity, testing effects of new caries prevention methods, and developing new caries-preventing products. Simulating the cariogenic challenges in the mouth, various demineralization-remineralization models have been used for cariology research. This review aimed to provide an overview of the common mechanistic studies on demineralization-remineralization for cariology research in recent literature. Most mechanistic studies were in vitro studies ($n = 294$, 84%) among the 350 cariology studies indexed in the Web of Science from 2014 to 2016. Among these in vitro studies, most studies (257/294, 87%) used chemical models that could be classified as simple mineralization models (159/257, 62%) or pH-cycling models (98/257, 38%). In vitro studies consumed less expense and time than in vivo studies. Furthermore, in vitro conditions were easier to control. However, they could hardly imitate the complex structures of oral cavities, the microbiological effect of oral biofilm, and the hydrodynamic instability of saliva. The advantages of chemical models included simplicity of the study, low cost, efficiency (time saving), reproducibility, and stability of experiments. However, the "caries" generated were not biological. Moreover, the chemical models were generally basic and could not mimic a carious lesion in the complex oral environment.

Keywords: demineralization; remineralization; fluoride; caries; review

1. Introduction

Dental caries is the localized destruction of dental hard tissues by acidic byproducts from bacterial fermentation of dietary carbohydrates [1]. It forms through a complex interaction over time between acid-producing bacteria and fermentable carbohydrates, and has many host factors including teeth and saliva. Despite many years of research and the availability of novel anti-caries products, dental caries is still one of the most prevalent chronic diseases affecting many people worldwide [2]. In the past decades, thousands of in vivo and in vitro studies on cariology have been published. Many of them are mechanistic studies that play an important role in cariology research in investigating caries pathogenicity, testing effects of new caries prevention methods (i.e., devices and drugs), and developing new caries-preventing products [2]. A mechanistic study can be defined as an experiment or test to analyze the biological and/or chemical events responsible for, or associated with, an observed effect (outcome). Mechanistic studies on demineralization-remineralization explore the molecular and physiological mechanisms by which substances exert their effects on teeth. The purpose of this review is to provide an overview of the common mechanistic studies on demineralization-remineralization in recent literature on cariology research.

2. Types of Mechanistic Studies in Recent Publications

A publication search was conducted using Web of Science, which is the first comprehensive scientific citation indexing database used by academics and researchers [3]. Web of Science is in a dominant position in the citation of academic references [4]. All the literature in the database has been published in journals with impact factors. A search using the keywords (demineralization OR remineralization) AND (dental caries) found 350 mechanistic studies from 2014 to 2016 using demineralization-remineralization models of enamel or dentin substrate (Figure 1). These mechanistic studies can be classified into three categories: in vitro studies (294 studies, 294/350, 84%); in situ studies including natural caries studies (53 studies, 53/350, 15%); and in vivo studies (3/350, 1%). Among the 294 in vitro studies, 257 used chemical models and 37 used biofilm models for the study of demineralization-remineralization of teeth (Figure 1). Since one common database with three main keywords were used, this review is not an exhaustive search and is not a systematic review. However, the results of the search provided an outline of common types of mechanistic studies on demineralization-remineralization for cariology research in recent literature.

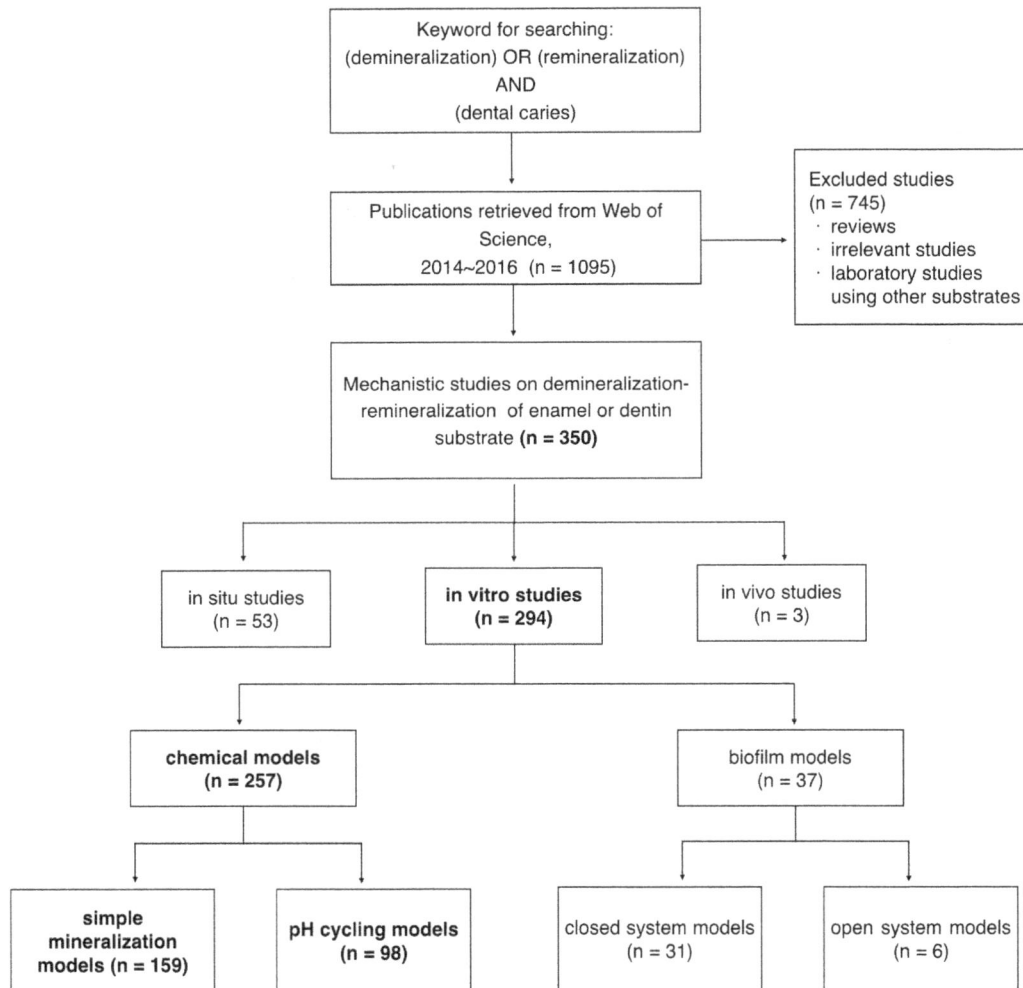

Figure 1. Mechanistic studies on demineralization-remineralization for cariology research published in Web of Science 2014–2016.

2.1. In Situ Studies

A small number (53/350, 15%) of the recent publications were in situ studies. In situ studies are proposed to make a balance of merits and limitations between in vitro and in vivo studies. Some in situ studies closely mimic the natural environment and process of dental caries formation in vivo. In situ studies examine dental caries exactly in place where they occur. They provide essential information about the physical-chemical characteristics of the dental ecosystem. In situ studies generally have four elements, which are human or animal tooth substrate, cariogenic dental biofilm, regular carbohydrate challenge, and valid reaction time according to the caries generation process and experimental design [5]. They can be used to study the interaction of anti-caries agents and environments.

Recent in situ studies have explored the process of demineralization and remineralization of enamel and/or dentine, or investigated the effectiveness of caries prevention agents or devices. The most common method of these studies was the use of palatal devices as the carrier of dental substrates. Some studies used extracted teeth with natural caries as specimens for evaluation. Unlike artificial caries, the formation of natural caries could not be controlled. Moreover, the position, type, depth, and other factors of the caries in different teeth were not similar. Therefore, it was difficult to use natural caries models to evaluate the effects of anti-caries agents because the parameters from different caries are incomparable.

The duration of the in situ studies was normally less than two months. The study designs, to some extent, were similar to in vivo studies. The substrates could be analyzed quantitatively to improve the sensitivity and validity of the methodology. Nevertheless, no actual carious deficiencies would be formed due to the short experimental period. The results, therefore, could not be comparable to those found in clinical situations. In situ studies normally recruited a small number of subjects. The results might not be representative because of individual variation. Furthermore, the results of the experiments highly relied on the compliance of the subjects [6].

2.2. In Vivo Studies

In vivo studies allow for the evaluation of the overall effects of an intervention on dental caries in the oral cavity. Rodents are animals commonly used in in vivo studies to study dental caries [7]. Animal studies provides higher scientific control and easier adaptability to calibration than in situ studies. Caries lesions induced in animal studies can greatly mimic the natural caries formation process [7]. Most aspects of caries formation, including such roles of diet, microbiological elements, tooth composition, and de-/remineralization processes, as well as their interactions can be simulated [8]. Smooth surface, fissure, and cervical caries can all be simulated with similar histological features to human caries. Despite the advantages mentioned above, animal studies do not predict clinical outcomes when it comes to anti-caries effect assessments for intervention such as fluoride application. Some animal studies exhibited different results from in vitro and in situ experiments [6]. Last but not least, the uncontrollable fluctuating oral environment and ethical problems associated with in vivo studies in humans made it difficult to study the mechanism of demineralization-remineralization of dental hard tissue [9].

Only a nonsignificant number (3/350, 1%) of the recent studies in this search were in vivo studies. These three studies were animal studies using rats as the subjects to test new anti-caries methods. The International Association Against Painful Experiments on Animals proclaimed that direct extrapolation from animals to humans was frequently invalid. This can be one of the main reasons that animal studies were uncommon in the recent studies [10].

2.3. In Vitro Studies

Researchers often use in vitro studies to study the demineralization-remineralization process in cariology research. In vitro studies simulate the oral environment from different perspectives and offer more controllable conditions than a natural environment. The designs of in vitro studies are often simple but can be complex according to the purposes of investigation. Even with a complex design, authors of in vitro studies find it almost impossible to mimic the complicated process of natural caries development. Hence, the design can be regarded as a compromise on the reality of the in vivo ecosystem. Nevertheless, researchers can still obtain meaningful and useful results.

The simplification of the in vitro study environment provides an alternative choice to conducting reproducible experiments in a controllable and simplified way [11].

The search suggested that in vitro studies were the most common mechanistic studies of cariology in recent years (294/350, 84%). In vitro studies consumed the least expense and time among all the laboratory studies. Furthermore, the conditions were simple and easy to control to meet the research requirements [6]. However, they can hardly imitate the complex structure of the oral cavity, the microbiological effect of oral biofilm, and the hydrodynamic instability of saliva. Different models were used in the in vitro studies. Each model had its own study design. The results can vary significantly because the conditions of caries formation and the characteristics of carious lesion can be very different from natural caries [10]. Moreover, the morphology and mineral loss created by the carious lesions vary significantly in different demineralization-remineralization models [12].

3. Demineralization-Remineralization Models Used for In Vitro Studies

The demineralization-remineralization models used for in vitro studies can be divided into biofilm models and chemical models. The biofilm models can be further divided into closed system models and open system models. The chemical models can be further divided into simple mineralization models and pH-cycling models.

3.1. Biofilm Models

Cariogenic bacteria were one of the key factors that influence the characteristics of carious lesions [13]. Some of the recent studies (37/294, 13%) used biofilm models with cariogenic bacteria. Nineteen out of 37 studies employed a pure culture system, which used a single strain of bacteria to provide cariogenic challenge. *Streptococcus mutans* was commonly used (18/19, 95%) as a single species within a pure culture system [14]. The structure and the composition of the mono-species biofilm is consistent. The bacteria cell growth and accumulation rate, as well as the physiological properties of the biofilm, can be accurately investigated. It also allows for the analysis of differences between or among different oral pathogenic species. However, interactions of bacteria, such as competition, cross-feeding, or succession of the colony are not considered [13]. Cariogenic consortia biofilms with a combination of two or more cariogenic bacteria were also used in seven studies. All of them were the co-cultivation of *streptococcus mutans* and *lactobacillus*, *bifidobacteria*, or *actinomyces.* The defined species consortia models give information on bacteria adhesion, accumulation, and competition. The simplified combination of cariogenic bacteria reduces the complexity and difficulty of measuring ecological phenomena. It produces metabolic data of the chosen species under an interactional circumstance. Microcosm biofilms evolved from dental plaque or saliva were used in 11 studies. They closely mimic the physiological and microbiological properties of natural dental plaque. The complexity, biodiversity, and heterogeneity of the natural cariogenic biofilm are well preserved [15]. Nevertheless, the bacterial populations of microcosm biofilms vary from different hosts, times, and environments.

Most of the recent studies used biofilm closed system models (31/37, 84%). Multi-well cell culture plates were used to incubate the cariogenic bacteria together with the enamel or dentin substrate in most studies (30/31, 97%) [16]. In a closed system model, a finite culture medium is provided in a sealed container such as plates or tubes. The growth conditions will change considerably with the consumption of the nutrients and the accumulation of metabolic products. Hence, the physiological and biological properties of the biofilm are not comparable with the natural ones. Closed system models were simple, repeatable, controllable, and inexpensive. A small number of the studies (6/37, 16%) used open system models such as the oral biofilm reactor [17–19] or artificial mouth model [20,21]. Open system models simulate the in vivo environment better than closed system models. They also allow for better regulation of biofilm growth rate and other variables. The continuous supply of nutrient medium and removal of waste metabolic products provide a steady state condition [22]. Nevertheless, the repeatability of the experimental result is low because of the heterogeneity of the biofilm in the open system. Besides, the possibility of contamination can be high due to the complexity of the construction.

3.2. Chemical Models

Among the 294 in vitro studies, most studies (257/294, 87%) used chemical models to generate artificial caries or demineralized lesions on enamel and/or dentin. Chemical models mimic the caries process through the use of acid or acid buffer to simulate demineralization and remineralization processes. When the acidity (pH) drops below a certain level (critical pH), saliva and plaque fluid cease to be saturated with calcium and phosphate. The enamel hydroxyapatite will dissolve and demineralization of enamel occurs. This is represented with a simplified chemical reaction: $Ca_{10}(PO_4)_6(OH)_2 + H^+ \leftrightarrow Ca^{2+} + HPO_4^{2-} + H_2O$. The left to right direction is demineralization. When calcium (Ca^{2+}), phosphate (PO_4^{3-}), and hydroxyl (OH^-) ions are accumulated, demineralization slows down to the moment when the saliva reaches saturation. When the pH goes up, re-deposition of minerals (remineralization) will occur and the reaction shifts from right to left.

Chemical models simplify the complex biofilm metabolism [23]. They aim to reflect the environment of the oral cavity to a chemical level rather than biological level [23]. The advantages of chemical models include simplicity of a study, low cost, efficiency (time saving), reproducibility, and stability of the experiment. A main disadvantage of chemical models is that they completely ignore the microbiological aspect of the caries formation.

4. Types of Chemical Models Used in Recent Studies

In this literature search, the chemical models used in recent studies could be further classified as simple mineralization models (159/257, 62%) and pH-cycling models (98/257, 38%).

4.1. Simple Mineralization Models

Simple mineralization models use simple demineralization agents of low pH value. This method cuts down the remineralization process to create demineralized lesions. Mild organic acids and acid buffers such as lactic acid and acetate acid are used to create demineralized lesions. These mild acids would create demineralized lesions that are more similar to natural caries than inorganic acids. Substrates such as enamel block are immersed in acidic solution to create a demineralization zone on the surface. Normally, one single solution with a stable pH value will be used in the process of caries generation. The optimal pH value to create a subsurface lesion ranges from 4.4 to 5.0 in most experimental designs. Hydrochloric acid, phosphate acid, and citric acid are used to create acid erosion models. These inorganic acids are more acidic than those used for cariology research, and their pH values can be as low as 1.0.

Some studies used substrates topped with an acidic gel to generate caries-like lesions. The two common acidic gels used are carboxymethylcellulose-based lactic acid gel and ethylenediaminetetraacetic (EDTA) acid gel [12]. The demineralization process will stop after mineral saturation is reached. In this status, the mineral gain and loss of the substrates will be in a dynamic balance. The amount and viscosity of the gel applied on the top of the substrate will affect the time of mineral saturation. The contact area of the tooth tissue and demineralization gel also has an impact on mineral saturation. For the carboxymethylcellulose-based lactic acid gel, the consistency of the gel provides a diffusion barrier on the surface of the substrates. The diffusion process of the ions is slower than the demineralization solutions [24]. In addition, the carboxymethylcellulose may combine with calcium and reduce the demineralizing activity of calcium [25]. With the same exposure time as methylcellulose gel on the surface of substrates, the lesions created by EDTA gel can be very deep and nearly all the mineral is eradicated. EDTA gel might not simulate subsurface lesions [12].

Many researchers use simple mineralization models because they minimize the time and operational steps of the experiments. These artificially created demineralized lesions mimicking caries lesions and acid erosion lesions are regarded as acceptable by some researchers [12]. Some studies added in a thermos-cycling protocol into a mineralization model to simulate the aging process of the specimens studied [26,27]. The extent of demineralization can be regulated by a number of factors such as acidity, time, temperature, mineral concentration, and mineral dissolution inhibitors [28]. By modifying these factors, the characteristics of lesions such as lesion depth, mineral loss ratio, and gradient of mineral lost can be controlled [12]. The demineralized lesions induced using simple mineralization models show a higher mineral loss ratio than natural caries [12]. Moreover, the study designs and the acid used in most recent studies are not the same. The physical and mechanical properties of the artificially created carious lesions are different. Hence, the results of these studies are not comparable and the conclusions drawn could be different [24]. It is important to interpret the results of these studies with caution.

4.2. PH-Cycling Model

The pH-cycling model was invented and first published in 1982 by Cate and Duijsters [29]. The model is based on a scheme in which a pH neutral environment was periodically interrupted by acid challenges. It intends to mimic the in vivo periodic alternation of pH, much as it occurs in the mouth when sugars are metabolized, to form a caries lesion. These combination experiments are designed to mimic the dynamics of mineral loss and gain involved in caries formation, which is an important advantage of the pH-cycling model. Other advantages include the high level of scientific control and the resulting lower variability intrinsic to in vitro models, as well as the smaller sample size required. Additionally, the response variables that can be employed in pH-cycling models are more sensitive than those available for use in a clinical situation [30]. The remineralization solution is often neutral in acidity (pH = 7). The pH used for demineralization solution varied from 4.4 to 5.5, depending on different substrates and demineralized acid. The duration of pH cycling ranges from a few days to months. pH-cycling models were often used to study dentin caries [31]. Dentin caries is a biochemical process characterized initially by the dissolution of the mineral part, thus exposing the organic matrix to breakdown by bacteria-derived and host-derived enzymes [32]. Solutions simulating plaque fluid conditions could be used to reduce the difference between pH cycling models and in vivo situations [33].

5. Conclusion

In conclusion, in vitro studies have been the most common method adopted for cariology research in recent studies. The easily controlled parameters of the models enabled the forthright regulation of model sensitivity to adapt to varied requirements of testing. In vitro studies have the advantages of simplicity, low cost, and efficiency (time saving). However, they cannot mimic all the factors affecting the caries formation process. The most common model used in in vitro studies was a chemical model. The advantages of chemical models include simplicity of the study, low cost, efficiency (time saving), reproducibility, and stability of the experiment. However, the caries generated are not biological and chemical models, and cannot mimic a carious lesion in the complex oral environment. Researchers should interpret the results and conclusions of these studies with caution. No study and model could suit all experimental designs. Different models have their own strengths and limitations when used for mechanistic studies on demineralization-remineralization. The criteria of selecting a model should meet the requirements of the experimental objectives.

Acknowledgments: This review was supported by HKU Seed Funding for Basic Research 201511159142.

Author Contributions: Ollie Yiru Yu did the literature search and drafted the manuscript. All other authors contributed equally.

References

1. Selwitz, R.H.; Ismail, A.I.; Pitts, N.B. Dental caries. *Lancet* **2007**, *369*, 51–59. [CrossRef]
2. ten Cate, J.M. Models and role models. *Caries Res.* **2015**, *49*, 3–10. [CrossRef] [PubMed]
3. Drake, M.A. *Encyclopedia of Library and Information Science*, 2nd ed.; Marcel Dekker: New York, NY, USA, 2003.
4. Falagas, M.E.; Pitsouni, E.I.; Malietzis, G.A.; Pappas, G. Comparison of pubmed, scopus, web of science, and google scholar: Strengths and weaknesses. *Faseb J.* **2008**, *22*, 338–342. [CrossRef] [PubMed]
5. Sung, Y.-H.; Kim, H.-Y.; Son, H.-H.; Chang, J. How to design in situ studies: An evaluation of experimental protocols. *Restor. Dent. Endod.* **2014**, *39*, 164–171. [CrossRef] [PubMed]
6. White, D.J. The comparative sensitivity of intra-oral, in vitro, and animal models in the 'profile' evaluation of topical fluorides. *J. Dent. Res.* **1992**, *71*, 884–894. [PubMed]
7. Klinge, B.; Jönsson, J. Animal models in oral health sciences. In *Handbook of Laboratory Animal Science, Volume II, Third Edition: Animal Models*; CRC Press: Boca Raton, FL, USA, 2011; p. 387.
8. Bowen, W.H. Rodent model in caries research. *Odontology* **2013**, *101*, 9–14. [CrossRef] [PubMed]
9. Tang, G.; Yip, H.K.; Cutress, T.W.; Samaranayake, L.P. Artificial mouth model systems and their contribution to caries research: A review. *J. Dent.* **2003**, *31*, 161–171. [CrossRef]
10. Bowen, W.H. Dental caries—Not just holes in teeth! A perspective. *Mol. Oral Microbiol.* **2016**, *31*, 228–233. [CrossRef] [PubMed]
11. Salli, K.M.; Ouwehand, A.C. The use of in vitro model systems to study dental biofilms associated with caries: A short review. *J. Oral Microbiol.* **2015**, *7*, 26149. [CrossRef] [PubMed]
12. Schwendicke, F.; Eggers, K.; Meyer-Lueckel, H.; Dorfer, C.; Kovalev, A.; Gorb, S.; Paris, S. In vitro induction of residual caries lesions in dentin: Comparative mineral loss and nano-hardness analysis. *Caries Res.* **2015**, *49*, 259–265. [CrossRef] [PubMed]
13. Bowden, G. The role of microbiology in models of dental caries: Reaction paper. *Adv. Dent. Res.* **1995**, *9*, 255–269. [CrossRef]
14. Chu, C.H.; Mei, L.; Seneviratne, C.J.; Lo, E.C.M. Effects of silver diamine fluoride on dentine carious lesions induced by streptococcus mutans and actinomyces naeslundii biofilms. *Int. J. Paediatr. Dent.* **2012**, *22*, 2–10. [CrossRef] [PubMed]
15. McBain, A.J. Chapter 4: In vitro biofilm models: An overview. *Adv. Appl. Microbiol.* **2009**, *69*, 99–132. [PubMed]
16. Mei, M.L.; Li, Q.L.; Chu, C.H.; Lo, E.C.M.; Samaranayake, L.P. Antibacterial effects of silver diamine fluoride on multi-species cariogenic biofilm on caries. *Ann. Clin. Microb. Anti.* **2013**, *12*, 4. [CrossRef] [PubMed]
17. Horie, K.; Shimada, Y.; Matin, K.; Ikeda, M.; Sadr, A.; Sumi, Y.; Tagami, J. Monitoring of cariogenic demineralization at the enamel-composite interface using swept-source optical coherence tomography. *Dent. Mater.* **2016**, *32*, 1103–1112. [CrossRef] [PubMed]
18. Zhou, Y.; Shimada, Y.; Matin, K.; Sadr, A.; Sumi, Y.; Tagami, J. Assessment of bacterial demineralization around composite restorations using swept-source optical coherence tomography (SS-OCT). *Dent. Mater.* **2016**, *32*, 1177–1188. [CrossRef] [PubMed]
19. Tezuka, H.; Shimada, Y.; Matin, K.; Ikeda, M.; Sadr, A.; Sumi, Y.; Tagami, J. Assessment of cervical demineralization induced by streptococcus mutans using swept-source optical coherence tomography. *J. Med. Imaging* **2016**, *3*, 014504. [CrossRef] [PubMed]
20. Schwendicke, F.; Diederich, C.; Paris, S. Restoration gaps needed to exceed a threshold size to impede sealed lesion arrest in vitro. *J. Dent.* **2016**, *48*, 77–80. [CrossRef] [PubMed]
21. Kramer, N.; Mohwald, M.; Lucker, S.; Domann, E.; Zorzin, J.I.; Rosentritt, M.; Frankenberger, R. Effect of microparticulate silver addition in dental adhesives on secondary caries in vitro. *Clin. Oral Investig.* **2015**, *19*, 1673–1681. [CrossRef] [PubMed]
22. Coenye, T.; Nelis, H.J. In vitro and in vivo model systems to study microbial biofilm formation. *J. Microbiol. Meth.* **2010**, *83*, 89–105. [CrossRef] [PubMed]
23. Skucha-Nowak, M.; Gibas, M.; Tanasiewicz, M.; Twardawa, H.; Szklarski, T. Natural and controlled demineralization for study purposes in minimally invasive dentistry. *Adv. Clin. Exp. Med.* **2015**, *24*, 891–898. [CrossRef] [PubMed]

24. Moron, B.M.; Comar, L.P.; Wiegand, A.; Buchalla, W.; Yu, H.; Buzalaf, M.A.R.; Magalhaes, A.C. Different protocols to produce artificial dentine carious lesions in vitro and in situ: Hardness and mineral content correlation. *Caries Res.* **2013**, *47*, 162–170. [CrossRef] [PubMed]

25. Lynch, R.J.M.; ten Cate, J.M. The effect of lesion characteristics at baseline on subsequent de- and remineralisation behaviour. *Caries Res.* **2006**, *40*, 530–535. [CrossRef] [PubMed]

26. Alsayed, E.Z.; Hariri, I.; Sadr, A.; Nakashima, S.; Bakhsh, T.A.; Shimada, Y.; Sumi, Y.; Tagami, J. Optical coherence tomography for evaluation of enamel and protective coatings. *Dent. Mater. J.* **2015**, *34*, 98–107. [CrossRef] [PubMed]

27. Ozgul, B.M.; Tirali, R.E.; Cehreli, S.B. Effect of biodentine on secondary caries formation: An in vitro study. *Am. J. Dent.* **2016**, *29*, 71–74. [PubMed]

28. Marquezan, M.; Correa, F.N.P.; Sanabe, M.E.; Rodrigues, L.E.; Hebling, J.; Guedes-Pinto, A.C.; Mendes, F.M. Artificial methods of dentine caries induction: A hardness and morphological comparative study. *Arch. Oral Biol.* **2009**, *54*, 1111–1117. [CrossRef] [PubMed]

29. ten Cate, J.M.; Duijsters, P.P.E. Alternating demineralization and remineralization of artificial enamel lesions. *Caries Res.* **1982**, *16*, 201–210. [CrossRef] [PubMed]

30. Buzalaf, M.A.R.; Hannas, A.R.; Magalhaes, A.C.; Rios, D.; Honorio, H.M.; Delbem, A.C.B. Ph-cycling models for in vitro evaluation of the efficacy of fluoridated dentifrices for caries control: Strengths and limitations. *J. Appl. Oral Sci.* **2010**, *18*, 316–334. [CrossRef] [PubMed]

31. Zhao, I.S.; Mei, M.L.; Li, Q.L.; Lo, E.C.; Chu, C.H. Arresting simulated dentine caries with adjunctive application of silver nitrate solution and sodium fluoride varnish: An in vitro study. *Int. Dent. J.* **2017**. [CrossRef] [PubMed]

32. Mei, M.L.; Lo, E.; Chu, C. Clinical use of silver diamine fluoride in dental treatment. *Compend Contin. Educ. Dent.* **2016**, *37*, 93–98.

33. Lynch, R.J.M.; Mony, U.; ten Cate, J.M. Effect of lesion characteristics and mineralising solution type on enamel remineralisation in vitro. *Caries Res.* **2007**, *41*, 257–262. [CrossRef] [PubMed]

11

Dental Pulp Stem Cell Recruitment Signals within Injured Dental Pulp Tissue

Charlotte Rombouts [1], Charlotte Jeanneau [1], Athina Bakopoulou [2] and Imad About [1,*

[1]   Aix Marseille Université, CNRS, ISM UMR 7287, 13288, Marseille, France; romboutscharlotte@gmail.com (C.R.); charlotte.jeanneau@univ-amu.fr (C.J.)

[2]   Department of Fixed Prosthesis & Implant Prosthodontics, School of Dentistry, Aristotle University of Thessaloniki, GR-54124, Thessaloniki, Greece; abakopoulou@dent.auth.gr

*   Correspondance: imad.about@univ-amu.fr;

Academic Editor: Louis M. Lin

Abstract: The recruitment of dental pulp stem cells (DPSC) is a prerequisite for the regeneration of dentin damaged by severe caries and/or mechanical injury. Understanding the complex process of DPSC recruitment will benefit future *in situ* tissue engineering applications based on the stimulation of endogenous DPSC for dentin pulp regeneration. The current known mobilization signals and subsequent migration of DPSC towards the lesion site, which is influenced by the pulp inflammatory state and the application of pulp capping materials, are reviewed. The research outcome of migration studies may be affected by the applied methodology, which should thus be chosen with care. Both the advantages and disadvantages of commonly used assays for investigating DPSC migration are discussed. This review highlights the fact that DPSC recruitment is dependent not only on the soluble chemotactic signals, but also on their interaction with neighboring cells and the extracellular matrix, which can be modified under pathological conditions. These are discussed to explain how these modifications lead to the stimulation of DPSC recruitment.

Keywords: dental pulp stem cells; chemotaxis; migration assay

1. Introduction

The discovery of dental pulp stem cells (DPSC) [1] has opened up a whole new research field that offers many possibilities in dentistry. Indeed, DPSC can differentiate into odontoblast-like cells and produce reparative dentin [2]. This was demonstrated *in vivo* by seeding DPSC onto human dentin slices implanted into immunocompromised mice. These cells synthesized reparative dentin on the implanted dentin surface [3]. Although other localizations, such as peripheral nerve-associated glia [4], cannot be excluded, DPSC mainly reside in the perivascular regions of the pulp [5]. An elegant *ex vivo* tooth model with pulp injury has demonstrated increased proliferation of DPSC in the perivascular area, followed by migration to the lesion site [6]. These phenomena were not observed with dentin injuries, indicating that the DPSC activation and migration signals are only initiated upon pulp injury with a damaged odontoblast layer. This review will discuss the different cues for DPSC recruitment in injured dental pulp and the methodologies used to investigate DPSC migration. This knowledge can be used for *in situ* tissue engineering purposes that engage the tooth's own cells in regenerating the lost or injured tissue. This is of particular interest in severe caries and cavity preparations with rotary instruments leading to pulp injury. In brief, bioactive molecules such as chemokines or growth factors encapsulated in scaffolds can be grafted into the lesion site where they will stimulate dentin pulp regeneration by enhancing the physiological activation and recruitment of endogenous DPSC. This approach offers several advantages over tissue engineering that involves the exogenous application of stem cells [7]. Indeed, the latter requires cell harvesting followed by *ex vivo* cultivation that is cost- and labor-intensive, and has a more complex clinical translation.

2. Migration of DPSC in Injured Pulp Microenvironment

2.1. Soluble Chemotactic Molecules

The migration of DPSC to the injured pulp site is a complex procedure that involves many processes which are not fully elucidated yet. To start with, DPSC need to be mobilized from their niche. In the literature, various DPSC mobilization signals have been reported which include growth factors (hepatocyte growth factor (HGF), basic fibroblast growth factor (FGF-2), transforming growth factor (TGFβ-1)), chemokines (monocyte chemoattractant protein-1 (MCP-1); chemokine (C-X-C motif) ligand 14 (CXCL14); stromal cell-derived factor 1 (SDF-1)), granulocyte-colony stimulating factor (G-CSF), sphingosine-1-phosphate (S1P), C5a and high mobility group box 1 (HMGB-1) [8–14]. These signals find their origin in different sources, including their release from the dentin matrix and their production by dental pulp cells. These sources are influenced by the local microenvironment defined by caries, the inflammatory state, mechanical injury and the application of restorative materials, as reviewed previously [15]. While these molecules are involved in DPSC recruitment, they can also be involved in other processes such as differentiation or inflammation (Table 1).

Table 1. Overview of migration signals for dental pulp stem cells (DPSC) with their corresponding receptors, and their specific roles in dentin pulp regeneration and inflammation.

Chemotactic Molecule	Receptor	Inflammation	Regeneration	Role	Reference
HGF	c-Met		x	Recruitment of DPSC	[13]
FGF-2	FGF receptors 1 and 2		x	Recruitment of DPSC and pulp cell proliferation	[9,16,17]
TGFβ-1	TGF-β1 receptors I and II		x	Recruitment of DPSC and odontoblastic differentiation	[9,16,18,19]
MCP-1	CCR2		x	Recruitment of DPSC and stem cell homing*	[10,20]
CXCL14	C-X-C chemokine receptor type 4 (CXCR4)	x	x	Recruitment of DPSC and mediator of immune cell migration*	[10,21]
G-CSF	G-CSF receptor	x	x	DPSC mobilization and anti-inflammatory properties	[12,22,23]
S1P	S1P receptor 1–3	x	x	Pleiotropic actions including recruitment of DPSC and inflammatory effects*	[9,24,25]
SDF-1	CXCR4		x	Recruitment of DPSC and stem cell homing*	[11,20,26,27]
C5a	C5a receptor	x	x	Recruitment of DPCS and inflammatory cells*	[8,28,29]
HMGB-1	receptor for advanced glycation end products (RAGE)	x	x	Recruitment of DPCS and production of inflammatory cytokines*	[14,30]

* Demonstrated outside dental pulp context.

2.2. Both Chemotaxis and Haptotaxis are Required for DPSC Migration

Next, DPSC need to move through the extracellular matrix (ECM) towards the lesion site. The details of this process are not clear, but one can assume that both chemotaxis and haptotaxis are involved. Chemotaxis is guidance by a gradient of soluble chemical cues such as chemokines and cytokines, and also differing pH or reactive oxygen species levels [31]. For instance, in the case of carious insult, an acidic dissolution of the mineralized dentin matrix occurs, leading to the release of various bioactive molecules that are immobilized and sequestered within the matrix [32]. Chemotactic factors sequestered in the dentin include HGF [13], TGFβ-1 [9,33,34] and FGF-2 [9,17,35]. Dental pulp cells migrated *in vitro* in response to dentin ECM extracts [36], which was dependent on an active Rho pathway. Indeed, using an inhibitor of the Rho pathway, the migration-inducing effects of the dentin ECM extracts were abolished. Increased gene expression of pluripotency and mesenchymal markers was observed in the migrated pulp cell populations, suggesting that these migrated cell populations include DPSC. Enhanced dental pulp cell migration was also observed in response to dentin chips [37]. Haptotaxis is guidance by a gradient of immobilized ligands on the ECM such as collagens, fibronectin, laminins, matrix-bound chemoattractants, and/or adhesion molecules present on encountered cells [31]. For example, pulp ECM components, including laminin, have been shown to induce DPSC migration [9,36].

2.3. Extracellular Matrix Remodeling and DPSC Migration

Controlled remodeling of the ECM is also involved in cellular migration and is ensured by the action of different protease systems, including matrix metalloproteinases (MMPs). MMPs produced by odontoblasts [38] are sequestered in the dentin matrix, which are released upon dentin dissolution. Indeed, an enhanced presence of MMPs has been observed at carious lesion sites [39]. These host-derived MMPs, together with bacteria-derived MMPs and other enzymes, will further promote matrix breakdown and the release of sequestered bioactive molecules [40]. After pulp injury, matrix metalloproteinase-3 (MMP3) was shown to be highly increased, which stimulated endothelial cell migration [41]. In addition, MMPs have been shown to activate several bioactive molecules including TGFβ-1 [42]. Since MMPs not only breakdown the ECM [43], but also control chemokine activity and chemotactic gradients [44], it can be assumed that they are essential for interstitial migration of DPSC in the pulp tissue. Nevertheless, direct evidence of MMP-induced migration of DPSC is lacking and further research such as that on bone marrow-derived mesenchymal stem cells is needed [45,46].

2.4. SDF-1/CXCR4 Axis in Injured Pulp

A recently investigated migration cue in dental pulp is the SDF-1/CXCR4 axis. It is hypothesized that there is an elevated production of SDF-1 in injured pulp tissue, which will recruit proliferating dental pulp stem cells expressing the CXCR4 receptor where they will contribute to reparative dentin formation [26,27]. CXCR4 receptor was expressed intracellularly in STRO1+ (mesenchymal stem cell marker) dental pulp stem cells of the apical papilla (SCAP). Nevertheless, *in vitro* 2D and 3D migration assays have demonstrated increased migration of these SCAP in response to SDF-1. It is suggested that in response to a spatiotemporal variation of SDF-1 concentrations, the CXCR4 receptor is externalized. Indeed, immunofluorescence staining of migrating SCAP showed CXCR4 expression, whereas no expression was seen on non-migrating cells [47]. Also, for migration, cells will adopt a suitable morphology via intracellular cytoskeletal changes and focal adhesion formations. In response to SDF-1, focal adhesion proteins such as paxillin and focal adhesion kinase (FAK) were phosphorylated in DPSC. Stress fiber assembly, together with focal adhesion formation at the cell periphery, was observed [11].

3. Influence of Inflammation

Inflammation and tissue regeneration are tightly linked, and the dental pulp is no exception. Indeed, the microenvironment of the inflamed pulp differs from the healthy pulp and emits various signals required for regeneration to proceed. For instance, IL-1β, which is present in inflamed pulp, has been shown to induce MCP-1 secretion by dental pulp cells [48], which was shown to stimulate dental pulp regeneration [10]. Dental pulp cells challenged with lipopolysaccharide (LPS), a Gram negative bacterial wall component, increased their expression of DPSC chemotactic factors including SDF-1, CXCR4, MCP-1, FGF-2 and TGF-β1. This was associated with increased DPSC migration and the specific inhibition of the SDF-1/CXCR4 axis demonstrated its importance in this LPS-mediated migration [49]. Toll-like receptor (TLR) signaling, a major component of the innate immune system, is also involved in DPSC migration following bacterial insult [50,51]. Both Gram positive and Gram negative bacteria were able to increase Toll-like receptor 4 (TLR4) receptor expression in DPSC, which was associated with increased cytokine expression [51]. LPS-induced migration of murine dental papilla-derived odontoblast-like cells was also dependent on TLR4 receptor signaling [52].

The complement system is another major component of innate immunity [53]. It is a proteolytic cascade of more than 40 plasma and cellular proteins that are activated during inflammation with the aim of pathogen removal. The anaphylatoxins C3a and C5a are well-known chemoattractants of leukocytes towards the site of complement activation. Interestingly, these anaphylatoxins have also been studied in the context of tissue regeneration [54]. In particular, C5a has demonstrated the potential to stimulate pulp tissue regeneration. Indeed, C5a was produced by dental pulp fibroblasts challenged with LPS and lipoteichoic acid (LTA), a component of the Gram-positive bacterial wall [28,29]. C5a has been shown to recruit DPSC, which express the C5a receptor, to the dental pulp lesion site [8].

Another example of a molecule traditionally known for its role in inflammation and with discovered chemotactic potential is HMGB-1. It is secreted in inflammatory conditions by dendritic cells, macrophages and monocytes, and increases the production of inflammatory cytokines [14]. HMGB-1 expression was observed in inflamed pulp tissue, both in the nuclear and cytoplasmic regions of fibroblasts, inflammatory and vascular endothelial cells. A chemotactic effect of HMGB-1 was observed with a reorganization of F-actin that accumulated in the cell periphery of dental pulp cells. Accordingly, the receptor that mediates the chemotactic effect of HMGB-1 was upregulated as well in inflamed dental pulp tissues [14]. In addition, HMGB-1 has also been shown to promote the proliferation and odontoblastic differentiation of DPSC [55].

4. Influence of Pulp Capping Materials

Several pulp capping materials, such as calcium silicate-based cements, have been shown to positively influence the dentin-pulp regenerative process [18,56]. This is mainly due to the release of Ca^{2+} ions, which are known to stimulate hard tissue formation [57–59]. The release of silicon ions from calcium silicate-based cements also induced odontoblastic differentiation of DPSC. It is suggested that silicon ions act through calcium channels and mitogen-activated protein kinase/extracellular signal-regulated kinases (MAPK/ERK) signaling [60,61]. Besides the established odontoblastic differentiation of DPSC, dental materials can also stimulate cellular migration. For instance, mineral trioxide aggregate (MTA) increased the early and short-term migration of SCAP [62]. BioAggregate and MTA increased DPSC migration in an *in vitro* scratch assay [63]. The bioceramic putty iRoot BP Plus induced dental pulp cell migration, which was associated with focal adhesion formation and stress fiber assembly [64]. Biodentine also induced DPSC migration, which was associated with an increased chemokine expression, such as CXCR4, MCP-1 and SDF-1 [65]. The released calcium can be held partially responsible for the increased cellular migration, as was shown for bone marrow-derived stem cells [66]. Besides this calcium release, calcium hydroxide and MTA were able to mobilize bioactive molecules sequestered in the dentin matrix [33,67], which can contribute to their migration-stimulating effects. Furthermore, Biodentine induced TGFβ-1 secretion by dental pulp fibroblasts [18], which has been shown to attract DPSC [16] (Figure 1). A recent study has demonstrated that fluoride-based restorative materials impact DPSC migration [68]. Indeed, the long-term release of low fluoride levels increased the migratory response of DPSC to the chemotactic factors SDF-1 and TGFβ-1.

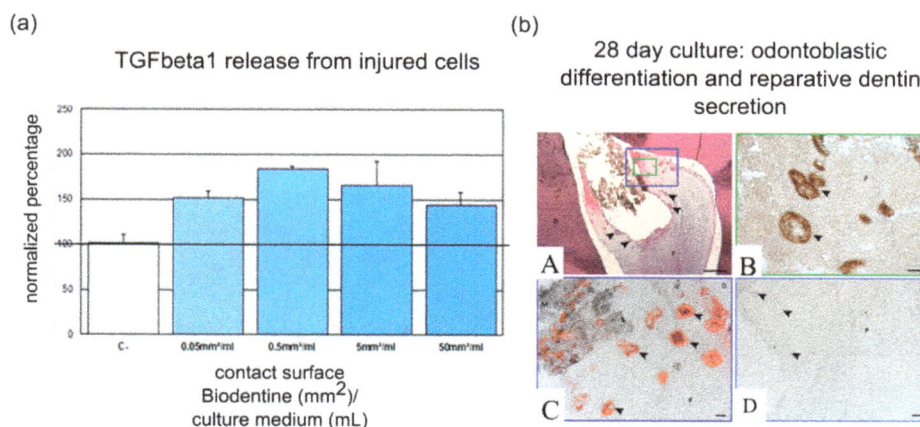

Figure 1. Biodentine and its effect on dental pulp regeneration. (**a**) Regardless of surface area, Biodentine induces TGFβ-1 release, a major chemoattractant for DPSC, from injured pulp cells; (**b**) Expression of odontoblast markers after pulp capping with Biodentine in entire tooth culture model. Numerous mineralization foci (arrowheads) can be viewed beneath the biomaterial after culture for two weeks and hematoxylin and eosin staining (**A**). Dentin sialoprotein (**B**) and nestin (**C**) are expressed in the mineralized foci, which represent an early form of reparative dentin (**D**). Abbreviations: D, dentin; P, pulp; M, biomaterial. Scale bars: A = 500 μm; B,C,D = 100 μm. Modified with permission from [18].

On the other hand, several materials demonstrated anti-migratory effects. For example, resin-based materials containing 2-hydroxyethyl methacrylate (HEMA) diminished DPSC migration [69]. HEMA has also been shown to decrease FGF-2 secretion by dental pulp cells [70], which may (partially) explain the decreased DPSC migration. An interesting study points out the importance of the local microenvironment, such as nutrient deprivation, in the pulp response to resin-based materials [71]. A concentration-dependent decrease in DPSC proliferation and migration was observed when exposed to TEGDMA (triethylene-glycol-dimethacrylate). Mineralization was also delayed when exposed to sub-toxic TEGDMA concentrations. A conditioned medium obtained from serum-deprived dental pulp cell cultures was able to attenuate these deleterious effects of sub-toxic TEGDMA concentrations, except for DPSC migration, which was attributed to increased FGF-2 and TGFβ-1 concentrations.

5. Methodologies Used to Study Dental Pulp Stem Cell Recruitment

5.1. In vitro *Boyden Chamber (Transwell Assay)*

The most commonly used chemotaxis assays are based on the Boyden chamber and are often referred to as Trans-well assays [72,73] (Figure 2a). In these assays, an insert with a porous membrane is used, with cells seeded on the upper site, which is placed into a culture well containing a medium with chemotactic factors. After a specific culture period, the cells on the upper site are swabbed away, leaving behind the cells that actively transmigrated to the other site of the membrane. The reproducibility and facility of this assay, together with its cost effectiveness, has made it a widely used tool to evaluate chemotactic potential of molecules. For instance, the chemotactic effect of SDF-1, S1P, EGF, FGF-2 and TGFβ-1 on DPSC has been demonstrated using a Trans-well assay [9,11]. The chemotactic potential of pulp and dentin ECM matrix extracts has been shown as well [36]. Haptotactic effects can be evaluated with a specific setting, as demonstrated for the so-called SIBLING molecules (small integrin-binding ligand, N-linked glycoproteins) [74]: dentin matrix protein-1 (DMP1), bone sialoprotein (BSP), and osteopontin (OPN). To this end, the porous membranes were coated with SIBLING solutions on the lower side, after which cells were seeded on the upper side. Haptotactic migration was observed with all three SIBLING proteins, which was dependent on the interaction between cellular αVβ3 integrin and the highly conserved integrin-binding tripeptide, RGD, on the protein.

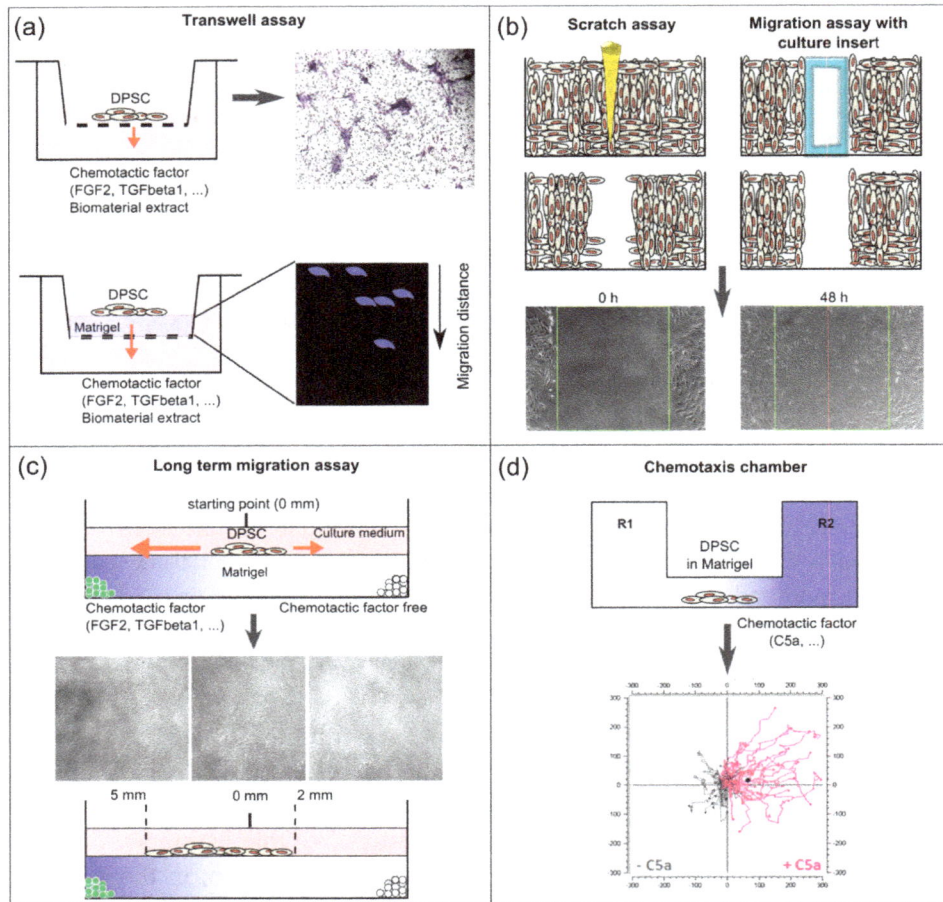

Figure 2. Schematic overview of the different *in vitro* assays used to study DPSC recruitment and migration. (**a**) On the upper panel, a classical Trans-well assay used to evaluate the chemotactic potential of bioactive molecules and biomaterials (extracts), with cells seeded on the upper side of the membrane. Results are obtained by swabbing the non-migrated cells from the upper side of the membrane followed by histological staining of the migrated cells on the lower side of the membrane. These can be counted and quantified. On the lower panel, a modified Trans-well assay where the porous membrane is coated with an extracellular matrix (ECM)-like gel (e.g., Matrigel, collagen), on which cells are seeded. Gels can be retrieved to evaluate the migrated distance of cells (e.g., by cell nuclear staining using 4',6-diamidino-2-phenylindole (DAPI) (blue) and confocal microscopy); (**b**) On the left, scratch assay to evaluate cellular migration. A scratch is made (usually using a pipette point) on confluent cell cultures. On the right, a modified assay to study cellular migration is represented. A culture insert is placed, around which cells are cultured. When the culture is confluent, the insert is removed leaving behind a reproducible cell-free zone with sharp borders, as opposed to the scratch assay. With both techniques, cellular migration into the cell-free zone is followed up microscopically and can be quantified using specialized software. A chemotactic gradient is absent in these assays; (**c**) Culture model to study long-term migration following the controlled release of chemotactic factors. Poly(lactic-co-glycolic acid) (PLGA) microspheres with or without chemotactic factors are embedded in Matrigel in a graduated tissue culture chamber. DPSC are seeded in the middle and their migration can be followed microscopically over long time periods (up to 10 days); (**d**) Specialized *in vitro* chemotaxis chamber. A stable chemotactic gradient is established by injecting a solution of chemotactic factor in one of the reservoirs. Cells are seeded in the observation area containing Matrigel in the middle of the chamber. Real-time monitoring of cellular migration can be performed up to 48 h. Quantitative evaluation is carried out by specialized software. Individual cells are tracked and the center of mass (CAM) is calculated. Trajectory plots can be presented graphically.

Various modifications of the Trans-well assay have been introduced over the past years. For example, the porous membrane can be coated with a gel that simulates the ECM, most often a collagen-based gel or Matrigel. In this way, one can get a step closer to the *in vivo* situation without too much effort. Indeed, chemotaxis *in vivo* is not only determined by the presence of a chemotactic gradient, but also by interaction between chemokines and the surrounding matrix and cellular interactions. In particular, the so-called mechanical tissue properties, stiffness and porosity, as well as chemokines, will together define the cell behavior, including intracellular signaling cytoskeletal changes, and integrin-focal interactions [75]. Adding a 3D-structure that cells need to migrate through requires cells to modify their shape and interact with the matrix, which forms both a barrier and a substrate [76]. Collagen is the most commonly used substrate for 3D migration assays. This is most likely because pulp ECM consists predominantly of collagen type I and III fibrils [77]. Suzuki and coauthors have used a modified Trans-well insert migration assay with 3D collagen to study the chemotactic potential of FGF-2, SDF-1 and bone morphogenetic protein 7 (BMP7) over a longer time period. DPSC were seeded onto the collagen gel in a Trans-well insert that was placed in culture medium with the respective molecules. After seven days, the collagen gels were retrieved, fixed and 4',6-diamidino-2-phenylindole (DAPI) stained for further analysis with confocal microscopy [17].

Several disadvantages associated with the Trans-well assay should be noted. Firstly, chemotactic gradients are diffusion-driven and thus rather unstable [7]. Secondly, this methodology does not allow for a real-time follow-up of the migration process. To respond to these limitations, *in vitro* chemotaxis chambers have been developed that allow for real-time monitoring of cellular migration [78] (Figure 2d). They are the size of a microscopic slide and have two reservoirs that are connected by an interstitial observational area where cells are seeded in Matrigel. These cells are subjected to a chemotactic gradient via a concentration-distribution of the solution injected into one of the reservoirs. With this approach, a more stable chemotactic gradient is established, and cells can be tracked for 48 h and over a longer distance with real-time microscopic imaging. This technique has been successfully applied to study the chemotactic potential of C5a on DPSC [8]. By calculating the displacement of the center of mass (CAM) of STRO1$^+$ cells over 48 h, a clear migration following the C5a gradient was shown. Another culture model to study cellular migration that has been developed is based on the use of graduated tissue culture chambers coated with Matrigel (Figure 2c). In this model, cells are seeded in a droplet in the middle. Microspheres with different molecules are embedded on opposite sides in the culture chamber and cellular migration can be followed microscopically. In this way, longer migration periods (up to 10 days) in response to the controlled release of FGF-2 and TGFβ-1 from microspheres have been studied in real-time [16].

5.2. In vitro *Scratch Assay*

Another cost-effective technique to study cell migration is the scratch assay, also referred to as the wound healing assay. A scratch is made in a confluent cell layer followed through the evaluation of cellular migration to close the cell-free gap. A modified version consists of growing cells around a culture insert which is removed when cells reach confluence, leaving behind a more reproducible gap with sharp edges (Figure 2b). This methodology does not allow the study of chemotaxis as a chemotactic gradient cannot be established. Nevertheless, it can give insight into the impact of different molecules or materials on cellular migration. This assay has mainly been used to study the influence of materials such as Biodentine, BioAggregate, ProRoot MTA and HEMA on DPSC migration [63,65,69].

5.3. Cell Migration Tracking *in vivo*

In vivo migration assays typically consist of tracking labeled transplanted cells into animal models by magnetic resonance imaging, optical fluorescence imaging, positron emission tomography and single-photon emission computed tomography [7]. These do not allow, however, for the assessment of endogenous cell recruitment, and require rather complex and expensive experimental procedures. End-point *in vivo* assays, on the other hand, can be used to study endogenous cell recruitment. These are based on the immunohistological identification of proliferating cells at different time points, following which the cellular migration route can be reconstructed. For example, a rat model was used to evaluate the spatio-temporal evolution of proliferating pulp cells in response to pulp injury treated with agarose beads containing bioactive ECM components [79]. Rats were sacrificed after 1, 3, 8, 15 and 30 days, and pulp tissues were immunostained using proliferating cell nuclear antigen (PCNA). Based on their findings, it could be deduced that cells migrated from the central part of the radicular pulp to the sub-odontoblast cell layer and then from the apical root to the crown. *Ex vivo* assays, based on the same approach, form a suitable alternative to study *in vivo* endogenous stem cell recruitment.

5.4. Ex vivo *Entire Tooth Culture Reproduces in vivo Migration Conditions*

For instance, an *ex vivo* culture model of entire human teeth has been developed [6] (Figure 3). Immature third molars extracted for orthodontic reasons are cleaned, and pulp injuries are made with sterilized instruments, after which they are put in culture medium as illustrated in Figure 3. This model has been used to investigate the migration of DPSC in response to pulp injury. To this end, teeth with a pulp cavity were cultured in medium containing 5-bromo-20-deoxyuridine (BrdU) for one day after pulp injury, after which teeth were cultured in culture medium without BrdU. In this way, it could be demonstrated that directly after pulp injury, proliferating cells were at the perivascular area, whereas after two weeks of culture these proliferating cells were detected in the vicinity of the cavity. This model is a cost-effective alternative to *in vivo* migration studies. Given that this is an entire tooth culture, it simulates the interaction of migrating cells with ECM components, reproduces interactions between the different pulp cell populations and the production of chemotactic factors by these cells. Nevertheless, some disadvantages can be noted, including the absence of a functional vascular system in the pulp and the limited simulation of all inflammatory reactions. Histological processing is also cumbersome, like for the above-mentioned *in vivo* assays.

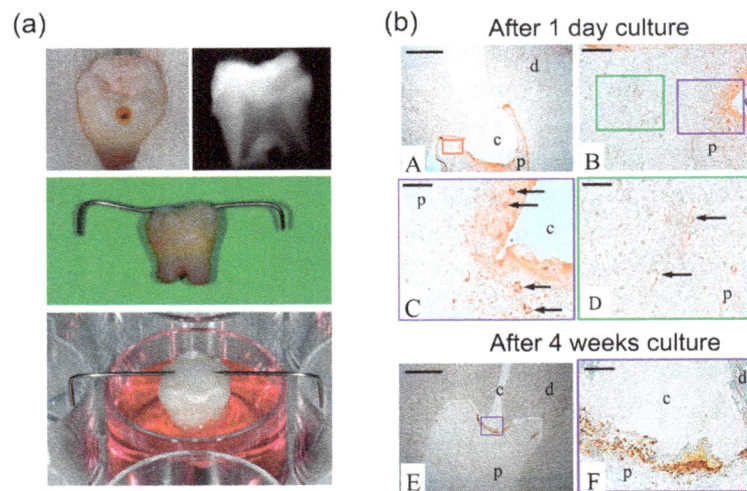

Figure 3. Overview of the *ex vivo* tooth model and its application for studying DPSC migration. (**a**) The pulp cavity was prepared in a clean immature third molar. X-ray imaging showed that the cavity is reaching the pulp. After cavity preparation, teeth were suspended with their root canals in culture medium with the aid of a steel wire fixed on the crown; (**b**) Representative histological images of teeth cultured with medium containing 5-bromo-20-deoxyuridine (BrdU) during one day after cavity preparation, followed with medium without BrdU for four weeks. After one day, the labelling was localized in the nuclei of cells in the perivascular area. The BrdU immunolabelling exhibited a gradient. It was strong in the blood vessels surrounding the cavity (**B** and **C**) and decreased in those away from the cavity (**B, D**). At four weeks, the immunolabelling was localized at the cavity area only (**E** and **F**). *Abbreviations*: c: cavity; d: dentin; p: pulp; arrows indicate vessels. Scale bars in (**A, E**) 1 mm; (**B, F**) 100 μm; (**C** and **D**) 50 μm. Modified with permission from [6].

6. Potential Use in Tissue Engineering

Three major processes can be discerned in tissue regeneration: the recruitment of stem/progenitor cells to the lesion site, the differentiation of these cells and the maturation of the newly formed tissue [80]. Tissue engineering approaches are aimed to optimize these processes. Here, we focus on the modulation of endogenous DPSC recruitment to the pulp lesion site, which can be categorized as *in situ* tissue engineering [20]. Specific chemotactic factors can be used to alter the host microenvironment and stimulate as such the migration of progenitor cells towards the lesion site [20]. Given that the majority of these soluble chemotactic factors have a rather short half-life and are expensive [81], appropriate delivery vehicles are required. Biodegradable microspheres are extensively investigated as they have promising properties including a controlled release of the bioactive molecule and ease of preparation, often with ground substances that are already clinically approved by the US Food and Drug Administration (e.g., poly(lactic-co-glycolic acid) (PLGA)) [82].

The SDF-1/CXCR4 migratory axis is being explored by various researchers for cell homing purposes. For example, poly-L-lactide scaffolds containing SDF-1, which were implanted between the skin and deep muscle of mice, induced stem cell recruitment [83]. Other chemotactic factors that have been investigated include FGF-2 and TGFβ-1, which are encapsulated in biodegradable PLGA microspheres [16]. It was observed that these growth factor-containing microspheres stimulate dental pulp cell proliferation and migration. An *in vivo* study has demonstrated the benefit of a composite material consisting of PLGA microspheres loaded with TGFβ-1 that have been incorporated in calcium phosphate cement [84]. This composite was used for pulp capping in goat incisors, and the subsequent histological evaluation showed that the composite with the highest TGFβ-1 concentration was able to stimulate odontoblastic differentiation of DPSC and associated tertiary dentin formation.

Besides exogenous application of chemotactic factors, other elements in pulp injury treatments can stimulate endogenous DPSC recruitment. For example, several pulp capping materials already used in the clinic will positively influence the dentin pulp regeneration process, partly by enhancing DPSC migration towards the lesion site. Interestingly, a recent study has showed a stimulating effect of magnetic nanocomposite scaffolds made of magnetite nanoparticles and polycaprolactone on DPSC migration [85]. Ethylenediaminetetraacetic acid (EDTA) preconditioning of dentin has also been demonstrated to increase DPSC migration [86], which can be attributed to the release of sequestered chemotactic factors in the dentin matrix.

In the clinic, DPSC recruitment to treat pulp injury will most likely include the application of a biodegradable device containing chemotactic factors overlaid with a bioactive pulp capping material.

7. Conclusions

Stem cell mobilization and recruitment appears as a complex process. It requires both soluble chemotactic factors and insoluble extracellular matrix and environmental factors, which constitute the pulp microenvironment. While some of these soluble factors are sequestered in the dentin, others originate from plasma or can be synthesized by pulp fibroblasts. Insoluble factors usually surround the stem cells and are necessary for the guided migration of these cells. Pathological conditions with moderate inflammation following pulp injury and after applying direct pulp capping bioactive materials lead to a modification of the pulp microenvironment. This modified microenvironment will promote the dental pulp stem cell recruitment that is required to replace the missing odontoblasts and to synthesize the pulp protective reparative dentin.

Knowledge of stem cell mobilization and migration signals from a variety of *in vitro*, *in vivo* and *ex vivo* methodologies show that each has specific advantages and disadvantages. While *in vitro* assays allow for a rapid and cost-effective evaluation of these signals, they should be considered as a first research step. Both *ex vivo* and *in vivo* assays will provide a more thorough understanding of stem cell mobilization and migration in the pulp.

These methodologies also serve the field of *in situ* tissue engineering that targets the tooth's own stem cells to stimulate dentin pulp regeneration. The explored treatment approaches include the controlled delivery of chemotactic factors from biodegradable devices such as microspheres. The ultimate goal of this procedure is to obtain reparative dentin formation by DPSC after their differentiation into odontoblast-like cells leading to dentin pulp regeneration, while preserving the pulp volume.

Acknowledgments: Supported by institutional funding from Aix-Marseille University and CNRS.

Abbreviations

The following abbreviations are used in this manuscript:

BMP	bone morphogenetic protein
BrdU	5-bromo-20-deoxyuridine
BSP	bone sialoprotein
CAM	center of mass
CXCL14	chemokine (C-X-C motif) ligand 14
CXCR4	C-X-C chemokine receptor type 4
DMP-1	dentin matrix protein-1
DPSC	dental pulp stem cells
DAPI	4',6-diamidino-2-phenylindole
ECM	extracellular matrix
EDTA	ethylenediaminetetraacetic acid
FAK	focal adhesion kinase
FGF-2	basic fibroblast growth factor
G-CSF	granulocyte-colony stimulating factor
HEMA	2-hydroxyethyl methacrylate
HGF	hepatocyte growth factor
HMGB-1	high mobility group box 1
LPS	lipopolysaccharide
LTA	lipoteichoic acid
MAPK/ERK	mitogen-activated protein kinase/extracellular signal-regulated kinases
MCP-1	monocyte chemoattractant protein 1
MMPs	matrix metalloproteinases
MMP3	matrix metalloproteinase-3
MTA	mineral trioxide aggregate
OPN	osteopontin
PLGA	poly(lactic-co-glycolic acid)
RAGE	receptor for advanced glycation end products
S1P	sphingosine-1-phosphatase
SCAP	dental pulp stem cells of the apical papilla
SDF-1	stromal cell-derived factor 1
SIBLING	small integrin-binding ligand, N-linked glycoproteins
TEGDMA	triethylene-glycol- dimethacrylate
TGFβ-1	transforming growth factor β 1
TLR	Toll-like receptor
TLR4	Toll-like receptor 4

References

1. Gronthos, S.; Mankani, M.; Brahim, J.; Robey, P.G.; Shi, S. Postnatal human dental pulp stem cells (DPSCs) in vitro and in vivo. *Proc. Natl. Acad. Sci. USA* **2000**, *97*, 13625–13630. [CrossRef] [PubMed]

2. About, I.; Bottero, M.J.; de Denato, P.; Camps, J.; Franquin, J.C.; Mitsiadis, T.A. Human dentin production in vitro. *Exp. Cell Res.* **2000**, *258*, 33–41. [CrossRef] [PubMed]

3. Batouli, S.; Miura, M.; Brahim, J.; Tsutsui, T.W.; Fisher, L.W.; Gronthos, S.; Robey, P.G.; Shi, S. Comparison of stem-cell-mediated osteogenesis and dentinogenesis. *J. Dent. Res.* **2003**, *82*, 976–981. [CrossRef] [PubMed]

4. Kaukua, N.; Shahidi, M.K.; Konstantinidou, C.; Dyachuk, V.; Kaucka, M.; Furlan, A.; An, Z.; Wang, L.; Hultman, I.; Ahrlund-Richter, L.; *et al.* Glial origin of mesenchymal stem cells in a tooth model system. *Nature* **2014**, *513*, 551–554. [CrossRef] [PubMed]

5. Shi, S.; Gronthos, S. Perivascular niche of postnatal mesenchymal stem cells in human bone marrow and dental pulp. *J. Bone Miner. Res.* **2003**, *18*, 696–704. [CrossRef] [PubMed]

6. Téclès, O.; Laurent, P.; Zygouritsas, S.; Burger, A.-S.; Camps, J.; Dejou, J.; About, I. Activation of human dental pulp progenitor/stem cells in response to odontoblast injury. *Arch. Oral Biol.* **2005**, *50*, 103–108. [CrossRef] [PubMed]

7. Andreas, K.; Sittinger, M.; Ringe, J. Toward in situ tissue engineering: chemokine-guided stem cell recruitment. *Trends Biotechnol.* **2014**, *32*, 483–492. [CrossRef] [PubMed]

8. Chmilewsky, F.; Jeanneau, C.; Laurent, P.; Kirschfink, M.; About, I. Pulp progenitor cell recruitment is selectively guided by a C5a gradient. *J. Dent. Res.* **2013**, *92*, 532–539. [CrossRef] [PubMed]

9. Howard, C.; Murray, P.E.; Namerow, K.N. Dental pulp stem cell migration. *J. Endod.* **2010**, *36*, 1963–1966. [CrossRef] [PubMed]

10. Hayashi, Y.; Murakami, M.; Kawamura, R.; Ishizaka, R.; Fukuta, O.; Nakashima, M. CXCL14 and MCP1 are potent trophic factors associated with cell migration and angiogenesis leading to higher regenerative potential of dental pulp side population cells. *Stem Cell Res. Ther.* **2015**, *6*, 111. [CrossRef] [PubMed]

11. Yang, J.-W.; Zhang, Y.-F.; Wan, C.-Y.; Sun, Z.-Y.; Nie, S.; Jian, S.-J.; Zhang, L.; Song, G.-T.; Chen, Z. Autophagy in SDF-1α-mediated DPSC migration and pulp regeneration. *Biomaterials* **2015**, *44*, 11–23. [CrossRef] [PubMed]

12. Murakami, M.; Horibe, H.; Iohara, K.; Hayashi, Y.; Osako, Y.; Takei, Y.; Nakata, K.; Motoyama, N.; Kurita, K.; Nakashima, M. The use of granulocyte-colony stimulating factor induced mobilization for isolation of dental pulp stem cells with high regenerative potential. *Biomaterials* **2013**, *34*, 9036–9047. [CrossRef] [PubMed]

13. Tomson, P.L.; Lumley, P.J.; Alexander, M.Y.; Smith, A.J.; Cooper, P.R. Hepatocyte growth factor is sequestered in dentine matrix and promotes regeneration-associated events in dental pulp cells. *Cytokine* **2013**, *61*, 622–629. [CrossRef] [PubMed]

14. Zhang, X.; Jiang, H.; Gong, Q.; Fan, C.; Huang, Y.; Ling, J. Expression of high mobility group box 1 in inflamed dental pulp and its chemotactic effect on dental pulp cells. *Biochem. Biophys. Res. Commun.* **2014**, *450*, 1547–1552. [CrossRef] [PubMed]

15. Chmilewsky, F.; Jeanneau, C.; Dejou, J.; About, I. Sources of dentin-pulp regeneration signals and their modulation by the local microenvironment. *J. Endod.* **2014**, *40*, S19–S25. [CrossRef] [PubMed]

16. Mathieu, S.; Jeanneau, C.; Sheibat-Othman, N.; Kalaji, N.; Fessi, H.; About, I. Usefulness of controlled release of growth factors in investigating the early events of dentin-pulp regeneration. *J. Endod.* **2013**, *39*, 228–235. [CrossRef] [PubMed]

17. Suzuki, T.; Lee, C.H.; Chen, M.; Zhao, W.; Fu, S.Y.; Qi, J.J.; Chotkowski, G.; Eisig, S.B.; Wong, A.; Mao, J.J. Induced Migration of Dental Pulp Stem Cells for *in vivo* Pulp Regeneration. *J. Dent. Res.* **2011**, *90*, 1013–1018. [CrossRef] [PubMed]

18. Laurent, P.; Camps, J.; About, I. Biodentine(TM) induces TGF-β1 release from human pulp cells and early dental pulp mineralization. *Int. Endod. J.* **2012**, *45*, 439–448. [CrossRef] [PubMed]

19. Sloan, A.J.; Couble, M.L.; Bleicher, F.; Magloire, H.; Smith, A.J.; Farges, J.C. Expression of TGF-beta receptors I and II in the human dental pulp by in situ hybridization. *Adv. Dent. Res.* **2001**, *15*, 63–67. [CrossRef] [PubMed]

20. Ko, I.K.; Lee, S.J.; Atala, A.; Yoo, J.J. *In situ* tissue regeneration through host stem cell recruitment. *Exp. Mol. Med.* **2013**, *45*, e57. [CrossRef] [PubMed]

21. Lu, J.; Chatterjee, M.; Schmid, H.; Beck, S.; Gawaz, M. CXCL14 as an emerging immune and inflammatory modulator. *J. Inflamm. (Lond).* **2016**, *13*, 1. [CrossRef] [PubMed]

22. Iohara, K.; Murakami, M.; Takeuchi, N.; Osako, Y.; Ito, M.; Ishizaka, R.; Utunomiya, S.; Nakamura, H.; Matsushita, K.; Nakashima, M. A novel combinatorial therapy with pulp stem cells and granulocyte colony-stimulating factor for total pulp regeneration. *Stem Cells Transl. Med.* **2013**, *2*, 521–533. [CrossRef] [PubMed]

23. Takeuchi, N.; Hayashi, Y.; Murakami, M.; Alvarez, F.J.; Horibe, H.; Iohara, K.; Nakata, K.; Nakamura, H.; Nakashima, M. Similar *in vitro* effects and pulp regeneration in ectopic tooth transplantation by basic fibroblast growth factor and granulocyte-colony stimulating factor. *Oral Dis.* **2015**, *21*, 113–122. [CrossRef] [PubMed]

24. Obinata, H.; Hla, T. Sphingosine 1-phosphate in coagulation and inflammation. *Semin. Immunopathol.* **2012**, *34*, 73–91. [CrossRef] [PubMed]

25. Pan, H.Y.; Yang, H.; Shao, M.Y.; Xu, J.; Zhang, P.; Cheng, R.; Hu, T. Sphingosine-1-phosphate mediates AKT/ERK maintenance of dental pulp homoeostasis. *Int. Endod. J.* **2015**, *48*, 460–468. [CrossRef] [PubMed]

26. Jiang, L.; Zhu, Y.-Q.; Du, R.; Gu, Y.-X.; Xia, L.; Qin, F.; Ritchie, H.H. The Expression and Role of Stromal Cell-derived Factor-1α-CXCR4 Axis in Human Dental Pulp. *J. Endod.* **2008**, *34*, 939–944. [CrossRef] [PubMed]

27. Jiang, L.; Peng, W.W.; Li, L.F.; Yang, Y.; Zhu, Y.Q. Proliferation and multilineage potential of CXCR4-positive human dental pulp cells in vitro. *J. Endod.* **2012**, *38*, 642–647. [CrossRef] [PubMed]

28. Chmilewsky, F.; Jeanneau, C.; Laurent, P.; About, I. Pulp fibroblasts synthesize functional complement proteins involved in initiating dentin-pulp regeneration. *Am. J. Pathol.* **2014**, *184*, 1991–2000. [CrossRef] [PubMed]

29. Chmilewsky, F.; Jeanneau, C.; Laurent, P.; About, I. LPS induces pulp progenitor cell recruitment via complement activation. *J. Dent. Res.* **2015**, *94*, 166–174. [CrossRef] [PubMed]

30. O'Callaghan, A.; Wang, J.; Redmond, H.P. HMGB1 as a key mediator of tissue response to injury: Roles in inflammation and tissue repair. *Eur. Surg. Acta Chir. Austriaca* **2006**, *38*, 283–292. [CrossRef]

31. Haeger, A.; Wolf, K.; Zegers, M.M.; Friedl, P. Collective cell migration: guidance principles and hierarchies. *Trends Cell Biol.* **2015**, *25*, 556–566. [CrossRef] [PubMed]

32. Smith, A.J.; Scheven, B.A.; Takahashi, Y.; Ferracane, J.L.; Shelton, R.M.; Cooper, P.R. Dentine as a bioactive extracellular matrix. *Arch. Oral Biol.* **2012**, *57*, 109–121. [CrossRef] [PubMed]

33. Tomson, P.L.; Grover, L.M.; Lumley, P.J.; Sloan, A.J.; Smith, A.J.; Cooper, P.R. Dissolution of bio-active dentine matrix components by mineral trioxide aggregate. *J. Dent.* **2007**, *35*, 636–642. [CrossRef] [PubMed]

34. Finkelman, R.D.; Mohan, S.; Jennings, J.C.; Taylor, A.K.; Jepsen, S.; Baylink, D.J. Quantitation of growth factors IGF-I, SGF/IGF-II, and TGF-β in human dentin. *J. Bone Miner. Res.* **1990**, *5*, 717–723. [CrossRef] [PubMed]

35. Roberts-Clark, D.; Smith, A. Angiogenic growth factors in human dentine matrix. *Arch. Oral Biol.* **2000**, *45*, 1013–1016. [CrossRef]

36. Smith, J.G.; Smith, A.J.; Shelton, R.M.; Cooper, P.R. Recruitment of dental pulp cells by dentine and pulp extracellular matrix components. *Exp. Cell Res.* **2012**, *318*, 2397–2406. [CrossRef] [PubMed]

37. Lymperi, S.; Taraslia, V.; Tsatsoulis, I.N.; Samara, A.; Velentzas, A.D.; Agrafioti, A.; Anastasiadou, E.; Kontakiotis, E. Dental Stem Cell Migration on Pulp Ceiling Cavities Filled with MTA, Dentin Chips, or Bio-Oss. *Biomed Res. Int.* **2015**, *2015*. [CrossRef] [PubMed]

38. Palosaari, H.; Pennington, C.J.; Larmas, M.; Edwards, D.R.; Tjäderhane, L.; Salo, T. Expression profile of matrix metalloproteinases (MMPs) and tissue inhibitors of MMPs in mature human odontoblasts and pulp tissue. *Eur. J. Oral Sci.* **2003**, *111*, 117–127. [CrossRef] [PubMed]

39. Jain, A.; Bahuguna, R. Role of matrix metalloproteinases in dental caries, pulp and periapical inflammation: An overview. *J. Oral Biol. Craniofacial Res.* **2015**, *5*, 212–218. [CrossRef] [PubMed]

40. Chaussain-Miller, C.; Fioretti, F.; Goldberg, M.; Menashi, S. The Role of Matrix Metalloproteinases (MMPs) in Human Caries. *J. Dent. Res.* **2006**, *85*, 22–33. [CrossRef] [PubMed]

41. Zheng, L.; Amano, K.; Iohara, K.; Ito, M.; Imabayashi, K.; Into, T.; Matsushita, K.; Nakamura, H.; Nakashima, M. Matrix metalloproteinase-3 accelerates wound healing following dental pulp injury. *Am. J. Pathol.* **2009**, *175*, 1905–1914. [CrossRef] [PubMed]

42. Mu, D.; Cambier, S.; Fjellbirkeland, L.; Baron, J.L.; Munger, J.S.; Kawakatsu, H.; Sheppard, D.; Broaddus, V.C.; Nishimura, S.L. The integrin alpha(v)beta8 mediates epithelial homeostasis through MT1-MMP-dependent activation of TGF-beta1. *J. Cell Biol.* **2002**, *157*, 493–507. [CrossRef] [PubMed]

43. Visse, R. Matrix Metalloproteinases and Tissue Inhibitors of Metalloproteinases: Structure, Function, and Biochemistry. *Circ. Res.* **2003**, *92*, 827–839. [CrossRef] [PubMed]

44. Gill, S.E.; Parks, W.C. Metalloproteinases and their inhibitors: regulators of wound healing. *Int. J. Biochem. Cell Biol.* **2008**, *40*, 1334–1347. [CrossRef] [PubMed]

45. Ho, I.A.W.; Yulyana, Y.; Sia, K.C.; Newman, J.P.; Guo, C.M.; Hui, K.M.; Lam, P.Y.P. Matrix metalloproteinase-1-mediated mesenchymal stem cell tumor tropism is dependent on crosstalk with stromal derived growth factor 1/C-X-C chemokine receptor 4 axis. *FASEB J.* **2014**, *28*, 4359–4368. [CrossRef] [PubMed]

46. Ries, C.; Egea, V.; Karow, M.; Kolb, H.; Jochum, M.; Neth, P. MMP-2, MT1-MMP, and TIMP-2 are essential for the invasive capacity of human mesenchymal stem cells: Differential regulation by inflammatory cytokines. *Blood* **2007**, *109*, 4055–4063. [CrossRef] [PubMed]

47. Liu, J.-Y.; Chen, X.; Yue, L.; Huang, G.T.-J.; Zou, X.-Y. CXC Chemokine Receptor 4 Is Expressed Paravascularly in Apical Papilla and Coordinates with Stromal Cell-derived Factor-1α during Transmigration of Stem Cells from Apical Papilla. *J. Endod.* **2015**, *41*, 1430–1436. [CrossRef] [PubMed]

48. Chang, M.-C.; Tsai, Y.-L.; Chang, H.-H.; Lee, S.-Y.; Lee, M.-S.; Chang, C.-W.; Chan, C.-P.; Yeh, C.-Y.; Cheng, R.-H.; Jeng, J.-H. IL-1β-induced MCP-1 expression and secretion of human dental pulp cells is related to TAK1, MEK/ERK, and PI3K/Akt signaling pathways. *Arch. Oral Biol.* **2016**, *61*, 16–22. [CrossRef] [PubMed]

49. Li, D.; Fu, L.; Zhang, Y.; Yu, Q.; Ma, F.; Wang, Z.; Luo, Z.; Zhou, Z.; Cooper, P.R.; He, W. The effects of LPS on adhesion and migration of human dental pulp stem cells in vitro. *J. Dent.* **2014**, *42*, 1327–1334. [CrossRef] [PubMed]

50. Akira, S.; Uematsu, S.; Takeuchi, O. Pathogen recognition and innate immunity. *Cell* **2006**, *124*, 783–801. [CrossRef] [PubMed]

51. Liu, Y.; Gao, Y.; Zhan, X.; Cui, L.; Xu, S.; Ma, D.; Yue, J.; Wu, B.; Gao, J. TLR4 Activation by Lipopolysaccharide and Streptococcus mutans Induces Differential Regulation of Proliferation and Migration in Human Dental Pulp Stem Cells. *J. Endod.* **2014**, *40*, 1375–1381. [CrossRef] [PubMed]

52. Park, J.H.; Kwon, S.M.; Yoon, H.E.; Kim, S.A.; Ahn, S.G.; Yoon, J.H. Lipopolysaccharide promotes adhesion and migration of murine dental papilla-derived MDPC-23 cells via TLR4. *Int. J. Mol. Med.* **2011**, *27*, 277–281. [PubMed]

53. Ricklin, D.; Hajishengallis, G.; Yang, K.; Lambris, J.D. Complement: a key system for immune surveillance and homeostasis. *Nat. Immunol.* **2010**, *11*, 785–797. [CrossRef] [PubMed]

54. Schraufstatter, I.U.; Khaldoyanidi, S.K.; DiScipio, R.G. Complement activation in the context of stem cells and tissue repair. *World J. Stem Cells* **2015**, *7*, 1090–1108. [CrossRef] [PubMed]

55. Qi, S.C.; Cui, C.; Yan, Y.H.; Sun, G.H.; Zhu, S.R. Effects of high-mobility group box 1 on the proliferation and odontoblastic differentiation of human dental pulp cells. *Int. Endod. J.* **2013**, *46*, 1153–1163. [CrossRef] [PubMed]

56. Nowicka, A.; Lipski, M.; Parafiniuk, M.; Sporniak-Tutak, K.; Lichota, D.; Kosierkiewicz, A.; Kaczmarek, W.; Buczkowska-Radlińska, J. Response of Human Dental Pulp Capped with Biodentine and Mineral Trioxide Aggregate. *J. Endod.* **2013**, *39*, 743–747. [CrossRef] [PubMed]

57. Matsumoto, S.; Hayashi, M.; Suzuki, Y.; Suzuki, N.; Maeno, M.; Ogiso, B. Calcium ions released from mineral trioxide aggregate convert the differentiation pathway of C2C12 cells into osteoblast lineage. *J. Endod.* **2013**, *39*, 68–75. [CrossRef] [PubMed]

58. An, S.; Gao, Y.; Ling, J.; Wei, X.; Xiao, Y. Calcium ions promote osteogenic differentiation and mineralization of human dental pulp cells: implications for pulp capping materials. *J. Mater. Sci. Mater. Med.* **2012**, *23*, 789–795. [CrossRef] [PubMed]

59. AbdulQader, S.T.; Kannan, T.P.; Rahman, I.A.; Ismail, H.; Mahmood, Z. Effect of different calcium phosphate scaffold ratios on odontogenic differentiation of human dental pulp cells. *Mater. Sci. Eng. C. Mater. Biol. Appl.* **2015**, *49*, 225–233. [CrossRef] [PubMed]

60. Wu, B.-C.; Kao, C.-T.; Huang, T.-H.; Hung, C.-J.; Shie, M.-Y.; Chung, H.-Y. Effect of verapamil, a calcium channel blocker, on the odontogenic activity of human dental pulp cells cultured with silicate-based materials. *J. Endod.* **2014**, *40*, 1105–1111. [CrossRef] [PubMed]

61. Liu, C.-H.; Hung, C.-J.; Huang, T.-H.; Lin, C.-C.; Kao, C.-T.; Shie, M.-Y. Odontogenic differentiation of human dental pulp cells by calcium silicate materials stimulating via FGFR/ERK signaling pathway. *Mater. Sci. Eng. C Mater. Biol. Appl.* **2014**, *43*, 359–366. [CrossRef] [PubMed]

62. Schneider, R.; Holland, G.R.; Chiego, D.; Hu, J.C.C.; Nör, J.E.; Botero, T.M. White mineral trioxide aggregate induces migration and proliferation of stem cells from the apical papilla. *J. Endod.* **2014**, *40*, 931–936. [CrossRef] [PubMed]

63. Zhu, L.; Yang, J.; Zhang, J.; Peng, B. A comparative study of bioaggregate and ProRoot MTA on adhesion, migration, and attachment of human dental pulp cells. *J. Endod.* **2014**, *40*, 1118–1123. [CrossRef] [PubMed]

64. Zhang, J.; Zhu, L.X.; Cheng, X.; Lin, Y.; Yan, P.; Peng, B. Promotion of Dental Pulp Cell Migration and Pulp Repair by a Bioceramic Putty Involving FGFR-mediated Signaling Pathways. *J. Dent. Res.* **2015**, *94*, 853–862. [CrossRef] [PubMed]

65. Luo, Z.; Li, D.; Kohli, M.R.; Yu, Q.; Kim, S.; He, W.X. Effect of Biodentine™ on the proliferation, migration and adhesion of human dental pulp stem cells. *J. Dent.* **2014**, *42*, 490–497. [CrossRef] [PubMed]

66. Aguirre, A.; González, A.; Planell, J.A.; Engel, E. Extracellular calcium modulates *in vitro* bone marrow-derived Flk-1+ CD34+ progenitor cell chemotaxis and differentiation through a calcium-sensing receptor. *Biochem. Biophys. Res. Commun.* **2010**, *393*, 156–161. [CrossRef] [PubMed]

67. Graham, L.; Cooper, P.R.; Cassidy, N.; Nor, J.E.; Sloan, A.J.; Smith, A.J. The effect of calcium hydroxide on solubilisation of bio-active dentine matrix components. *Biomaterials* **2006**, *27*, 2865–2873. [CrossRef] [PubMed]

68. Calarco, A.; Di Salle, A.; Tammaro, L.; De Luca, I.; Mucerino, S.; Petillo, O.; Riccitiello, F.; Vittoria, V.; Peluso, G. Long-Term Fluoride Release from Dental Resins Affects STRO-1+ Cell Behavior. *J. Dent. Res.* **2015**, *94*, 1–7. [CrossRef] [PubMed]

69. Williams, D.W.; Wu, H.; Oh, J.-E.; Fakhar, C.; Kang, M.K.; Shin, K.-H.; Park, N.-H.; Kim, R.H. 2-Hydroxyethyl methacrylate inhibits migration of dental pulp stem cells. *J. Endod.* **2013**, *39*, 1156–1160. [CrossRef] [PubMed]

70. Tran-Hung, L.; Laurent, P.; Camps, J.; About, I. Quantification of angiogenic growth factors released by human dental cells after injury. *Arch. Oral Biol.* **2008**, *53*, 9–13. [CrossRef] [PubMed]

71. Paschalidis, T.; Bakopoulou, A.; Papa, P.; Leyhausen, G.; Geurtsen, W.; Koidis, P. Dental pulp stem cells' secretome enhances pulp repair processes and compensates TEGDMA-induced cytotoxicity. *Dent. Mater.* **2014**, *30*, e405–e418. [CrossRef] [PubMed]

72. Chen, H.-C. Boyden chamber assay. *Methods Mol. Biol.* **2005**, *294*, 15–22. [PubMed]

73. Motasim, K.S.; Nystrom, M.L.; Thomas, G.J. Cell migration and invasion assays. *Methods Mol. Biol.* **2011**, *731*, 333–343.

74. von Marschall, Z.; Fisher, L.W. Dentin matrix protein-1 isoforms promote differential cell attachment and migration. *J. Biol. Chem.* **2008**, *283*, 32730–32740. [CrossRef] [PubMed]

75. Rhee, S. Fibroblasts in three dimensional matrices: cell migration and matrix remodeling. *Exp. Mol. Med.* **2009**, *41*, 858–865. [CrossRef] [PubMed]

76. Kramer, N.; Walzl, A.; Unger, C.; Rosner, M.; Krupitza, G.; Hengstschläger, M.; Dolznig, H. *In vitro* cell migration and invasion assays. *Mutat. Res.* **2013**, *752*, 10–24. [CrossRef] [PubMed]

77. Goldberg, M.; Smith, A.J. Cells and extracellular matrices of dentin and pulp: A biological basis for repair and tissue engineering. *Crit. Rev. Oral Biol. Med.* **2004**, *15*, 13–27. [CrossRef] [PubMed]

78. Zengel, P.; Nguyen-Hoang, A.; Schildhammer, C.; Zantl, R.; Kahl, V.; Horn, E. μ-Slide Chemotaxis: A new chamber for long-term chemotaxis studies. *BMC Cell Biol.* **2011**, *12*, 21. [CrossRef] [PubMed]

79. Hirata, A.; Dimitrova-Nakov, S.; Djole, S.-X.; Ardila, H.; Baudry, A.; Kellermann, O.; Simon, S.; Goldberg, M. Plithotaxis, a collective cell migration, regulates the sliding of proliferating pulp cells located in the apical niche. *Connect. Tissue Res.* **2014**, *55* Suppl 1, 68–72. [CrossRef] [PubMed]

80. Vanden Berg-Foels, W.S. In situ tissue regeneration: Chemoattractants for endogenous stem cell recruitment. *Tissue Eng. Part B Rev.* **2014**, *20*, 28–39. [CrossRef] [PubMed]

81. Yun, Y.-R.; Won, J.E.; Jeon, E.; Lee, S.; Kang, W.; Jo, H.; Jang, J.-H.; Shin, U.S.; Kim, H.-W. Fibroblast growth factors: biology, function, and application for tissue regeneration. *J. Tissue Eng.* **2010**, *2010*, 218142. [CrossRef] [PubMed]

82. Lü, J.-M.; Wang, X.; Marin-Muller, C.; Wang, H.; Lin, P.H.; Yao, Q.; Chen, C. Current advances in research and clinical applications of PLGA-based nanotechnology. *Expert Rev. Mol. Diagn.* **2009**, *9*, 325–341. [CrossRef] [PubMed]

83. Ko, I.K.; Ju, Y.M.; Chen, T.; Atala, A.; Yoo, J.J.; Lee, S.J. Combined systemic and local delivery of stem cell inducing/recruiting factors for in situ tissue regeneration. *FASEB J.* **2012**, *26*, 158–168. [CrossRef] [PubMed]

84. Zhang, W.; Walboomers, X.F.; Jansen, J.A. The formation of tertiary dentin after pulp capping with a calcium phosphate cement, loaded with PLGA microparticles containing TGF-β1. *J. Biomed. Mater. Res. Part A* **2008**, *85*, 439–444. [CrossRef] [PubMed]

85. Yun, H.-M.; Lee, E.-S.; Kim, M.; Kim, J.-J.; Lee, J.-H.; Lee, H.-H.; Park, K.-R.; Yi, J.-K.; Kim, H.-W.; Kim, E. Magnetic Nanocomposite Scaffold-Induced Stimulation of Migration and Odontogenesis of Human Dental Pulp Cells through Integrin Signaling Pathways. *PLoS ONE* **2015**, *10*, e0138614. [CrossRef] [PubMed]

86. Galler, K.M.; Widbiller, M.; Buchalla, W.; Eidt, A.; Hiller, K.-A.; Hoffer, P.C.; Schmalz, G. EDTA conditioning of dentine promotes adhesion, migration and differentiation of dental pulp stem cells. *Int. Endod. J.* **2015**, 1–10. [CrossRef] [PubMed]

12

Knowledge, Attitudes, and Practices of Mothers of Preschool Children About Oral Health in Qatar: A Cross-Sectional Survey

Asmaa Alkhtib [1] and Abdul Morawala [2,*] 🄳

[1] Oral Health Division Operations, Primary Health Care Corporation, Doha 26555, Qatar; drasmaaalkhtib@gmail.com

[2] Department of Dentistry, Primary Healthcare Corporation, Specialist Pediatric Dentist, Doha 26555, Qatar

* Correspondence: akmpedo@gmail.com;

Abstract: Health-related behaviors are influenced by knowledge and awareness, with oral health being no exception. It is well-known that oral diseases are influenced by social determinants. There is an association between the oral health knowledge of mothers and the status of their children's oral health. In Qatar, the knowledge and practices of oral health in preschool children have not been previously reported. The aim of this study was to assess the knowledge, attitude, and related practices of mothers of preschool children about oral health in Qatar. A total of 400 questionnaires were distributed by the principals of kindergarten to mothers of children attending 16 government kindergartens in Qatar. The questionnaire included 38 close-ended questions grouped into nine categories, addressing different aspects of knowledge and practices related to early childhood oral health. The questionnaire was constructed in English, before being translated into Arabic, which is the local language in Qatar. The questionnaire instrument was pre-tested on mothers with demographic characteristics matching the main population. These participants were not included in the main study. The questionnaire study was associated with a clinical epidemiological study to assess dental caries and enamel defects of the sampled children. The dmft caries index (decayed, missing and filled teeth) was used for that purpose according to the World Health Organization criteria. For the questionnaire administered to mothers with clinical survey variables, a binary logistic regression analysis was performed to determine the associations between the measures of oral health status (dmft, Dental index) and mothers' oral health knowledge and practices. A total of 48% mothers thought that children should have their teeth brushed from the age of three years and 42% chose younger than two years as a starting age for brushing. More than half (54%) of the mothers thought that children should not have their teeth flossed. In general, no significant statistical association was found between dmft and any other variables, except for whether or not the child had visited the dentist. Logistic regression analyses were performed to determine the association between the measures of oral health status (dmft, DI) and mothers' oral health knowledge and practices. After controlling for the other independent variables included in this model, the test of the model was not statistically significant, which indicated that none of the variables represent a significant risk for occurrence of caries. The only exception was whether or not the child had visited the dentist (odds ratio = 2.51, 95% confidence interval 1.091–5.774). Despite the existence of good knowledge of oral health care, there were deficiencies in the oral health care provided to children. This may reflect that seeking dental care is either not very important or it is challenging to obtain access to a child-friendly dentist in the public health system in Qatar. The results of this study suggest that there is a need for an oral health promotion program to fill the gaps in knowledge for mothers regarding oral health care for young children.

Keywords: dental caries; knowledge; mother; oral health; preschool children; Qatar

---

1. Introduction

Health-related behaviors are influenced by knowledge and awareness, with oral health being no exception. There is an association between oral health knowledge, age, and the education level of mothers, which are directly linked to the status of their children's oral health [1–4]. Oral health is an integral component of general health that plays an essential role in the life of a child. Dental caries are one of the pertinent oral health problems that are universally present. In most developing countries, the levels of dental caries are steadily rising. Countries in the Middle East have demonstrated a high prevalence of early childhood caries (ECC) [5,6]. A recent study in Qatar showed that the prevalence of ECC is 89% and the dmft caries index (decayed, missing and filled teeth) is 7.6.

In Qatar, the oral health knowledge and practices of mothers in relation to the oral health of their children have not been reported previously. Hence, the aim of the study was to assess the knowledge, attitude, and related practices of mothers of preschool children about oral health in Qatar.

2. Materials and Methods

Ethical clearance was obtained from the Human Ethics Research Committee at the University of Melbourne (#1034161) and the Medical Research Centre at Hamad Medical Corporation in Qatar (#10097). The Government of Qatar authorized this study involving pre-school children aged 3–4 years in the public kindergartens. A questionnaire assessing the knowledge and attitude of mothers toward the oral health of preschool children was developed based upon the primary researcher's knowledge as a pediatric dentist [7]. The questionnaire included 38 close-ended questions grouped into 9 categories, addressing different aspects of knowledge and practices related to early childhood oral health. The questionnaire was constructed in English before being translated into Arabic, which is the local language in Qatar. The questionnaire instrument was pre-tested on a sample of 7 mothers with demographic characteristics similar to those of the test population. These participants were excluded from the main study. The sample for this study aimed to be representative of children attending governmental kindergartens in Qatar. The total number of children in governmental kindergartens in the school year of 2011–2012 was 6374, so the sampled children represented about 4% of the eligible population at the time of the study.

The questionnaire was part of an information package that the family received from the kindergarten principals. Written consent was obtained from all participants. Dental caries of the children were also recorded using the dmft index according to the World Health Organization criteria (1997) [8]. The questionnaire data were entered into Microsoft® Excel 2003 spreadsheets (Microsoft Corporation, Seattle, WA, USA) and exported to SPSS 20.0™ for Windows® (SPSS, Chicago, IL, USA). Inferential statistics were used to examine any possible associations between dependent variables and independent variables. The outcome measures (dependent variables) included the oral health knowledge of mothers in general and the knowledge pertaining to their children's oral health, the oral health practices of mothers and those provided to their children, and the dietary habits of the children. The independent variables were early feeding habits, dietary habits, oral hygiene practices, and oral health care provided to children and mothers.

For the questionnaire administered to mothers and the clinical survey variables, a binary logistic regression analysis was performed to determine the associations between the measures of oral health status (dmft, Dental Index) and mothers' oral health knowledge and practices. Such analyses were used to assess the association between the potential risk factors and the development of caries, which may assist in developing a prediction model. All explanatory variables in the set within the model (the so-called "enter method") were fitted into a single model, where each variable was considered a potential confounder and the data were analyzed with and without controlling for the potential confounder. Results with p-values less than 0.05 were considered statistically significant.

3. Results

Most mothers returned the questionnaires, as there was a high response rate of 316/400 (79%). Table 1 shows the demographic data of the study participants.

Table 1. (a) Distribution of caries in Qatari children by gender (dmft) and (b) the demographic data of the participants.

(a)					
Caries Experience Distribution:	Sex		Total n = 250 (%)	Mean ($\pm$SD)	Range
	Female n (%) *	Male n (%) *			
Decayed teeth	110 (44)	113 (45)	223 (89)	7 (5.0)	0–20
Missing teeth	16 (6)	23 (9)	39 (15)	0.3 (0.8)	0–6
Filled teeth	18 (7))	19 (8)	37 (15)	0.3 (0.8)	0–7
dmft * ($\pm$SD)	7.6 ($\pm$5.3)	7.6 ($\pm$4.9)	-	7.6 ($\pm$5.0)	0–20
SiC * ($\pm$SD)	-	-	-	13.6 ($\pm$2.5)	
Caries prevalence	44%	45%	89%		
Caries free	13 (5)	14 (6)	27 (11)	-	-
Soft tissue (abscessed teeth)	9 (3)	14 (6)	23 (9)	-	-

(b)		
Demographics	Number	Percentage
Sex of children		
Male	146	46
Female	169	53
Total	315	100
Nationality		
Qatari	305	96
Non Qatari	10	04
Total	315	100
Mother's education level (n = 298) *		
Primary level	23	7
High school	145	46
University	130	41
Age group of mother (n = 298) *		
16–25 years	36	11
26–34 years	181	57

* Percentage calculated out of total participants.

The majority of the children were breast-fed (71%) and bottle-fed (83%). Interestingly, 24% of the children were never breast-fed at all. Thirty-six percent of the children went to sleep with a milk bottle. The most common (40%) content of the bottle was cow's milk. Around 37% of mothers provided on-demand breast-feeding and 30% provided on-demand bottle-feeding. When mothers were asked to rate several types of food and snacks for their potential effect on teeth, their overall knowledge was reasonable. Most mothers (63–90%) knew that all types of sweets (sugar, candies, and chocolate), retentive carbohydrates (potato chips), and soft drinks were bad for teeth and that healthy food items (vegetables, fruits, milk, and cheese) were good for teeth. However, there was less than optimal knowledge about the potential harmful effects of orange juice on teeth, as 85% of mothers thought it was good for the teeth (Table 2).

Table 2. Distribution of the study participants based upon their dietary knowledge ($n = 315$).

Impact of Food Stuff on the Child's Oral Health	Missing	Good	Bad	I Do Not Know
Sweets				
Sugar	20 (6)	24 (8)	254 (80)	18 (6)
Candies	18 (6)	9 (3)	284 (90)	5 (1)
Chocolates	18 (6)	14 (4)	277 (88)	7 (2)
Retentive carbohydrates (potato chips)	19 (6)	41 (13)	200 (63)	56 (18)
Sweetened drinks				
Soft drink	19 (6)	1 (0.3)	285 (90)	11 (3)
Orange juices	21 (7)	269 (85)	14 (5)	12 (3)
Healthy foodstuff				
Vegetables	17 (5)	296 (94)	1 (0.3)	2 (1)
Fruits	17 (5)	297 (94)	0	2
Milk	17 (5)	296 (94)	0	3
Cheese	20 (6)	294 (94)	0	2

More than half (61%) of the mothers reported that they had tooth decay or gum problems. In terms of visiting the dentist, only 38% reported that they would go every six months and 18% would go every year. A striking finding was that 25% of mothers did not remember "when was the last time you went to the dentist?" despite most (78%) of the mothers having stated that they brushed their teeth twice per day. A total of 48% thought that children should have their teeth brushed from the age of three years and 42% chose younger than two years as a starting age for brushing. More than half (54%) of the mothers thought that children should not have their teeth flossed (Table 3).

Table 3. Knowledge of mothers related to the child's oral health.

	Replied (%)	Missing (%)
How often do you think people should see the dentist?		
When they have dental problem (e.g., toothache)	49 (16)	
Every 5 years	0	
Every 2 years	4 (1)	14 (5)
Every year	33 (10)	
Every 6 months	216 (68)	
At what age should children first be taken to the dentist?		
Older than 6 years of age	104 (33)	
At 6 years	56 (18)	19 (6)
At 3 years	136 (43)	
Younger than 2 years	1 (0.3)	
At what age should children have their teeth brushed?		
Older than 6 years of age	3 (1)	
At 6 years	12 (4)	16 (5)
At 3 years	152 (48)	
Younger than 2 years	133 (42)	
Do you think children should have their teeth flossed?		
No	172 (54)	26 (9)
Yes	118 (37)	
If yes, at what age children should floss their teeth?		
Older than 6 years of age	13 (4)	
At 6 years	44 (14)	193 (61)
At 3 years	46 (15)	
Younger than 2 years	20 (6)	

Half of the children had not yet visited the dentist, and of those who did (43%), most (61%) of their mothers did not answer the question about when the child first had visited the dentist. Of the children who visited the dentist, only 10% went for a regular checkup. More children visited the dentist when a problem occurred, such as having a toothache (14%) or having a cavity and needing a filling (16%). The mean age of commencing tooth brushing was three (±0.9) years. More than half (53%) of the children brushed their teeth by themselves and 48% had parental assistance in brushing. There were 248 cases for which the results from both the clinical examination and the mother's questionnaire were available. This allowed us to examine the association between the survey results and the dental caries experience. In general, no significant statistical association was found between dmft and any other variables, except for whether or not the child had visited the dentist. Table 4 shows the association between the knowledge of the mother and the frequency of caries of the child based on the dmft index.

Table 4. Association between caries experience of the child and mother's knowledge.

Oral Health Knowledge and Practices of Mothers	No or Low Caries n (Valid %)	Severe Caries n (Valid %)	Sig. (2-Sided Exact Test)
Mother's age (n = 232)			
16–34 years	48 (21)	119 (51)	0.133
35 years or older	12 (5)	53 (23)	
Mothers' education (n = 235)			
Primary/high school	35 (15)	106 (45)	
University	26 (11)	68 (29)	0.651
Has the child visited the dentist (n = 235)			
No	43 (18)	87 (37)	
Yes	19 (8)	86 (36.6)	0.011 *
Rate orange juice for effect on teeth (n = 234)			
Good	60 (26)	154 (66)	
Bad/I don't know	2 (1)	18 (8)	0.111
Was the child bottle-fed (n = 235)			
No	6 (3)	25 (11)	
Yes	56 (24)	148 (63)	0.390

* = statistically significant.

Logistic regression analyses were performed to determine the association between the measures of oral health status (dmft, DI) and mothers' oral health knowledge and practices. After controlling for the other independent variables included in this model, the test of the model was not statistically significant, which indicated that none of the variables represent a significant risk for occurrence of caries, except for whether or not the child had visited the dentist (odds ratio (OR) = 2.51, 95% confidence interval (CI) 1.091–5.774).

4. Discussion

Parental knowledge, attitude, and practices can have an impact on children's oral health. Children under the age of five years generally spend most of their time with parents and guardians. These early years involve "primary socialization", during which the earliest childhood routines and habits are acquired [9,10]. During the first three years during the pre-school period, the role of parents is important in maintaining the good oral health of the child [11]. The present study findings focused on mothers' knowledge, attitudes, and practices toward the oral health of preschool children in Qatar that have not previously been reported. These results are comparable to other results conducted in similar cohorts of mothers in the USA [12] and Saudi Arabia [13–15]. In the current study, the findings highlighted some practices that are considered to increase the risk of dental caries. Around one-third (36%) of the children went to bed with a bottle that mostly contained milk (40%). There was no differentiation in the questionnaire between formula or cow's milk, which is the most commonly used milk in Qatar. Over one-third (42%) of the children were reported to snack frequently and the preferred snacks were mostly cariogenic. Frequent consumption of sweetened drinks and starchy food (cariogenic diet) has been found to be associated with the occurrence of tooth decay in several studies [16–18]. In a study carried out in Nepal, only 29% of the respondents had knowledge that prolonged and frequent bottle-feeding affects dental health [19]. The results of this study were similar to the results of studies conducted by Moulana et al. [20], Wyne et al. [21], Kamolmatyakul and Saiong [22], and Chan et al. [23], in which the majority of the mothers were aware that consumption of sugary items can lead to dental caries. However, there was little awareness about the different forms of sugary items, apart from chocolates, that are harmful to the teeth. This has shed light on inadequate knowledge about the relationship between the different forms of sugar consumption and dental caries. All these findings are suggestive of poor knowledge about oral health and indicates the need for effective oral health education programs.

Several independent studies and the American Academy of Pediatric Dentistry have recommended early dental visits for children, which should ideally take place before one year of age or within six months of the eruption of primary teeth. This is strongly supported by the American Dental Association [24–28]. The study by Chabra et al. found that only 15.2% of the parents were aware that the first dental visit of the child should occur before the age of one [29], whereas Hussein et al. reported even lower awareness among parents (12.5%) in terms of this knowledge [30].

Many mothers (61%) had oral health problems and a quarter of them could not remember the last time they visited the dentist. This may provide an indication that seeking dental care is not a priority for these mothers or there might be difficulties in accessing dental care despite dental services in Qatar being readily available in each suburb. Despite the good knowledge about oral health care, there was a significant deficiency in the oral health care and oral hygiene provided to children. Many mothers did not answer critical questions about the dental care provided to their child: 61% did not answer the question "When did your child visit the dentist?", 59% did not answer "Why did your child visit the dentist?", and 57% did not answer "What type of treatment was provided to the child when the child visited the dentist?". This may reflect that seeking dental care is either not important for them or it is challenging to obtain access to a child-friendly dentist in the public health system in Qatar.

In our study, we observed that although knowledge of the various aspects of oral health and dental decay was present, the attitudes of a number of the mothers toward oral health practices were found to be unhealthy and would set a bad precedent for the growing child. This indicates that they were unable to translate their knowledge into habit. This needs to be further discussed and scrutinized. The literacy rate among Qatari women is 97.6%. Although the majority of mothers had sound knowledge about oral health in children, low motivation, low enthusiasm, and the lack of practical training could be a result of a poor implementation of knowledge [31–34]. Parents should be considered key persons in ensuring the well-being of young children. In addition, appreciating their knowledge, attitude, and practices about their children's oral health may help the dental community to understand some of the reasons why children do not receive the dental care that they need [32].

This study had limitations, including sampling bias. The sample was obtained exclusively from government kindergartens, which cater only to Qatari children. Qatari nationals represent about 20% of the population and the remaining 80% are from Arabic and non-Arabic ex-patriates. If private kindergartens were included in the sampling frame and non-Qatari children were sampled, the results may have been different. The general cultural perception about Qatari children is that they are spoiled in many ways and indulging their diet is one of them. Therefore, these results may represent the "tip of the iceberg". Furthermore, in this study, children who did not attend kindergartens were not included in the sample. Mothers of children who do not attend kindergarten may have different views from those who send their children to kindergarten. Another bias is the non-response bias: the 21% of mothers that did not respond may have had different perspectives than those who responded to the questionnaire. Finally, the self-reported responses might not represent mothers' true knowledge and behaviors. Mothers may report what they think should be the correct practice or knowledge rather than the truth. The statistically significant association between the occurrence of caries and whether the child visited the dentist might be a random finding or may reflect the fact that only children with dental caries visit the dentist.

5. Conclusions

The results of the questionnaire reflected that the oral health knowledge of mothers is reasonable, although there is room for improvement in oral health messages on the starting age for brushing and the importance of flossing. The general dietary knowledge of mothers was good, except for their knowledge about the harmful effects of orange juice on teeth. Despite the good knowledge about oral health care, there was a significant deficiency in the oral health care and oral hygiene provided to children. This also reinstates the urgent need to plan and conduct appropriate oral health programs targeting the two different groups through strategies that are tailored to their understanding and requirements. More emphasis should be placed on improving their level of knowledge, which would ultimately be reflected in their oral health behavior. Health education should focus on parental responsibility for oral health and mothers should be encouraged to provide practical and emotional support to their children with regard to oral hygiene habits. This may reflect the fact that seeking dental care is either not important for them or it is challenging to obtain access to a child-friendly dentist in the public health system in Qatar. The results of this study suggest that there is a need for an oral health promotion program to fill the gaps in knowledge for mothers regarding oral health care for young children.

Author Contributions: Conceptualization, Methodology, by A.A.; Formal Writing-Original & Draft Preparation by A.M.; Writing-Review & Editing, Visualization by A.A. and A.M.

References

1. Petersen, P.E.; Bourgeois, D.; Ogawa, H.; Estupinan-Day, S.; Ndiaye, C. The global burden of oral diseases and risks to oral health. *Bull. World Health Organ.* **2005**, *83*, 661–669. [PubMed]
2. Dentistry, A.A.P. Policy on Early Childhood Caries (ECC): Classifications, Consequences, and Preventive Strategies. *Pediatr. Dent.* **2014**, *37*, 50–52.
3. Abiola Adeniyi, A.; Ogunbodede, O.E.; Jeboda, O.S.; Folayan, O.M. Do maternal factors influence the dental health status of Nigerian pre-school children? *Int. J. Paediatr. Dent.* **2009**, *19*, 448–454. [CrossRef] [PubMed]
4. Suresh, B.S.; Ravishankar, T.L.; Chaitra, T.R.; Mohapatra, A.K.; Gupta, V. Mother's knowledge about pre-school child's oral health. *J. Indian Soc. Pedod. Prev. Dent.* **2010**, *28*, 282–287. [PubMed]
5. Jain, R.; Oswal, K.; Chitguppi, R. Knowledge, attitude and practices of mothers toward their children's oral health: A questionnaire survey among subpopulation in Mumbai (India). *J. Dent. Res. Sci. Dev.* **2014**, *1*, 40–45. [CrossRef]
6. Mani, S.A.; John, J.; Ping, W.Y.; Ismail, N.M. Knowledge, attitude and practice of oral health promoting factors among caretakers of children attending day-care centers in Kubang Kerian, Malaysia: A preliminary study. *J. Indian Soc. Pedod. Prev. Dent.* **2010**, *28*, 78–83. [CrossRef] [PubMed]
7. Macintosh, A.C.; Schroth, R.J.; Edwards, J.; Harms, L.; Mellon, B.; Moffatt, M. The impact of community workshops on improving early childhood oral health knowledge. *Pediatr. Dent.* **2010**, *32*, 110–117. [PubMed]
8. World Health Organization. *Oral Health Surveys—Basic Methods*; WHO: Geneva, Switzerland, 1997.
9. Featherstone, J.D. The caries balance: The basis for caries management by risk assessment. *Oral Health Prev. Dent.* **2004**, *2*, 259–264. [PubMed]
10. Holm, A.K. Caries in the preschool child international trends. *J. Dent.* **1990**, *18*, 291–295. [CrossRef]
11. Elham, B.; Hajizamani, A.; Mohammadi, T.M. Oral health behaviour of parents as a predictor of oral health status of their children. *ISRN Dent.* **2013**, *2013*, 741783.
12. Al-Hussyeen, A.A.; Al-Sadhan, S. Feeding practices and behavior of Saudi children with early childhood caries and dental knowledge of mothers. *Saudi Dent. J.* **2000**, *14*, 112–117.
13. Ashkanani, F.; Al-Sane, M. Knowledge, attitudes and practices of caregivers in relation to oral health of preschool children. *Med. Princ. Pract.* **2013**, *22*, 167–172. [CrossRef] [PubMed]
14. Divaris, K.; Lee, J.Y.; Baker, A.D.; Vann, W.F., Jr. Caregivers' oral health literacy and their young children's oral health-related quality-of-life. *Acta Odontol. Scand.* **2012**, *70*, 390–397. [CrossRef] [PubMed]

15. Akpabio, A.; Klausner, C.P.; Inglehart, M.R. Mothers'/guardians' knowledge about promoting children's oral health. *J. Dent. Hyg./Am. Dent. Hyg. Assoc.* **2008**, *82*, 12.

16. Ghanim, A.; Adenubi, A.; Wyne, K. Caries prediction model in pre-school children in Riyadh, Saudi Arabia. *Int. J. Paediatr. Dent.* **1998**, *8*, 115–122. [CrossRef] [PubMed]

17. Hashim, R.; Williams, S.; Thomson, W.M. Severe early childhood caries and behavioural risk indicators among young children in Ajman, United Arab Emirates. *Eur. Arch. Paediatr. Dent.* **2011**, *12*, 205–210. [CrossRef] [PubMed]

18. Seow, W.K.; Clifford, H.; Battistutta, D.; Morawska, A.; Holcombe, T. Case-control study of early childhood caries in Australia. *Caries Res.* **2009**, *43*, 25–35. [CrossRef] [PubMed]

19. Khanal, K.; Shrestha, D.; Ghimire, N.; Younjan, R.; Sanjel, S. Assessment of Knowledge Regarding Oral Hygiene among Parents of Pre-School Children Attending Pediatric Out Patient Department in Dhulikhel Hospital. *Kathmandu Univ. Med. J.* **2015**, *49*, 38–43. [CrossRef]

20. Moulana, S.A.; Yashoda, R.; Puranik, M.P.; Hiremath, S.S.; Gaikwad, R. Knowledge, attitude and practices towards primary dentition among the mothers of 3–5 year old pre-school children in Bangalore city. *J. Indian Assoc. Public Health Dent.* **2012**, *19*, 83–92.

21. Wyne, A.H.; Chohan, A.N.; Alrowily, F.H.; Shehri, B.M. Oral health knowledge, attitude and practices by parents of the children attending KSUCD clinics. *Pak. Oral Dent. J.* **2004**, *24*, 145–148.

22. Kamolmatyakul, S.; Saiong, S. Oral health knowledge, attitude and practices of parents attending Prince of Songkla University Dental Hospital. *Int. J. Health Promot. Educ.* **2007**, *45*, 111–113. [CrossRef]

23. Chan, S.C.; Tsai, J.S.; King, N.M. Feeding and oral hygiene habits of preschool children in Hong Kong and their caregivers' dental knowledge and attitudes. *Int. J. Paediatr. Dent.* **2002**, *12*, 322–331. [CrossRef] [PubMed]

24. Widmer, R. The first dental visit: An Australian perspective. *Int. J. Paediatr. Dent.* **2003**, *13*, 270. [CrossRef] [PubMed]

25. Rayner, J.A. The first dental visit: A UK viewpoint. *Int. J. Paediatr. Dent.* **2003**, *13*, 269. [CrossRef] [PubMed]

26. Nainar, S.M.; Straffon, L.H. Targeting of Year One dental visit for Unite States children. *Int. J. Paediatr. Dent.* **2003**, *13*, 258–263. [CrossRef] [PubMed]

27. Douglass, J.M.; Douglass, A.B. Infant oral health education for pediatric and family practice residents. *Pediatr. Dent.* **2005**, *27*, 284–291. [PubMed]

28. AAPD. Policy of Dental Home, Oral Health Policies, AAPD—Reference Manual 2004–2005. Available online: http://www.aapd.org/advocacy/dentalhome/ (accessed on 1 September 2015).

29. Chhabra, N.; Chhabra, A. Parents knowledge, attitudes and cultural belief regarding oral health and dental care of preschool children in an Indian population. *Eur. Arch. Paediatr. Dent.* **2012**, *13*, 76–82. [CrossRef] [PubMed]

30. Hussein, A.S.; Abu-Hassan, M.I.; Schroth, R.J.; Ghanim, A.M. Parent's Perception on the Importance of their Children's First Dental Visit (A cross-sectional Pilot Study in Malaysia). *J. Oral Res.* **2013**, *1*, 17–25.

31. Togoo, R.A.; Luqman, M.; Al-Hammadi, A.A.; Al-Rabai, N.A.; Ahmasani, S.M.; Al-Qahtani, B.D. Caregivers' knowledge, attitudes, and oral health practices for infants attending day-care centers in two cities in southern Saudi Arabia. *Gulf Med. J.* **2017**, *6*, 35–41.

32. Al-Oufi, A.A.; Omar, O.M. Oral Health Knowledge and Practices of Mothers toward Their Children's Oral Health in Al Madinah. *Br. J. Med. Med. Res.* **2016**, *15*, 1–10. [CrossRef]

33. Singhal, D.K.; Acharya, S.; Thakur, A.S. Maternal Knowledge, attitude and practices regarding oral health of preschool children in Udupi taluk, Karnataka, India. *J. Int. Dent. Med. Res.* **2017**, *10*, 270–277.

34. Ministry of Development, Planning and Statistics. *Annual Statistical Abstract*; Education Chapter, Training Chapter; Ministry of Development, Planning and Statistics: Doha, Qatar, 2015.

13

Dental Biofilm and Laboratory Microbial Culture Models for Cariology Research

Ollie Yiru Yu, Irene Shuping Zhao, May Lei Mei, Edward Chin-Man Lo and Chun-Hung Chu *

Faculty of Dentistry, The University of Hong Kong, Hong Kong, China; yuyiru@hku.hk (O.Y.Y.);
irenezhao110@gmail.com (I.S.Z.); mei1123@hku.hk (M.L.M.); hrdplcm@hkucc.hku.hk (E.C.-M.L.)
* Correspondence: chchu@hku.hk;

Abstract: Dental caries form through a complex interaction over time among dental plaque, fermentable carbohydrate, and host factors (including teeth and saliva). As a key factor, dental plaque or biofilm substantially influence the characteristic of the carious lesions. Laboratory microbial culture models are often used because they provide a controllable and constant environment for cariology research. Moreover, they do not have ethical problems associated with clinical studies. The design of the microbial culture model varies from simple to sophisticated according to the purpose of the investigation. Each model is a compromise between the reality of the oral cavity and the simplification of the model. Researchers, however, can still obtain meaningful and useful results from the models they select. Laboratory microbial culture models can be categorized into a closed system and an open system. Models in the closed system have a finite supply of nutrients, and are also simple and cost-effective. Models in the open system enabled the supply of a fresh culture medium and the removal of metabolites and spent culture liquid simultaneously. They provide better regulation of the biofilm growth rate than the models in the closed system. This review paper gives an overview of the dental plaque biofilm and laboratory microbial culture models used for cariology research.

Keywords: biofilm; dental plaque; demineralization; remineralization; caries; review

1. Introduction

Dental caries is the localized destruction of dental hard tissues by acidic byproducts from dental plaque containing acid-producing bacteria. Cariology research allows the investigation of caries' pathogenicity, testing the effects of new caries-prevention methods (i.e., some devices and drugs) and developing new caries-preventing products. This review paper gives an overview of the dental plaque biofilm and in vitro biofilm models used for cariology research. It aims to provide essential and instructive information for researchers who seek to plan and design cariology research.

2. The Dental Plaque Biofilm

Dental plaque is an oral microbial biofilm that is found on exposed tooth surfaces in the mouth. It has a large diversity of species and consists of densely packed bacteria embedded in a matrix of organic polymers of bacterial and salivary origin. Dental plaque is the causal agent of dental caries in the presence of sugar and time. In the oral cavity, the formation of dental plaque on the tooth surface follows a similar sequence to that of biofilms in other natural ecosystems. A biofilm is formed by bacteria sticking to each other and, often, adhering to a surface. The bacteria are embedded within a self-produced matrix of extracellular polymeric substance. In dental biofilm, *streptococcus mutans* is a major bacterium producing the extracellular polysaccharide matrix in dental biofilms. The bacterial cells growing in a biofilm are physiologically distinct from planktonic cells which float or swim in a liquid medium. Bacteria in the plaque biofilm can respond to many factors, such as cellular recognition of specific or non-specific attachment sites on a surface and nutritional signals. Marsh and Martin [1] divided the formation and growth of oral biofilm into five stages (Figure 1).

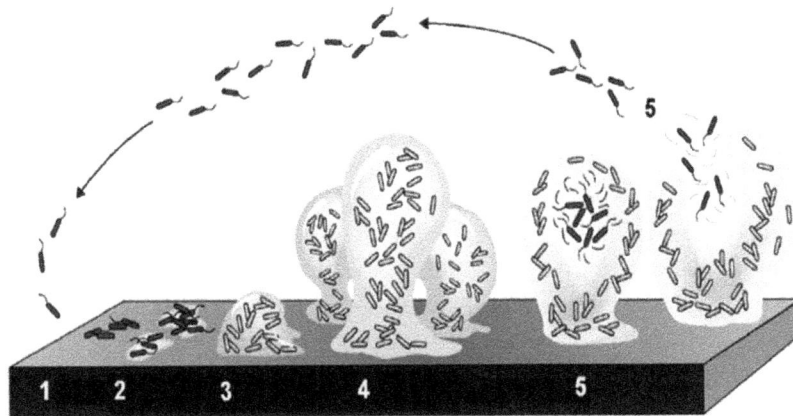

Figure 1. Five stages of biofilm formation and growth (adapted from Stoodley et al., 2002 [2])

Oral biofilms can form on almost any surface present in the oral cavity including enamel, dentin, cementum, gingiva, oral mucosa, carious lesion, restoration, dental implant, and denture. Dental plaque will colonize rapidly, not only the coronal enamel surface but also the exposed root surface. The growth of microbiota on the exposed root surface proceeds more rapidly than that on the smooth enamel surface because of the irregular surface topography of the exposed root dentin surface. The organization and structure of dental plaque vary considerably according to the sites where plaque forms [1]. The growth of microorganisms on specific oral niches is affected by various factors such as acidity (pH) of the environment, availability of nutrients, presence of antimicrobial agents, and host defense.

Surface-bound microorganisms have a survival and/or selective advantage over their planktonic phases [1]. Bacteria in dental plaque have stronger resistance to antimicrobial agents than planktonic bacteria. Bacterial extracellular polysaccharides prevent the perfusion of antimicrobial agents to bacterial targets; this acts as a barrier to protect the plaque bacteria against certain environmental threats such as antibiotics, antibodies, surfactant, bacteriophage, and white blood cells [3]. Resistance of biofilm bacteria to antimicrobial agents may also develop. As a result, the minimum inhibitory concentration of antimicrobial agents against bacteria in biofilm is significantly higher (up to 1000-fold) than that in liquid [1].

Though there are many bacteria associated with dental caries, a few groups of cariogenic bacteria such as *streptococci*, *actinomycetes,* and *lactobacilli* are found to be more closely associated than the others. These groups of bacteria often dominantly proliferate in the dental biofilm collected from the carious lesions of teeth. *Streptococcus* is the predominant species in cariogenic microbe. It colonizes clean tooth surfaces at an early stage, and it also relates to root caries. The predominant coccal isolated from carious dentin in root caries are *S. mutans, S. sanguis,* and *S. mitis* [4]. *S. mutans* and *S. sobrinus* are difficult to distinguish. Hence, these two species are always lumped together and regarded as *mutans streptococci. Mutans streptococci* can adapt to acidic environments, which is the key factor contributing to its cariogenic potential. *Actinomycetes* is an initial colonizer of human root surfaces. *A. naeslundii* and *A. viscosus* can induce root surface caries [5]. *Actinomycetes* is often isolated from subgingival microflora and from plaque associated with root caries [6] (they have long surface appendages named fibrils, or fimbriae). The fibrils allow *actinomycetes* to adhere to the surface of tooth roots. Fibrils also improve the attachment of *actinomycetes* to other bacteria in dental plaque. *Lactobacilli* are aciduric bacteria, including *L. acidophilus, L. rhamnosus, L. casei,* and *L. oris* [7]. Patients with caries have higher counts of *lactobacilli* than those with no caries. Evaluating the amount of *Lactobacilli* in saliva is used as a caries-activity testing method in clinical assessment [8]. *Lactobacilli* is difficult to grow and mature as a mono-species biofilm. However, it can be a predominate species in a substantial biofilm in the presence of *S. mutans* [9]. A potential relationship was found among some species of *lactobacilli, streptococci,* and *actinomycetes* in the root caries formation process [10].

3. Laboratory Microbial Culture Models

Laboratory microbial culture models simulate the oral environment for cariology study. Unlike in vivo studies, they do not have problems relating to the uncontrollable fluctuating locus-specific of the oral environment [11,12]. Two complementary microbiological approaches can be taken to generate biofilm in microbial culture models. The first is the evolution of a plaque microcosm from natural oral microflora. A microcosm is defined as "a laboratory subset of the natural system from which it originates and from which it also evolves" [13]. Microcosm plaques are similar in composition, growth, acidity (pH) behavior, biochemical properties, and (probably) in complexity to natural plaque.

The second approach is the construction of defined-species biofilm consortia with major plaque species, or a mixture of different species of the acquired oral bacteria (such as the American Type Culture Collection (ACTT) bacteria). Consortia are simpler than plaque microcosms; they have the advantage of incorporating individual bacterial species. Even in a simple batch culture method, oral multispecies consortia can develop complex biofilms on enamel and dentin that can induce carious lesions similar to those in vivo. The designs of laboratory microbial culture models vary according to the purpose of the laboratory studies. They can be classified as closed system and open system. Each system is a compromise between the reality of the in vivo ecosystem and the simplification of the system. However, a well-designed model and study allow researchers to obtain meaningful and useful results [13].

3.1. The Closed System

Microbial culture models in the closed system have a finite supply of nutrients. The growth rates of the biofilm are rapid at the beginning of the cultivation when there are ample nutrients. However, this is uncommon in the natural growth of biofilm [14,15]. The growth conditions will change considerably with consumption of the nutrients and the accumulation of metabolic products. Hence, the physiological and biological properties of the biofilm are not comparable with the natural ones. Researchers used closed system models because of their simplicity, high productivity, repeatability, controllability of the experimental conditions, less contamination, and cost-effective properties. The agar plate and microtiter biofilm models are two examples of the common microbial culture models in closed system.

3.1.1. The Agar Plate

The agar plate is one of the simplest laboratory microbial culture models (Figure 2). The nutrient supply is not continuous. Bacteria growth on the surface of the agar can only be supported until the finite nutrient is exhausted. Thus, results of studies using this simplistic model should be interpreted with caution. This situation is different from bacterial growth on a hard tissue surface, because the biofilm consumes nutrients from the substrate. It resembles biofilms associated with soft tissue infections or growing in an extracellular matrix. This model has been used to test the susceptibility of oral biofilm to various antimicrobials, especially some light active chemicals [16,17]. The disc-diffusion method is not an ideal way to predict the therapeutic effects of antimicrobial [18]. The effects of the antibacterial agents can be misinterpreted because the cationic antibacterial agents may combine with the anionic agar polysaccharide gel [19].

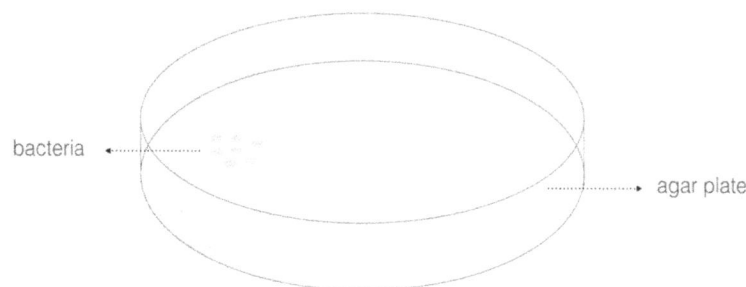

Figure 2. Agar plate.

3.1.2. The Microtiter Biofilm Model

The microtiter biofilm model is made of a multiple-well microtiter plate. A microtiter plate is commonly made of polystyrene, but it can be manufactured in a variety of materials. A microtiter plate is a flat plate with multiple "wells" (used as small test tubes). A standard definition of a microtiter plate was developed by the Society for Laboratory Automation and Screening (SLAS) and published by the American National Standards Institute (ANSI). Henceforth, the microplate standards are known as ANSI/SLAS standards. A configuration of a 96-well microtiter is shown in Figure 3. Each well of a microplate typically holds several milliliters of liquid. The microplate is regarded as a standard tool in cariology research, allowing the biofilm to grow independently in each well.

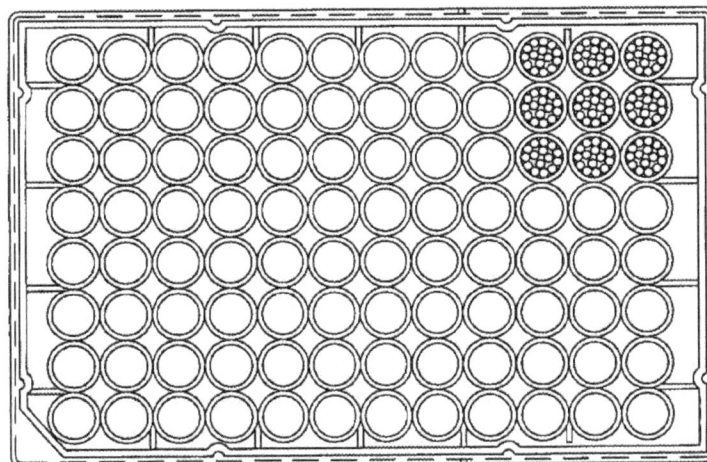

Figure 3. Configuration of the 96-well microtiter.

3.2. The Open System

The open system can be described as a continuous culture system. It enables the supply of a fresh culture medium and the removal of metabolites and spent culture liquid simultaneously. Hence, the concentration of bacteria and metabolic products remains constant [20]. Moreover, the biofilms can stay in a stable state or keep in a dynamic balance [21]. Nevertheless, the repeatability of the experimental result is low because of the heterogeneity of the biofilm in the open system. Besides, the possibility of contamination can be high due to the complexity of the construction.

The open system simulates the in vivo environment better than the closed system. It also allows better regulation of the biofilm growth rate and other variables. Common microbial culture models in the open system include the chemostat model, the flow cell biofilm model, the constant depth film fermenter model, the drip flow biofilm reactor, the multiple Sorbarod model, and the multiple artificial mouth model.

3.2.1. Chemostat

Chemostat is preferred for biofilm experiments because the continuous culture of chemostat can provide homogeneity and a steady environment (Figure 4). The experimental parameters can be investigated independently in the highly-controlled conditions [22]. Oral bacteria grow planktonically in a conventional chemostat. A fresh cultural medium is provided at the same rate as the culture waste liquid removal rate. Planktonic bacteria have the tendency to form biofilm at a solid-liquid interface in a chemostat. A substrate such as a tooth slice can be suspended in the chemostat to provide a surface for bacterial colonization and biofilm or dental plaque formation. Chemostat is generally expensive and space-consuming in laboratory. Precaution is needed to prevent excessive bacteria growth in chemostat, which can block the tubing [23].

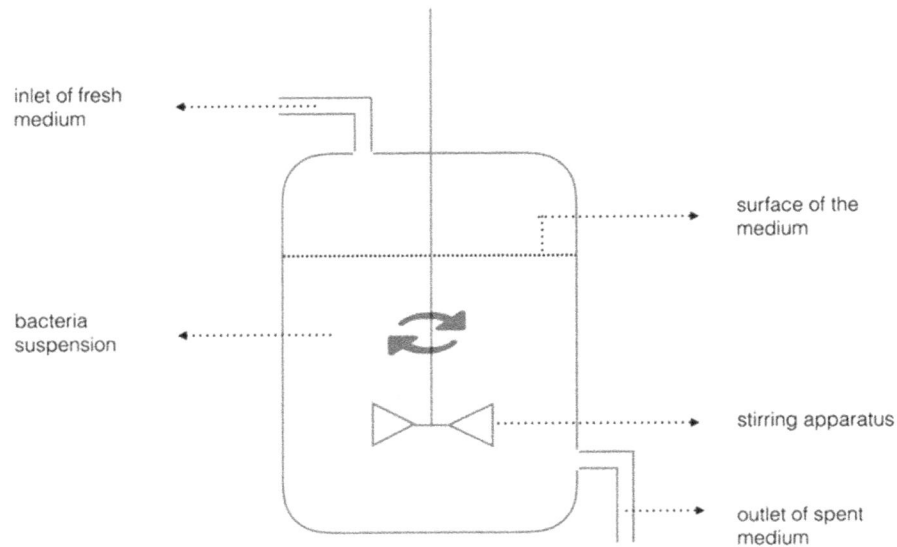

Figure 4. Schematic diagram of chemostat.

3.2.2. The Flow Cell Biofilm Model

The flow cell biofilm model is used as perfusion chambers to observe the initial growth and physiology of stationary bacterial cells [24]. The culture fluid passes through a tube and biofilms are cultured in a flow reactor where the substratum is placed. Biofilms can grow on the surface of tooth blocks [25], microscopy glass slides, or glass rods [26]. The flow cell biofilm model is shown in Figure 5. Bacteria suspension stored in a chemostat (A) and bacteria-free medium (B) are stirred or pumped (D) to a mixed chamber (C) and go through the flow reactor (E) to create a flow. Therefore, the shear force will work on the microbe when the culture fluid passes through the surface of the biofilm. The outside chemostat in the flow cell biofilm model allows external biofilm growth, which means the growth condition can be controlled and the biofilm can grow for an extended period. Other advantages are flexibility of sample configuration, presence of fluid dynamics, plaque monitoring. and the possibility of extra experimental treatments.

The flow cell biofilm model simulates the in situ situation of undisturbed biofilm communities. The constant environment is provided with laminar flow [24]. The model has been adopted frequently in the evaluation of the effects of antimicrobial agents because it is convenient to make comparisons of viability of microbes among different experimental groups [27]. In addition, the continuous flow system simulates the clearance of antimicrobial agents in the mouth. A limitation of this device is that the laminar fluid flows through the biofilm instead of across its surface. It mimics the flow of saliva on the surface of mucosal, but the pathways of saliva flowing on hard-surface biofilms are different. Flow cell biofilm models are also expensive and space consuming.

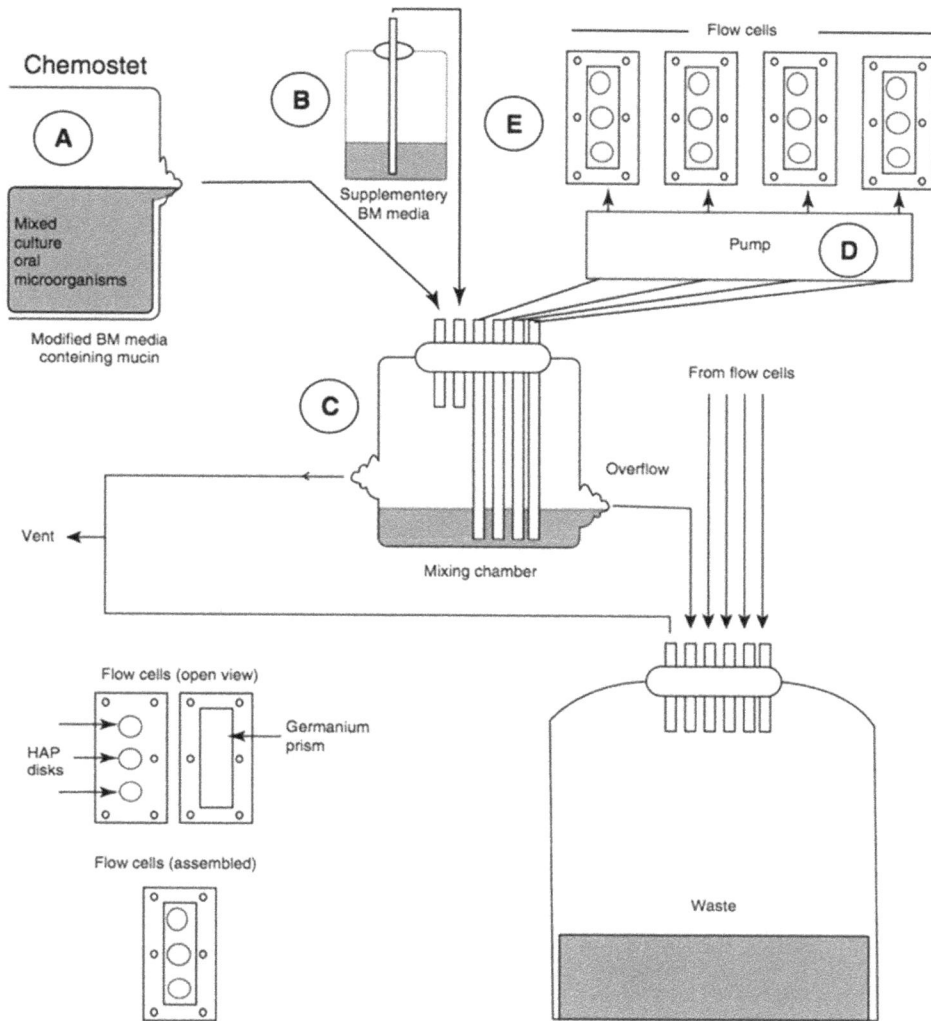

Figure 5. Configuration of the flow cell biofilm model (adapted from Herles et al., 1994 [28]

3.2.3. The Constant Depth Film Fermenter Model

The major components of the constant depth film fermenter (CDFF) model are plugs, a rotating stainless steel disk, and static scarper blades [23]. The plugs allow the growth of biofilm. The rotating stainless steel disk holds the samples. The static scarper blades control the depth of the biofilm. These components are put into a glass container where a fresh cultural medium is provided and culture waste liquid is removed. The configuration of CDFF is shown in Figure 6.

The thickness of biofilms is controlled to a predetermined depth by mechanically removing the excess biofilm. This simulates the tongue movement over the teeth. The thickness of biofilms can be 200 μm [29,30] to mimic dental plaques. The properties of biofilms that are developed are relatively constant over time. The CDFF model supports restrained growth and produces a number of replicate biofilms. Since the thickness of the biofilms is predetermined, subsampling and effluent analysis are limited to some extent [31]. The model was used to study etiology of caries [32], to assess antimicrobial effect on biofilm [33], and to investigate the structure of biofilm [34].

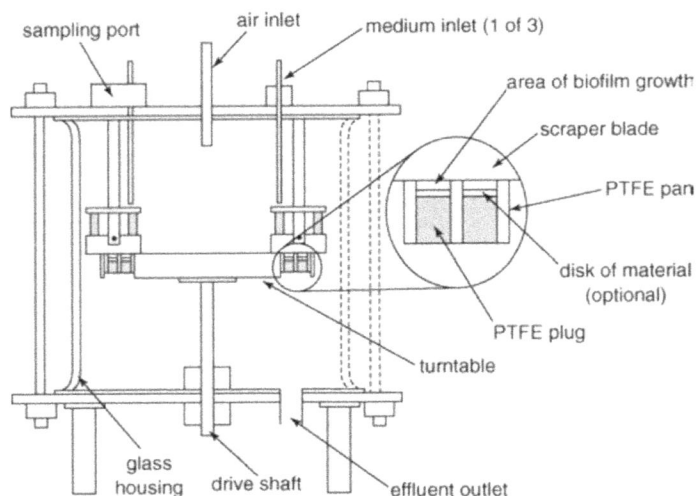

Figure 6. Configuration of the constant depth film fermenter (adapted from Pratten et al., 2007 [35]

3.2.4. The Drip Flow Biofilm Reactor

The drip flow biofilm model is often used to grow and establish solid-liquid or solid-air interface biofilms. The model usually contains four chambers in an adjustable inclined fermenter. The schematic diagram of drip-flow biofilm model is shown in Figure 7.

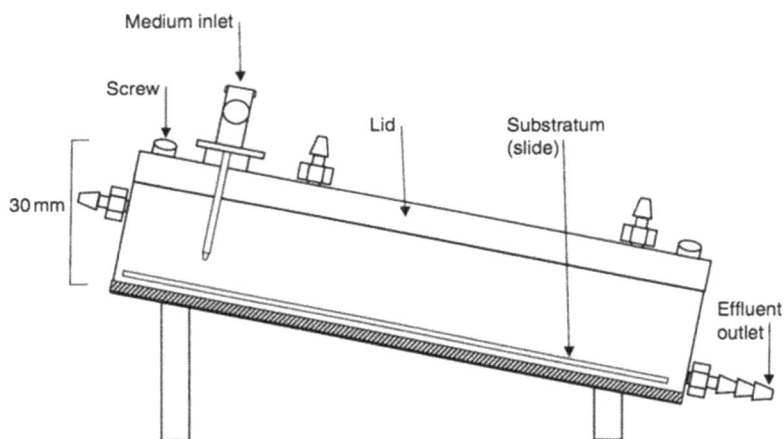

Figure 7. Schematic diagram of a drip flow biofilm reactor (adapted from McBain et al., 2009 [15]

The biofilms grow on angled tooth surfaces, which are continuously irrigated with small volumes of fresh medium from the inlet. The incline of the fermenter enables the medium to flow over the tooth surface with biofilm, providing a low-shear environment for the biofilm.

The model allows plaque to grow on the tooth surface and to stabilize for longer periods, which enables relatively stable development of microbial communities [36]. However, as the medium flow on the surface of the substrata might not be always consistent, aerial heterogeneity over the surface of substratum may exist [15]. This model is commercially available (Biosurfaces Technologies Corporation, Bozeman, MT, USA), and thus is commonly used by researchers. This model was used to test disinfection efficacy [37], to investigate the effect of powered tooth brushing on removal of biofilm [38], and to compare the antibacterial effects of anti-caries agents [36].

3.2.5. The Multiple Sorbarod Model

The multiple Sorbarod model uses a permeable Sorbarod membrane as the substratum. The fresh medium is supplied by continuous perfusion through the membrane. The exfoliated bacterial cells and metabolic wastes will be removed with spent culture medium. The schematic diagram of the multiple Sorbarod model is shown in Figure 8.

In this model, the flow rate of the medium can be controlled. Therefore, the growth rate of the biofilm is controllable [15]. The multiple Sorbarod model was used to investigate the effect of oral hygiene activities on anaerobic oral biofilms [39] and to assess the plaque-control effects of some specific enzymes [40]. An advantage of this model is that the growth rate of the biofilm can be controlled. Another advantage is that the detached bacterial cells in the spent culture medium can be studied to evaluate the biological effect of experimental treatment [36]. Since the model develops heterogeneous biofilm, it cannot be used in study design where homogeneity of the biofilm is important [15].

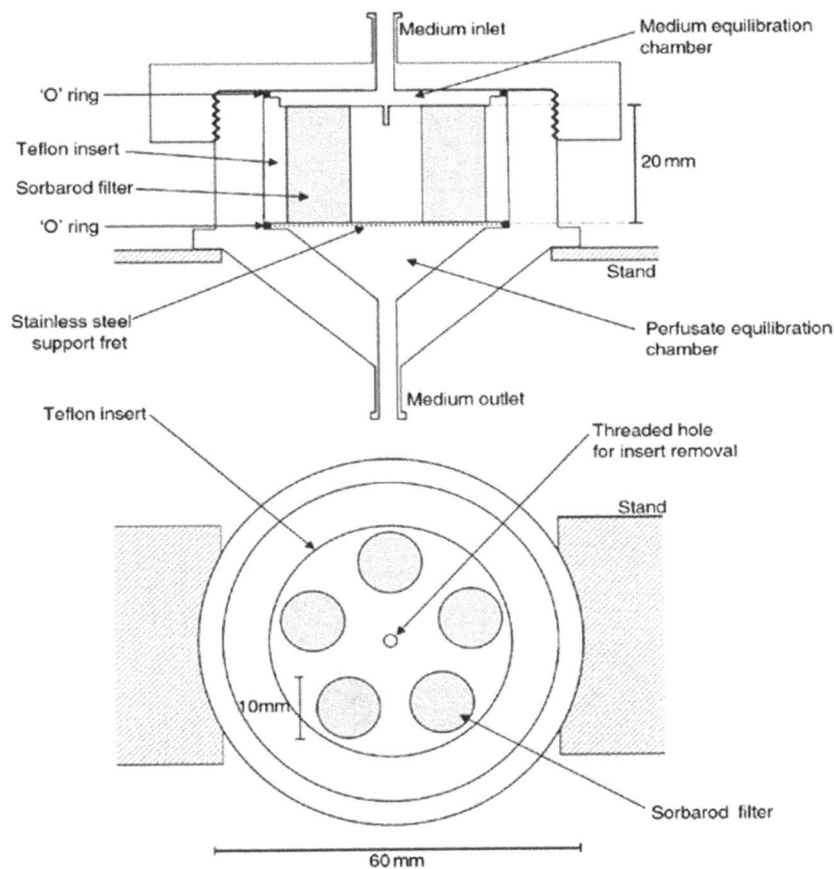

Figure 8. A schematic diagram of a multiple Sorbarod device (adapted from McBain et al., 2005 [41]

3.2.6. The Multiple Artificial Mouth

The multiple artificial mouth (MAM) is a computer-controlled, multiple-station model. It has a more complicated construction than the models discussed above.

A MAM can accurately simulate an in vivo environment using computer-controlled facilities [42]. It has several microstations, which are relatively independent to one other (Figure 9). Different experimental conditions can be applied simultaneously in different microstations.

Environmental variables can be easily controlled in the MAM. This allows analysis of the biofilm during its development, without contaminating other samples. Acidity can be monitored using a pH electrode and a micro-reference electrode [12]. These well-controlled conditions improve the standardization and flexibility of the MAM, and therefore enhance its ability to culture biofilms similar to natural oral flora. Sissons et al. found that biofilms developed in this system exhibited metabolic and pH behavior that resembled typical natural plaques [42]. The MAM has been adopted in different studies, such as biodiversity of plaques [43], fluoride and phosphate assay [44], plaque calcium level measurement [45], and the generation of consortia using major plaque species [46]. The biofilm samples in this model were exposed to the same temperature and gas-phase fluctuation. The MAM aims to mimic the oral environment. Therefore, saliva substitutes play an important role in the model. Approximate laminar flows are applied to simulate the situations in the oral cavity, instead of turbulent flow in chemostat.

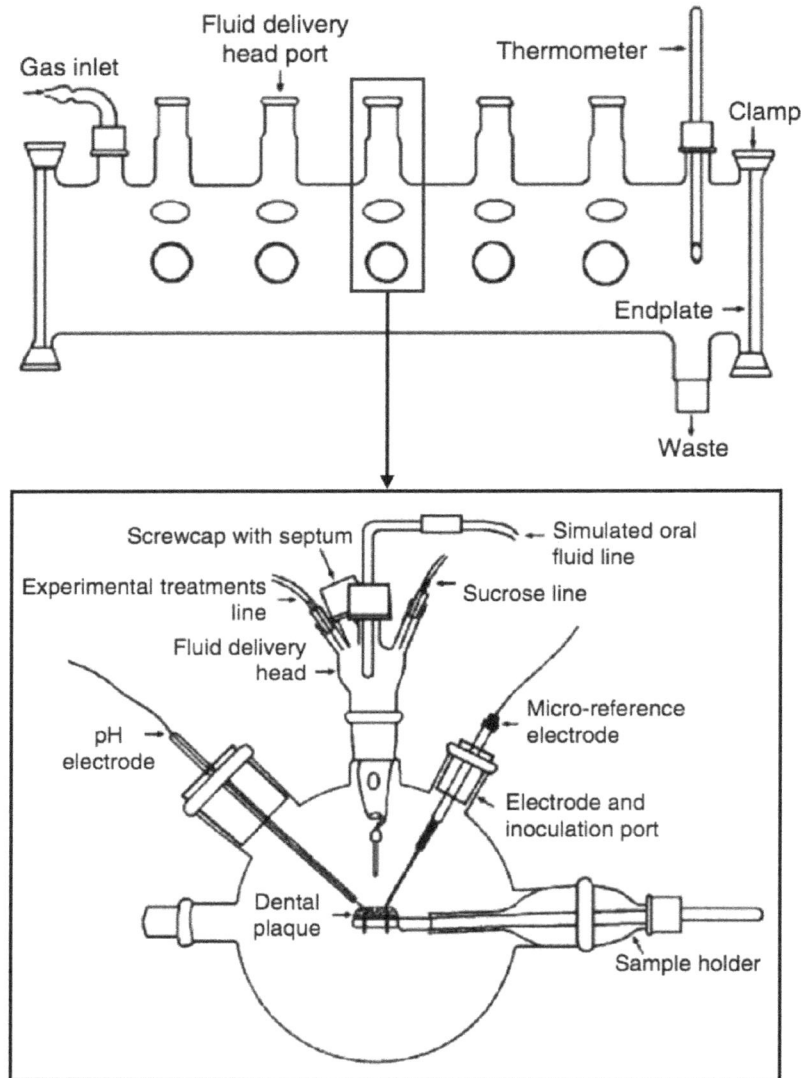

Figure 9. Schematic diagram of a multiple artificial mouth (adapted from Sissons et al., 2000 [47])

4. Summary

Dental biofilm is an essential factor in the etiology of dental caries. Cariogenic bacteria *streptococci*, *actinomycetes,* and *lactobacilli* are found to be more closely associated with dental caries. Laboratory microbial culture models can provide a steady and controllable environment for cariology research.

The models play an important role in cariology research in investigating caries pathogenicity, testing effects of new caries prevention methods, and developing new caries-preventing products. Each model has its advantages and disadvantages from both experimental design and experiment cost. Table 1 shows a comparison of the discussed in vitro biofilm systems.

Table 1. Characteristics of common microbial culture models for cariology research.

Parameter	Agar Plate	Microtiter	Chemostat	Flow Cell	CDFF	Drip Flow	MSD	MAM
Duration	Hours to days	Hours to days	Hours to days	Hours to days	Days to weeks	Days to weeks	Days to weeks	Days to weeks
Planktonic phase	Controlled	Controlled	Controlled	Controlled	None	None	None	None
Growth control by media	None	Via planktonic phase	Yes	Yes	Yes	Yes	Yes	Yes
Fluid flow	No	No	Turbulent	Laminar	Laminar	Drop	Laminar	Drop
Shear force	No	No	Yes	Yes	Yes	No	Yes	No
Defined thickness	No	No	Achievable	Achievable	Yes	No	No	No
Timed reagents	No	Manually	Yes	Pulse	Yes	Yes	Yes	Computer control
Alternative substrate	No	Yes	Yes	Yes	Yes	Yes	No	Yes
Different conditions	No	No	No	No	No	Yes	No	Yes
Subsampling during growth	Yes	Yes	Yes	Yes	Yes	Yes	Yes	Yes

CDFF = Constant depth film fermenter; MSD = Multiple Sorbarod device; MAM = Multiple artificial mouth.

The designs of the biofilm models that are included vary from simple to sophisticated according to the purposes of investigation. Agar plate and microtiter are microbial culture models in the closed system that are low-cost and simple to manage. Microbial culture models in the open system are more complex and the biofilms generated are closer to natural dental plaque. Selection of the type of model used for a biofilm study depends on the growth conditions, requirements for the specific biofilm, and purposes of the study.

Acknowledgments: This review is supported by HKU Seed Funding for Basic Research 201511159142.

Author Contributions: Ollie Yiru Yu did the literature search and prepared the first draft of this manuscript. All authors contributed equally in order to finish this manuscript.

References

1. Marsh, P.; Martin, M. Chapter 5: Dental plaque. In *Marsh and Martin's Oral Microbiology*, 6th ed.; Elsevier: Edinburgh, UK; New York, NY, USA, 2016; pp. 81–111.
2. Stoodley, P.; Sauer, K.; Davies, D.G.; Costerton, J.W. Biofilms as complex differentiated communities. *Annu. Rev. Microbiol.* **2002**, *56*, 187–209. [CrossRef] [PubMed]
3. Costerton, J.W.; Cheng, K.J.; Geesey, G.G.; Ladd, T.I.; Nickel, J.C.; Dasgupta, M.; Marrie, T.J. Bacterial biofilms in nature and disease. *Annu. Rev. Microbiol.* **1987**, *41*, 435–464. [CrossRef] [PubMed]
4. Sumney, D.L.; Jordan, H.V. Characterization of bacteria isolated from human root surface carious lesions. *J. Dent. Res.* **1974**, *53*, 343–351. [CrossRef] [PubMed]
5. Van Houte, J.; Jordan, H.V.; Laraway, R.; Kent, R.; Soparkar, P.M.; DePaola, P.F. Association of the microbial flora of dental plaque and saliva with human root-surface caries. *J. Dent. Res.* **1990**, *69*, 1463–1468. [CrossRef] [PubMed]

6.   Newbrun, E. *Cariology*; Quintessence: Chicago, IL, USA, 1989.

7.   Samaranayake, L.P. Lactobacilli, corynbacteria and propionibacteria. In *Essential Microbiology for Dentistry*; Samaranayake, L.P., Ed.; Michael Parkinson: New York, NY, USA, 2006; p. 105.

8.   Silverstone, L.M.; Johnson, N.W.; Hardie, J.M.; Willimas, R.A.D. The microbiology of dental caries. In *Dental Caries Aetiology, Pathology and Prevention*; Macmillan: London, UK, 1981; p. 10.

9.   Filoche, S.K.; Anderson, S.A.; Sissons, C.H. Biofilm growth of lactobacillus species is promoted by actinomyces species and streptococcus mutans. *Oral Microbiol. Immunol.* **2004**, *19*, 322–326. [CrossRef] [PubMed]

10. Bowden, G.H.; Ekstrand, J.; McNaughton, B.; Challacombe, S.J. Association of selected bacteria with the lesions of root surface caries. *Oral Microbiol. Immunol.* **1990**, *5*, 346–351. [CrossRef] [PubMed]

11. Sissons, C.H. Artificial dental plaque biofilm model systems. *Adv. Dent. Res.* **1997**, *11*, 110–126. [CrossRef] [PubMed]

12. Tang, G.; Yip, H.K.; Cutress, T.W.; Samaranayake, L.P. Artificial mouth model systems and their contribution to caries research: A review. *J. Dent.* **2003**, *31*, 161–171. [CrossRef]

13. Wimpenny, J.W. The validity of models. *Adv. Dent. Res.* **1997**, *11*, 150–159. [CrossRef] [PubMed]

14. Coenye, T.; Nelis, H.J. In vitro and in vivo model systems to study microbial biofilm formation. *J. Microbiol. Methods* **2010**, *83*, 89–105. [CrossRef] [PubMed]

15. McBain, A.J. Chapter 4: In vitro biofilm models: An overview. *Adv. Appl. Microbiol.* **2009**, *69*, 99–132. [PubMed]

16. Dobson, J.; Wilson, M. Sensitization of oral bacteria in biofilms to killing by light from a low-power laser. *Arch. Oral Biol.* **1992**, *37*, 883–887. [CrossRef]

17. O'Neill, J.F.; Hope, C.K.; Wilson, M. Oral bacteria in multi-species biofilms can be killed by red light in the presence of toluidine blue. *Lasers Surg. Med.* **2002**, *31*, 86–90. [CrossRef] [PubMed]

18. Bayston, R.; Ashraf, W.; Barker-Davies, R.; Tucker, E.; Clement, R.; Clayton, J.; Freeman, B.J.C.; Nuradeen, B. Biofilm formation by propionibacterium acnes on biomaterials in vitro and in vivo: Impact on diagnosis and treatment. *J. Biomed. Mater. Res. Part A* **2007**, *81*, 705–709. [CrossRef] [PubMed]

19. Sutherland, I.W. The biofilm matrix—An immobilized but dynamic microbial environment. *Trends Microbiol.* **2001**, *9*, 222–227. [CrossRef]

20. Marsh, P.D. Host defenses and microbial homeostasis—Role of microbial interactions. *J. Dent. Res.* **1989**, *68*, 1567–1575.

21. Sim, C.P.C.; Dashper, S.G.; Reynolds, E.C. Oral microbial biofilm models and their application to the testing of anticariogenic agents. *J. Dent.* **2016**, *50*, 1–11. [CrossRef] [PubMed]

22. Bowden, G. The role of microbiology in models of dental caries: Reaction paper. *Adv. Dent. Res.* **1995**, *9*, 255–269. [CrossRef]

23. Xuelian, H.; Qiang, G.; Biao, R.; Yuqing, L.; Xuedong, Z. Models in caries research. In *Dental Caries*; Springer: Berlin, Germany, 2016; pp. 157–173.

24. Palmer, R.J., Jr. Microscopy flowcells: Perfusion chambers for real-time study of biofilms. *Methods Enzymol.* **1999**, *310*, 160–166. [PubMed]

25. Hodgson, R.J.; Lynch, R.J.; Watson, G.K.; Labarbe, R.; Treloar, R.; Allison, C. A continuous culture biofilm model of cariogenic responses. *J. Appl. Microbiol.* **2001**, *90*, 440–448. [CrossRef] [PubMed]

26. Foster, J.S.; Kolenbrander, P.E. Development of a multispecies oral bacterial community in a saliva-conditioned flow cell. *Appl. Environ. Microbiol.* **2004**, *70*, 4340–4348. [CrossRef] [PubMed]

27. Leung, K.P.; Crowe, T.D.; Abercrombie, J.J.; Molina, C.M.; Bradshaw, C.J.; Jensen, C.L.; Luo, Q.; Thompson, G.A. Control of oral biofilm formation by an antimicrobial decapeptide. *J. Dent. Res.* **2005**, *84*, 1172–1177. [CrossRef] [PubMed]

28. Herles, S.; Olsen, S.; Afflitto, J.; Gaffar, A. Chemostat flow cell system: An in vitro model for the evaluation of antiplaque agents. *J. Dent. Res.* **1994**, *73*, 1748–1755. [PubMed]

29. McBain, A.J.; Bartolo, R.G.; Catrenich, C.E.; Charbonneau, D.; Ledder, R.G.; Gilbert, P. Effects of triclosan-containing rinse on the dynamics and antimicrobial susceptibility of in vitro plaque ecosystems. *Antimicrob. Agents Chemother.* **2003**, *47*, 3531–3538. [CrossRef] [PubMed]

30. Metcalf, D.; Robinson, C.; Devine, D.; Wood, S. Enhancement of erythrosine-mediated photodynamic therapy of streptococcus mutans biofilms by light fractionation. *J. Antimicrob. Chemother.* **2006**, *58*, 190–192. [CrossRef] [PubMed]

31. McBain, A.J.; Bartolo, R.G.; Catrenich, C.E.; Charbonneau, D.; Ledder, R.G.; Gilbert, P. Growth and molecular characterization of dental plaque microcosms. *J. Appl. Microbiol.* **2003**, *94*, 655–664. [CrossRef] [PubMed]

32. Deng, D.M.; ten Cate, J.M. Demineralization of dentin by streptococcus mutans biofilms grown in the constant depth film fermentor. *Caries Res.* **2004**, *38*, 54–61. [CrossRef] [PubMed]

33. Deng, D.M.; Buijs, M.J.; ten Cate, J.M. The effects of substratum on the ph response of streptococcus mutans biofilms and on the susceptibility to 0.2% chlorhexidine. *Eur. J. Oral Sci.* **2004**, *112*, 42–47. [CrossRef] [PubMed]

34. Pratten, J.; Andrews, C.S.; Craig, D.Q.; Wilson, M. Structural studies of microcosm dental plaques grown under different nutritional conditions. *FEMS Microbiol. Lett.* **2000**, *189*, 215–218. [CrossRef] [PubMed]

35. Pratten, J. Growing oral biofilms in a constant depth film fermentor (CDFF). *Curr. Protoc. Microbiol.* **2007**. [CrossRef]

36. Ledder, R.G.; McBain, A.J. An in vitro comparison of dentifrice formulations in three distinct oral microbiotas. *Arch. Oral Biol.* **2012**, *57*, 139–147. [CrossRef] [PubMed]

37. Buckingham-Meyer, K.; Goeres, D.M.; Hamilton, M.A. Comparative evaluation of biofilm disinfectant efficacy tests. *J. Microbiol. Methods* **2007**, *70*, 236–244. [CrossRef] [PubMed]

38. Adams, H.; Winston, M.T.; Heersink, J.; Buckingham-Meyer, K.A.; Costerton, J.W.; Stoodley, P. Development of a laboratory model to assess the removal of biofilm from interproximal spaces by powered tooth brushing. *Am. J. Dent.* **2002**, *15*, 12B–17B. [PubMed]

39. Ledder, R.G.; Sreenivasan, P.K.; DeVizio, W.; McBain, A.J. Evaluation of the specificity and effectiveness of selected oral hygiene actives in salivary biofilm microcosms. *J. Med. Microbiol.* **2010**, *59*, 1462–1468. [CrossRef] [PubMed]

40. Ledder, R.G.; Madhwani, T.; Sreenivasan, P.K.; de Vizio, W.; McBain, A.J. An in vitro evaluation of hydrolytic enzymes as dental plaque control agents. *J. Med. Microbiol.* **2009**, *58*, 482–491. [CrossRef] [PubMed]

41. McBain, A.J.; Sissons, C.; Ledder, R.G.; Sreenivasan, P.K.; de Vizio, W.; Gilbert, P. Development and characterization of a simple perfused oral microcosm. *J. Appl. Microbiol.* **2005**, *98*, 624–634. [CrossRef] [PubMed]

42. Sissons, C.H.; Cutress, T.W.; Hoffman, M.P.; Wakefield, J.S. A multi-station dental plaque microcosm (artificial mouth) for the study of plaque growth, metabolism, ph, and mineralization. *J. Dent. Res.* **1991**, *70*, 1409–1416. [CrossRef] [PubMed]

43. Rasiah, I.A.; Wong, L.; Anderson, S.A.; Sissons, C.H. Variation in bacterial dgge patterns from human saliva: Over time, between individuals and in corresponding dental plaque microcosms. *Arch. Oral Biol.* **2005**, *50*, 779–787. [CrossRef] [PubMed]

44. Pearce, E.I.; Sissons, C.H.; Coleman, M.; Wang, X.; Anderson, S.A.; Wong, L. The effect of sucrose application frequency and basal nutrient conditions on the calcium and phosphate content of experimental dental plaque. *Caries Res.* **2002**, *36*, 87–92. [CrossRef] [PubMed]

45. Wong, L.; Sissons, C.H. Human dental plaque microcosm biofilms: Effect of nutrient variation on calcium phosphate deposition and growth. *Arch. Oral Biol.* **2007**, *52*, 280–289. [CrossRef] [PubMed]

46. Shu, M.; Wong, L.; Miller, J.H.; Sissons, C.H. Development of multi-species consortia biofilms of oral bacteria as an enamel and root caries model system. *Arch. Oral Biol.* **2000**, *45*, 27–40. [CrossRef]

47. Sissons, C.H.; Wong, L.; An, Y.H. Laboratory culture and analysis of microbial biofilms. In *Handbook of Bacterial Adhesion*; Springer: New York, NY, USA, 2000; pp. 133–169.

14

Behavior Assessment in Children Following Hospital-Based General Anesthesia versus Office-Based General Anesthesia

LaQuia A. Vinson [1],*, Matthew L. Rasche [2], Brian J. Sanders [1], James E. Jones [1], Mark A. Saxen [3], Angela M. Tomlin [4] and James A. Weddell [1]

[1] Department of Pediatric Dentistry Indiana University School of Dentistry, James Whitcomb Riley Hospital for Children Indianapolis, Indiana, IN 46202, USA; bjsander@iu.edu (B.J.S.); jej7@iu.edu (J.E.J.); jweddell@iu.edu (J.A.W.)

[2] Private Practice, Bloomington, IN 47401, USA; mrasche@gmail.com

[3] Department of Oral Pathology, Medicine, and Radiology, Indiana University School of Dentistry Indianapolis, Indiana, IN 46202, USA; msaxen93@gmail.com

[4] Department of Pediatrics Indiana University School of Medicine, James Whitcomb Riley Hospital for Children Indianapolis, Indiana, IN 46202, USA; atomlin@iu.edu

* Correspondence: laqawalk@iu.edu; .

Academic Editor: Barbara Cvikl

Abstract: The purpose of this study was to determine if differences in behavior exist following dental treatment under hospital-based general anesthesia (HBGA) or office-based general anesthesia (OBGA) in the percentage of patients exhibiting positive behavior and in the mean Frankl scores at recall visits. This retrospective study examined records of a pediatric dental office over a 4 year period. Patients presenting before 48 months of age for an initial exam who were diagnosed with early childhood caries were included in the study. Following an initial exam, patients were treated under HBGA or OBGA. Patients were followed to determine their behavior at 6-, 12- and 18-month recall appointments. Fifty-four patients received treatment under HBGA and 26 were treated under OBGA. OBGA patients were significantly more likely to exhibit positive behavior at the 6- and 12-month recall visits ($p = 0.038$ & $p = 0.029$). Clinicians should consider future behavior when determining general anesthesia treatment modalities in children with early childhood caries presenting to their office.

Keywords: behavior management; hospital denistry; general anesthesia; infant oral health; early childhood caries

1. Introduction

Administration of general anesthesia has historically served an important role in the practice of dentistry by allowing specific patient populations such as young children greater access to comprehensive dental care [1,2]. In recent years, behavior management techniques used by pediatric dentists have evolved toward increased use of general anesthesia in accordance with changing parenting philosophies, expectations, and safe outcomes [3]. Parents have become more willing to accept dental treatment of their children using general anesthesia over other behavior management techniques [4]. The use of general anesthesia allows both the practitioner and patient a modality in which safe, comprehensive treatment can be performed under optimal conditions [5–7]. It has been suggested that treatment performed under general anesthesia is of higher quality than treatment performed during other forms of behavior management [8]. However, rising costs and scheduling difficulties of traditional hospital-based general anesthesia (HBGA) services have resulted in increased use of office-based general anesthesia (OBGA) services for dental treatment [5,9,10].

The American Dental Association's guidelines on the use of sedation and general anesthesia by dentists define general anesthesia as a drug-induced loss of consciousness during which patients cannot be aroused, even from painful stimulation [2]. General anesthesia can be obtained through different pharmacologic routes of administration while hospital-based general anesthesia (HBGA) is obtained primarily from the administration of inhalation medications. It is common for office-based general anesthesia (OBGA) to be obtained primarily from parenteral intravenous drug administration.

Classifying pediatric dental patients' behavior has been historically reported using the Frankl method of classification, and managing these patients with sedation is widely accepted among dental practitioners [11]. A number of studies have reported on patients' behavior during subsequent recall visits following different forms of sedation. Kupietzky and Blumenstyk reported data using the Frankl scale on behavior of patients following treatment under general anesthesia versus oral conscious sedation [12]. The 1998 study reported no difference in patients' behavior at subsequent recall visits between patients treated under conscious sedation versus general anesthesia for children receiving dental treatment at a young age. O'Sullivan et al. performed a retrospective study of 80 children treated under general anesthesia that were followed for at least 2 years post treatment [13]. Of the children requiring additional restorative dental treatment, 80% readily accepted dental care using local anesthesia without the assistance of conscious or general sedation techniques. Peretz et al. evaluated children receiving dental treatment under conscious sedation and general anesthesia from the Hebrew University-Hadassah School of Medicine pediatric dental clinic. They reported similar behavior between the two groups as evidenced by Frankl scores 13 months postoperatively between children that had been treated for early childhood caries (ECC) by the use of oral conscious sedation or general anesthesia [14].

Fuhrer et al. reported on patient behavior during three subsequent recall visits following dental treatment rendered under conscious sedation and general anesthesia in 80 patients from a pediatric dental office [15]. Patients included those who presented before 36 months of age with ECC for an initial exam. Following treatment, patients were followed to determine behavior at 6-, 12-, and 18-month preventive recall appointments. Positive behavior was defined as a Frankl score of 3 or 4. They concluded that patients who were treated under general anesthesia, as opposed to conscious sedation, were approximately four times more likely to exhibit positive behavior at the 6 month recall appointment. Behavior at 12- and 18-month recall appointments, although not statistically significant, trended towards positive behavior. They also concluded that clinicians should consider future behavior when determining treatment modalities for children.

Treatment performed under general anesthesia has been shown to have many benefits for both the patient and dental team [1,7,8,13]. Currently, there have been no studies that have evaluated future behavior after treatment of patients with hospital based general anesthesia versus office-based general anesthesia. The purpose of the present study was to assess behavior and determine if there were differences in the percentage of patients exhibiting positive behavior following hospital based general anesthesia (HBGA) versus office based general anesthesia (OBGA).

2. Materials and Methods

This retrospective study was approved by the Institutional Review Board of Indiana University (Study #EX1002-16). Records of patients who received dental treatment under HBGA and OBGA from a pediatric dental office over a four-year period were reviewed. Inclusion criteria included patients who presented to the pediatric dental office for an oral exam and were diagnosed with early childhood caries (ECC). Early childhood caries is defined by the American Academy of Pediatric Dentistry (AAPD) as a patient having at least 1 carious lesion, 1 tooth missing due to caries or 1 dental restoration prior to 48 months of age [16]. Information was collected from the patient's clinical notes concerning age, race, gender, behavior at the initial and recall exams, and existing medical conditions of each patient. Patients who had medical conditions that could potentially influence behavior were included. The Frankl behavior scale was used to assess patient's behavior in this investigation [17] (Table 1).

Table 1. Definition of the Frankl Scale.

Frankl Scale	Rating	Description
Definitely Negative	1	Refusal of treatment, forceful crying, fearfulness, or any other overt evidence of extreme negativism.
Negative	2	Reluctance to accept treatment, uncooperativeness, some evidence of negative attitude but not pronounced (sullen, withdrawn).
Positive	3	Acceptance of treatment; cautious behavior at times; willingness to comply with the dentist, at times with reservation, but patient follows the dentist's direction cooperatively.
Definitely Positive	4	Good rapport with the dentist, interest in the dental procedures, laughter and enjoyment.

A retrospective chart review was performed of the patients' previously recorded behavior. Behavior scores were recorded by one of the three pediatric dentists who had examined the patient at the time of their initial visit and were determined to be a 1, 2, 3 or 4 according to the Frankl scale. Positive Behavior was defined as a Frankl Score of 3 or 4. In this study, the decision to use one form of pharmacologic behavior management over another was not a randomized assignment: the decision to use either method was determined by the pediatric dentist who examined the patient at their initial visit. To account for possible biases in the data between the two groups, Frankl score baseline behavior, comorbidities (asthma, sensory disabilities, heart murmurs, etc.), age, gender, race, severity of dental problems, and all other collected factors were examined and adjusted for in the analyses. For example, if most children with autism were given HBGA then the analyses needed to account for autism since there may be differences in behavior between children with or without autism.

The patients treated under HBGA all received care at a pediatric outpatient surgery center under the supervision of a pediatric anesthesiologist. The patients treated under OBGA all received care at a dental office under the supervision of a dentist anesthesiologist. Patients in both groups were treated and released with no unexpected outcomes. The patients' Frankl scores were recorded following treatment under HBGA or OBGA at the 6-, 12-, and 18-month preventive recall appointments. Groups were tested for differences in the percentages exhibiting positive behavior at the 6-, 12-, and 18-month recall appointments.

The HBGA and OBGA groups were compared for differences in age, number of treated teeth, and initial-visit Frankl score using two-sample *t*-tests and for differences in sex, race, presence of any comorbidities, presence of asthma, and initial-visit positive behavior (Frankl score 3 or 4) using chi-square tests. Associations of subsequent 6-, 12-, and 18-month recall visits, Frankl scores with age, number of treated teeth, and initial visit Frankl scores were evaluated using correlation coefficients and with each anesthesia group, sex, race, and presence of any comorbidities using one-way ANOVA. Associations of recall-visit positive behavior with age and number of treated teeth were evaluated using two-sample *t*-tests and with each anesthesia group, sex, race, and presence of any comorbidities using chi-square tests. Multiple-variable analyses of Frankl scores were performed using analysis of covariance, while multiple-variable analyses of positive behavior were performed using logistic regression.

3. Results

Fifty-four patients fitting the inclusion criteria treated under HBGA were identified and 26 were identified as treated under OBGA. Subject characteristics are shown in (Table 2).

Table 2. Subject characteristics and demographics.

Category	HBGA, N (%)	OBGA
Male	33 (61)	14 (54)
Female	21 (39)	12 (46)
Total	54	26
African American	17 (31)	13 (50)
Asian	2 (4)	1 (4)
Caucasian	12 (22)	6 (23)
Hispanic Origin	23 (43)	6 (23)
Age, mean $\pm$ SD	2.8 $\pm$ 0.8	3.0 $\pm$ 0.7
Asthma	7 (13)	2 (8)
Any Comorbidity	11 (20)	4 (15)
# Treated Teeth, mean $\pm$ SD	10.8 $\pm$ 3.6	8.2 $\pm$ 3.0

The hospital-based general anesthesia group had significantly more treated teeth than the office-based general anesthesia group ($p = 0.002$). There were no other statistically significant differences between the two groups at the initial visit. Behavior at the initial exam showed a relationship with behavior at the recall exams, so behavior at the initial exam was included as a covariate in the analyses comparing the behaviors between anesthesia groups. No other variables were significantly associated with positive behavior or Frankl scores at the recall visits.

The associations of anesthesia administration with the behavior outcomes were analyzed using multiple-variable models that included number of treated teeth and behavior at the initial exam as covariates. A significantly higher proportion of OBGA patients had positive behavior than HBGA patients at the six-month recall visit ($p = 0.038$) and 12-month recall visit ($p = 0.028$) (Figure 1).

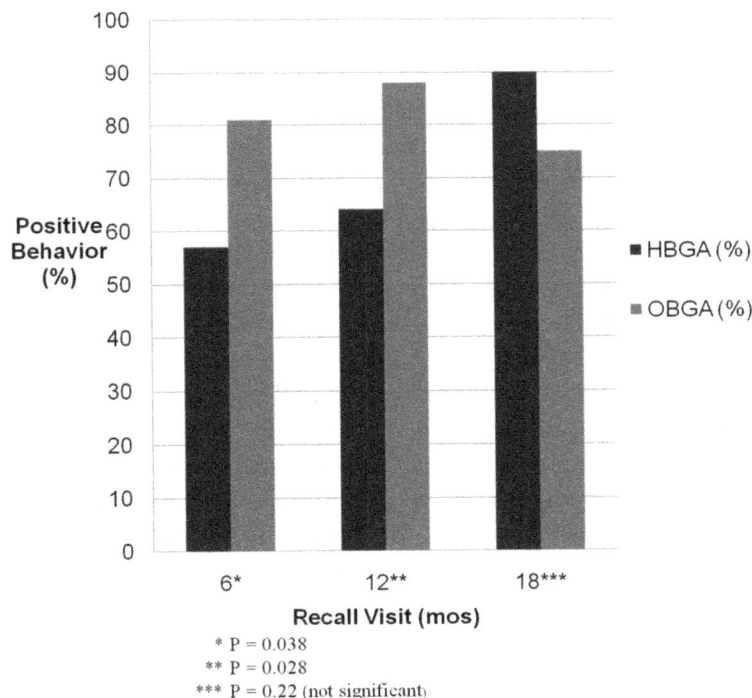

* P = 0.038
** P = 0.028
*** P = 0.22 (not significant)

Figure 1. Percentage of postive behavior at follow up visits.

The difference was not statistically significant at the eighteen-month recall visit ($p = 0.22$). The mean Frankl scores were significantly higher for the HBGA patients than for the OBGA patients at the eighteen-month recall visit ($p = 0.019$) (Table 3).

Table 3. Mean Frankl scores at follow-up visits.

Recall Appointment Interval	HBGA Mean (SD)	OBGA Mean (SD)	p-Value
6 months	2.5 (1.2)	3.0 (0.8)	$p = 0.19$
12 months	2.9 (1.2)	3.4 (1.0)	$p = 0.08$
18 months *	3.4 (0.9)	2.9 (1.2)	$p = 0.019$

* Data is statistically significant ($p = 0.019$). Due to large number of subjects without this data, it is unknown whether this is 'real' or just due to which subjects remained and had data at 18 months.

4. Discussion

In this study, the majority of the patients exhibited baseline behavior that was classified as either definitely negative to negative at the initial visit. To minimize influences of prior dental experiences, this study included patients who were selected before the age of 48 months. Children in this age group would be most likely to have positively affected behavior at follow-up visits. In this study, patients were more likely to exhibit positive behavior following dental treatment for ECC under OBGA than HBGA at their 6- and 12-month recall appointments. The trend toward a higher Frankl score at subsequent recall visits also follows a natural progression of young patients to exhibit improved behavior over time as they grow and mature.

A significant dropout rate occurred between the 6- and 12-month to the 18-month recall appointments. This may lead to careful interpretation of the 18-month data as there are a large number of subjects without this data. The Frankl score means at 6- and 12-months showed that the HBGA had lower Frankl scores at these exams but higher scores at 18-months. This may be a non-significant trend as the tests were not statistically significant. Unfortunately, disparity in maintaining routine dental visits is a consistent finding among patients of lower socioeconomic status, which may contribute to the dropout rate that was seen in this study [18].

O'Sullivan's retrospective study of 80 children treated under general anesthesia with greater than 2 year follow-up appointments revealed that patients readily accepted dental care chair side using local anesthesia [13]. The present study revealed an increase in mean Frankl score at follow-up appointments with both general anesthesia groups that may be consistent with findings from the O'Sullivan study. Although there was not a large sample size, the findings of this study suggest there was a difference in behavior within the general anesthesia group as patients in the OBGA group were more likely to exhibit positive behavior than patients in the HBGA group at 6- and 12-month recall appointments. Nonetheless, this likelihood of future positive behavior may influence a clinician and parent to be more apt to select OBGA over HBGA for dental treatment.

By their nature, retrospective studies can portray an inherent amount of bias associated with their findings. An attempt was made to limit bias by creating a tailored study design and using specific inclusion criteria. In this study patients were seen by different practitioners at their appointments, which may have limited the consistency of recorded behavior due to different interpretations of the Frankl scale. All patients treated under OBGA received care in the same office from the same dental anesthesiologist to control the protocol and limit bias of the retrospective study. Patients treated under HBGA were all treated in the same outpatient setting under the care of a pediatric anesthesiologist consistent with the standard hospital protocols. As a retrospective study, it was not possible to create a "blind" environment for the data collector. A larger sample size may be warranted necessary to draw stronger conclusions and future studies may be needed to reveal potential influences of comorbidities or other differences between each groups' behavior following general anesthesia.

Advanced pharmacologic behavioral management techniques utilizing general anesthesia have received increased acceptance in contemporary society concurrent with changes in parenting practices [3,4]. Dentists perceive that children have worse behavior due to changes in parenting [3]. Even so, hospital-based general anesthesia has traditionally filled an important niche in pediatric dentistry. Office-based general anesthesia has emerged in recent years as a valuable and safe alternative approach for dental treatment [5,9,10]. Office-based general anesthesia may allow for increased convenience, ease of scheduling, and cost savings as compared to hospital-based general anesthesia for both patients and dentists [5]. The future of OBGA appears robust as organized dentistry and state legislatures react to economic conditions and public demands for safe, convenient cost-effective anesthesia care [9,19,20].

5. Conclusions

1. Pediatric dental patients were more likely to exhibit positive behavior at the 6- and 12-month recall appointments following dental treatment for early childhood caries under OBGA than HBGA.

2. Clinicians may consider future behavior of dental patients when determining general anesthesia treatment modalities in children with early childhood caries presenting to their office.

References

1. American Dental Association. *Policy Statement: The Use of Conscious Sedation, Deep Sedation, and General Anesthesia in Dentistry*; American Dental Association: Chicago, IL, USA, 2012; pp. 1–3.

2. American Dental Association. *Guidelines for the Use of Conscious Sedation, Deep Sedation, and General Anesthesia for Dentists*; American Dental Association: Chicago, IL, USA, 2012; pp. 1–14.

3. Sheller, B. Challenges of managing child behavior in the 21st century dental setting. *Pediatr. Dent.* **2004**, *26*, 111–113. [PubMed]

4. Eaton, J.J.; McTigue, D.J.; Fields, H.W., Jr.; Beck, M. Attitudes of contemporary parents toward behavior management techniques used in pediatric dentistry. *Pediatr. Dent.* **2005**, *27*, 107–113. [PubMed]

5. Caputo, A.C. Providing deep sedation and general anesthesia for patients with special needs in the dental office-based setting. *Spec. Care Dent.* **2009**, *29*, 26–30. [CrossRef] [PubMed]

6. American Academy of Pediatric Dentistry Reference Manual. Guideline on behavior guidance for the pediatric dental patient. *Pediatr. Dent.* **2015–2016**, *32*, 147–155.

7. Vinckier, F.; Gizani, S.; Declerck, D. Comprehensive dental care for children with rampant caries under general anesthesia. *Int. J. Paediatr. Dent.* **2001**, *11*, 25–32. [CrossRef] [PubMed]

8. Eidelman, E.; Faibis, S.; Peretz, B. A comparison of restorations for children with early childhood caries treated under general anesthesia or conscious sedation. *Pediatr. Dent.* **2000**, *22*, 33–37. [PubMed]

9. Yagiela, J.A. Office-based anesthesia in dentistry. Past, present, and future trends. *Dent. Clin. N. Am.* **1999**, *43*, 201–215. [PubMed]

10. Nick, D.; Thompson, L.; Anderson, D.; Trapp, L. The use of general anesthesia to facilitate dental treatment. *Gen. Dent.* **2003**, *51*, 464–468. [PubMed]

11. Frankl, S.N.; Shiere, F.; Fogels, H.R. Should the parent remain with the child in the dental operatory? *J. Dent. Child.* **1962**, *29*, 150–153.

12. Kupietzky, A.; Blumenstyk, A. Comparing the behavior of children treated using general anesthesia with those treated using conscious sedation. *ASDC J. Dent. Child.* **1998**, *65*, 122–127. [PubMed]

13. O'Sullvan, E.A.; Curzon, M.E. The efficacy of comprehensive dental care for children under general anesthesia. *Br. Dent. J.* **1991**, *171*, 56–58. [CrossRef]

14. Peretz, B.; Faibis, S.; Ever-Hadani, P.; Eidelman, E. Children with baby bottle tooth de cay treated under general anesthesia or sedation: Behavior in a follow-up visit. *ASDC J. Dent. Child.* **2000**, *24*, 97–101.

15. Fuhrer, C.T.; Weddell, J.A.; Sanders, B.J.; Jones, J.E.; Dean, J.A.; Tomlin, A. Effect on behavior of dental treatment rendered under conscious sedation and general anesthesia in pediatric patients. *Pediatr. Dent.* **2009**, *31*, 389–394.

16. American Academy of Pediatric Dentistry Reference Manual. Policy on early childhood caries (ECC): Classifications, consequences, and preventative strategies. *Pediatr. Dent.* **2015–2016**, *37*, 50–52.

17. Edelstein, B.L.; Chinn, C.H. Update on disparities in oral health and access to dental care for America's children. *Acad. Pediatr.* **2009**, *9*, 415–419. [CrossRef] [PubMed]

18. Stigers, J.I. Nonpharmacologic management of children's behaviors. In *McDonald and Avery's Dentistry for the Child and Adolescent*, 10th ed.; Dean, J.A., Ed.; Mosby Elsevier: Maryland Heights, MO, USA, 2015; pp. 286–302.

19. Hicks, C.G.; Jones, J.E.; Saxen, M.A.; Maupome, G.; Sanders, B.J.; Walker, L.A.; Weddell, J.A.; Tomlin, A. Demand in Pediatric Dentistry for Sedation and General Anesthesia by Dentists Anesthesologists: A Survey of Directors of Dentist Anesthesiologist and Pediatric Dentistry Residencies. *Anesth. Prog.* **2012**, *59*, 3–11. [CrossRef] [PubMed]

20. Olabi, N.F.; Jones, J.E.; Saxen, M.A.; Sanders, B.J.; Walker, L.A.; Weddell, J.A.; Schrader, S.M.; Tomlin, A.M. The Use of Office-Based Sedation and General Anesthesia by Board Certified Pediatric Dentists Practicing in the United States. *Anesth. Prog.* **2012**, *59*, 12–17. [CrossRef] [PubMed]

15

Effect of Violet-Blue Light on *Streptococcus mutans*-Induced Enamel Demineralization

Grace Gomez Felix Gomez [1,*] **ⓘ**, Frank Lippert [2], Masatoshi Ando [2], Andrea Ferreira Zandona [3], George J. Eckert [4] and Richard L. Gregory [1,*]

[1]   Department of Biomedical and Applied Sciences, Indiana University School of Dentistry, Indianapolis, IN 46202, USA

[2]   Department of Cariology, Operative Dentistry and Dental Public Health, Indiana University School of Dentistry, Indianapolis, IN 46202, USA; flippert@iu.edu (F.L.); mando@iu.edu (M.A.)

[3]   Department of Operative Dentistry, University of North Carolina, Chapel Hill, NC 27599, USA; azandona@email.unc.edu

[4]   Department of Biostatistics, Indiana University, Indianapolis, IN 46202, USA; geckert@iu.edu

*   Correspondence: gfelixgo@iupui.edu (G.F.G.); rgregory@iu.edu (R.L.G.)

Abstract: Background: This in vitro study determined the effectiveness of violet-blue light (405 nm) on inhibiting *Streptococcus mutans*-induced enamel demineralization. Materials and Methods: *S. mutans* UA159 biofilm was grown on human enamel specimens for 13 h in 5% CO_2 at 37 °C with/without 1% sucrose. Wet biofilm was treated twice daily with violet-blue light for five minutes over five days. A six-hour reincubation was included daily between treatments excluding the final day. Biofilms were harvested and colony forming units (CFU) were quantitated. Lesion depth (L) and mineral loss (ΔZ) were quantified using transverse microradiography (TMR). Quantitative light-induced fluorescence Biluminator (QLF-D) was used to determine mean fluorescence loss. Data were analyzed using one-way analysis of variance (ANOVA) to compare differences in means. Results: The results demonstrated a significant reduction in CFUs between treated and non-treated groups grown with/without 1% sucrose. ΔZ was significantly reduced for specimens exposed to biofilms grown without sucrose with violet-blue light. There was only a trend on reduction of ΔZ with sucrose and with L on both groups. There were no differences in fluorescence-derived parameters between the groups. Conclusions: Within the limitations of the study, the results indicate that violet-blue light can serve as an adjunct prophylactic treatment for reducing *S. mutans* biofilm formation and enamel mineral loss.

Keywords: violet-blue light; phototherapy; *Streptococcus mutans*; dental caries

1. Introduction

Dental caries is a biofilm-mediated disease; therefore, biofilm is indispensable for caries initiation. There are a multitude of factors involved in the initiation and progression of caries [1]. Dental caries is preventable by controlling a few of the many factors involved in the development of the disease [2]. Since disease management is more effective in the early stages, the dogma has been to detect carious lesions at its initial stage to prevent its progression to cavitation. Currently, various preventive strategies ranging from natural products to nanotechnological approaches are under development focusing on biofilm modulation. One novel method is phototherapy to inactivate oral biofilm formation [3]. *S. mutans* is considered a primary cariogenic bacterium and has the capacity to form biofilm, produce and resist acidic conditions [4].

Light therapy studies have been applied for several oral microorganisms [5]. *S. mutans* had been studied widely with photodynamic therapy using exogenous photosensitizers such as Erythrosine, Rose Bengal, Toluidine Blue, and Malachite Green, among others [6–9]. Few studies have focused on phototherapy without the presence of exogenous photosensitizers [10–13]. Photosensitizers or photoactivable compounds can be either added exogenously, or present endogenous, within the bacterium. These photosensitizers absorb light of a specific wavelength or a range of wavelengths, get activated, and undergo a transition of energy from a ground state to an excited singlet state. Subsequently the transfer of energy from the excited photosensitizer with the available molecular oxygen produces reactive oxygen species (ROS), mediating bacterial destruction [5–12]. Preliminary studies have shown the photo inhibitory effects of violet-blue light on *S. mutans* biofilm [14]. The aim of this in vitro study was to determine the effect of violet-blue light at the surface level of the tooth, namely enamel, and on the *S. mutans* biofilm.

2. Materials and Methods

2.1. Study Design

Sixty enamel specimens were used in this experiment. From this sample pool, 48 specimens were randomly selected for randomization into 4 intervention groups that included violet-blue light treated and non-treated control groups. Group 1 ($n = 12$) consisted of biofilms grown with Tryptic Soy Broth (TSB) with 0% sucrose and treated with violet-blue light; Group 2 ($n = 12$) consisted of biofilms grown in TSBS with 1% sucrose and treated with violet-blue light; Group 3 ($n = 12$) consisted of biofilms grown with TSB not treated with violet-blue light; and Group 4 ($n = 12$) consisted biofilms grown with TSBS not treated with violet-blue light. Analysis of specimens from the intervention group was done at the end of a 5-day treatment period [13]. The remaining 12 specimens were used for baseline measurements at the end of 13 h period before the intervention. Baseline samples ($n = 6$ each) for both TSB and TBSS were used. Baseline measurements before treatment provide information on the actual effect of the treatment. Groups 1 and 2 were treated with violet-blue light (13 mW/cm^2; ~4 J/cm^2) for 5 min, 2 times a day, 4 days a week; but only once on the 5th day of the treatment. Quantification of biofilm cells was performed to obtain a baseline measurement at 13 h and on the final day of the treatment period. Additionally, all 60 of the enamel specimens were imaged for fluorescence loss using QLF-D and sectioned to determine mineral loss and lesion depth through TMR (Figure 1).

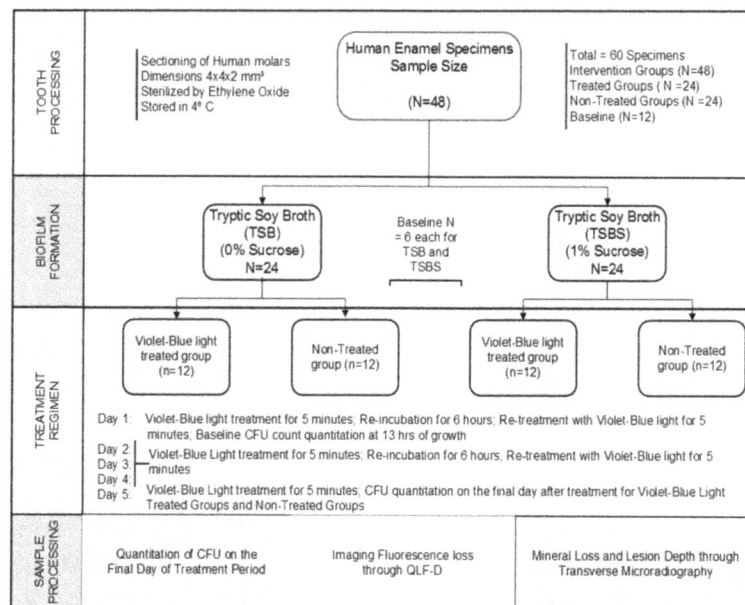

Figure 1. Flowchart of the study design.

2.2. Bacterial Culture Conditions

S. mutans (UA159, serotype c strain) stored at $-80\ °C$ with glycerol was used in this study. The bacteria were cultured on mitis salivaris sucrose bacitracin (MSSB, Anaerobe Systems, Morgan Hill, CA, USA) agar plates. *S. mutans* was grown in 5 mL of Tryptic Soy Broth (TSB, Acumedia, Baltimore, MD, USA) for 24 h in a 5% CO_2 incubator at $37\ °C$ [15].

2.3. Enamel Specimen Preparation

Sixty enamel specimens were prepared from extracted human molars without any cracks, fractures or caries (Institutional Review Board (IRB) approval (# NS0911-07). A Lap Craft L'il Trimmer^{TM} (Powell, OH, USA) was used to decoronate the crown portion of the tooth. Enamel specimens with dimensions of $4 \times 4 \times 2\ mm^3$ were cut using a Isomet saw (Buehler, Lake Bluff, IL, USA). Specimens were ground sequentially with 500, 1200, 2400 and 4000 grit silicon carbide paper with a RotoPol-31/RotoForce-4polishing/grinding machine (Struers, Cleveland, OH, USA). Specimens were ground with each sandpaper grit for 4 s and the specimen thickness was reduced to 2 mm. The actual thickness ranged from 1.6 to 2.1 mm. Clear nail varnish was used to coat all sides and the bottom of the enamel specimens. Approximately one third of the top surface of the enamel specimens was covered with nail varnish. Quality assurance of the specimens was done with a microscope at $20\times$ magnification to determine absence of cracks, fractures or fissures. Compromised specimens were excluded [16] (modified from Lippert and Juthani, 2015).

2.4. Specimen Sterilization

Human enamel specimens were rinsed for 3 min, sonicated for 3 min, and again rinsed for 3 min with deionized water. The specimens were placed in moist cotton gauze, sealed in a whirl pak bag (Sigma-Aldrich, St. Louis, MO, USA), and sterilized with ethylene oxide gas [17].

2.5. Biofilm Formation

Overnight bacterial broth cultures were diluted 1:100 with TSB or TSBS. *S. mutans* biofilm cells were grown in sterile 96-well microtiter plates (Fisher Scientific, Co., Newark, DE, USA) with ($n = 12$) and without ($n = 12$) enamel specimens [18]. The biofilm cells were incubated for 13 h in a 5% CO_2 incubator at $37\ °C$ to reach the logarithmic phase of growth. A gap of one well was left in between the biofilm samples and a 2-well distance was maintained between TSB and TSBS groups.

2.6. Violet-Blue LIGHT source

The light emitted from the quantitative light-induced fluorescence (QLF-clin, Inspektor Research Systems^{TM} BV, Amsterdam, The Netherlands) was used as a light source for the treatment of *S. mutans* biofilm cells in this study. It employs a 35-Watt Xenon arc lamp, and violet-blue light is filtered through a high-pass band filter. The spectral range of the violet-blue light is within a range of 380 to 450 nm with a peak wavelength at 405 nm [14].

2.7. Treatment with Violet-Blue Light

Before irradiation, planktonic or supernatant liquid was removed from above the biofilm cells and the wet biofilm was exposed to violet-blue light continuously for 5 min. The pH of each of the supernatants were measured. The distance between the bottom of the microtiter plate and the light source was kept constant at 2.0 cm. A black background was used to avoid scattering of light. Seal mate was placed as a barrier between the sample and the light source opening. Immediately after exposure, freshly prepared TSB or TSBS growth medium was added to each well. The treated biofilm cells were reincubated for 6 h in a 5% CO_2 incubator at $37\ °C$ [14]. After 6 h, the biofilm cells were again treated with violet-blue light for 5 min and reincubated with fresh TSB or TSBS for 13 h, until the next treatment on the following consecutive day. The procedure was repeated for 5 days, except on the final day, when only one treatment was provided without the 6 h reincubation.

2.8. Quantification of Colony-Forming Units

At the end of fifth day of the experiment, supernatant liquid was removed for pH measurements. Baseline CFUs of the 13 h biofilm with TSB and TSBS on the first day before the treatment were also obtained. CFUs of violet-blue light treated and non-treated groups in TSB and TSBS were obtained from the final day of the treatment regimen. Biofilm at the bottom of the plate was gently washed once with 0.9% saline. Enamel specimens were carefully removed from the microtiter plate and placed in 1 mL of saline solution in mini centrifuge tubes, vortexed for 10 s, sonicated on ice for 20 s, and again vortexed for 10 s [14,19]. Serial dilutions of the bacterial samples were prepared with 0.9% saline and plated in duplicates on Tryptic Soy Agar (TSA) plates using a spiral plater (Spiral System™, Cincinnati, OH, USA). TSA agar plates were incubated for 48 h at 37 °C in a 5% CO_2 incubator, and the colony-forming units (CFUs) were counted by an automated colony counter using Protocol™ (Synbiosis Inc., Frederick, MD, USA) software.

2.9. Quantitative Light-Induced Fluorescence

A quantitative light-induced fluorescence biluminator (QLF-D) was used to acquire images of the enamel specimens. A jig was prepared to secure the enamel specimen with silicone rubber (Oomo-30). The images were acquired through an illumination tube fitted on a SLR camera with white and blue light-emitting diodes (LED) under dark conditions. Fluorescence images of enamel specimens were obtained using a C3 proprietary software on QLF-D. The images were digitally archived for further analysis of mineral loss or lesion depth through QA2 analysis software. The QLF-D parameters mean fluorescence loss, delta F (ΔF); maximum fluorescence loss (ΔF_{max}); lesion volume, delta Q (ΔQ); and lesion area (Area) were collected [20].

2.10. Transverse Microradiography

Enamel specimens were treated briefly with 70% ethyl alcohol and stored under moistened conditions with deionized water (diH_2O). Enamel specimens were superglued to acrylic rods and enamel sections of 100 ± 20 μm thickness were prepared with a hard tissue microtome. One section per specimen was selected to be imaged. The enamel sections were placed on an ultra-resolution flat plate sized $5 \times 5 \times 2$ mm^3 (Microchrome Technology Inc., San Jose, CA, USA). Calibration of the TMR PSL Imaging System (Thermo-Kevex PXS5-928WB-LV, Tube 48934, Photonic Science Limited, East Sussex, UK) with respect to its absorption coefficient was done with an aluminum step wedge for an acceptable correlation of 0.99970. Imaging of the enamel specimens were obtained through X-ray source with a 45 kV voltage and a current of 45 μA. The obtained images were read and processed using TMRD1 5.0.01 software and finally analyzed through TMR2006 software v.3.0.0.18 (Inspektor Research Systems BV, Amsterdam, The Netherlands). Mineral loss (ΔZ) and lesion depth (L) were determined.

2.11. pH Measurements

A pH meter (Accumet, Fisher Scientific, Pittsburgh, PA, USA) was used to measure the pH of the pooled samples of every group. The supernatant containing planktonic cells on top of the biofilm was removed before light irradiation for pH measurement. The pH was measured on the first day before the treatment and on the fifth or final day of the treatment regimen.

2.12. Statistical Analysis

One-way ANOVA was performed for TSB and TSBS groups, followed by pairwise group comparisons for baseline, violet-blue light treated and non-treated groups, to determine any difference in CFU. QLF-D parameters such as fluorescence loss (ΔF), lesion area (Area), lesion volume (ΔQ) and lesion depth (L) and mineral loss (ΔZ) were obtained through transverse microradiography (TMR).

3. Results

3.1. Photoinhibition of S. mutans Biofilm on Human Enamel Specimens

Baseline ($n = 6$) *S. mutans* biofilm grown in the absence of sucrose with TSB had statistically lower CFU numbers than the violet-blue light treated groups ($p < 0.001$) and also with non-treated groups ($p < 0.0001$). Baseline *S. mutans* biofilm grown in the presence of sucrose with TSBS had statistically higher CFU numbers than the violet-blue light treated groups ($p < 0.0001$) and the non-treated groups ($p = 0.0149$). Baseline CFU was obtained at 13 h for TSB and TSBS, and was compared against the CFU obtained on the final day of the intervention for the treated and non-treated groups within their respective media (Figure 2).

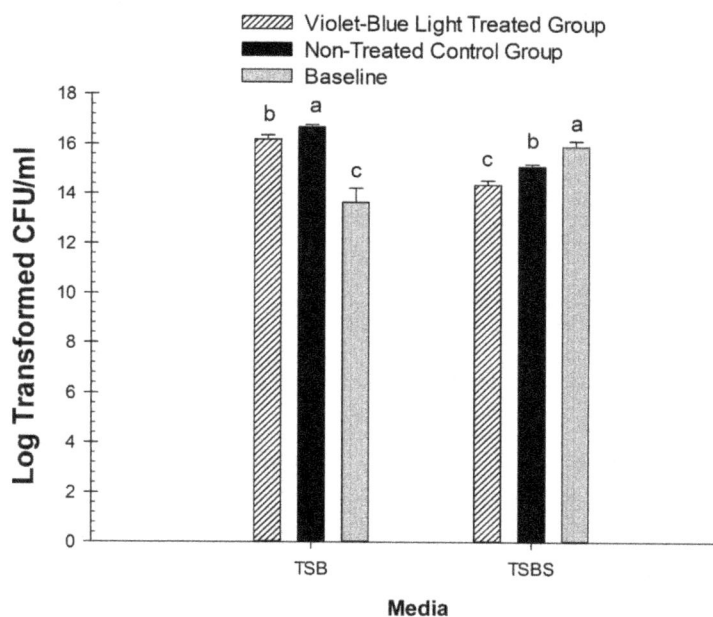

Figure 2. Comparison of baseline *S. mutans* biofilm CFU with treated and non-treated TSB and TSBS groups. The Log CFUs of the violet-blue light treated and non-treated group on the 5th day of the treatment were compared with the baseline counts at 13 h for TSB and TSBS. Different lower-case letters represent significant differences between groups, with comparisons performed separately within each media.

3.2. Effect of Violet-Blue Light on the Viability of S. mutans Biofilm Cells

The results of the photoinhibition of violet-blue light at the end of the treatment demonstrated that violet-blue light treated groups ($n = 12$) had significantly lower CFUs than the non-treated control groups ($n = 12$) with TSB ($p = 0.0333$) and similar significantly different results were obtained with TSBS ($p = 0.0008$). There was an approximately 28% reduction of bacterial numbers in TSB and 48% in TSBS (Figure 2).

3.3. Effect of Violet-Blue Light on the Lesion Depth by Fluorescence Image Analysis of Enamel Specimens through QLF-D

With respect to QLF-D parameters, there were no differences between the baseline value, violet-blue light treated and non-treated groups, ($p = 0.37$ for ΔF, $p = 0.40$ for ΔF_{max}, $p = 0.40$ for ΔQ, $p = 0.41$ for lesion area, $p = 0.12$) on human enamel specimens with *S. mutans* biofilm with TSB

(Table 1). Enamel specimens subjected to *S. mutans* biofilm in TSBS demonstrated that there were significant differences between the baseline and the violet-blue light treated groups and non-treated control groups. ΔF, ΔF_{max}, ΔQ, Area were significantly lower for baseline values than the violet-blue light and non-treated control groups ($p < 0.0001$). The photoinhibitory effect of the violet-blue light treated and non-treated groups indicated that there were no significant differences in TSBS ($p > 0.08$) (Table 1).

Table 1. Log transformation of QLF-D parameters on the effect of violet-blue light on the lesion depth by image analysis of loss of fluorescence on human enamel specimens by *S. mutans* biofilm grown in TSB or TSBS through QLF-D. *S. mutans* in TSB had no significant group differences for any of the QLF-D parameters. TSBS baseline had significantly lower QLF-D parameters than Blue ($p < 0.001$) and No Blue ($p < 0.0001$), while Blue and No Blue were not significantly different from one another ($p > 0.08$).

Log Transformed QLF-D Parameters	Media	Baseline		Violet-Blue Light		Non-Treated Light	
		N	Mean (SE)	N	Mean (SE)	N	Mean (SE)
delta *F*	TSB	6	0.61 (0.93)	12	1.50 (0.52)	12	1.86 (0.40)
	TSBS	6	0.52 (0.90)*	12	3.08 (0.17)	12	3.52 (0.09)
delta *F*$_{max}$	TSB	6	0.91 (1.03)	12	1.90 (0.58)	12	2.25 (0.45)
	TSBS	6	0.75 (0.97)*	12	3.48 (0.15)	12	3.82 (0.07)
delta *Q*	TSB	6	4.52 (2.25)	12	7.16 (1.31)	12	7.50 (1.11)
	TSBS	6	4.23 (2.13)*	12	10.70 (0.28)	12	11.22 (0.28)
Area	TSB	6	3.16 (1.81)	12	5.29 (1.04)	12	5.46 (0.90)
	TSBS	6	2.95 (1.72)*	12	7.62 (0.12)	12	7.70 (0.20)

Asterisk (*) represents statistical significance ($p < 0.05$).

3.4. Effect of Violet-Blue Light on Mineral Loss and Lesion Depth through Transverse Microradiography

The photoinibitory properties of violet-blue light was effective with *S. mutans* biofilm exhibiting less ΔZ ($p = 0.0293$) with TSB (Figure 3). However, there was no significant difference in ΔZ found in *S. mutans* biofilm formed with TSBS ($p = 0.09$) (Figure 3). Violet-blue light treated groups and non-treated control groups did not have significantly different lesion depths (L) in TSB or TSBS ($p > 0.14$). Baseline enamel specimens had less ΔZ and (L) compared to violet-blue light treated ($p < 0.001$) and non-treated control groups ($p \leq 0.0001$).

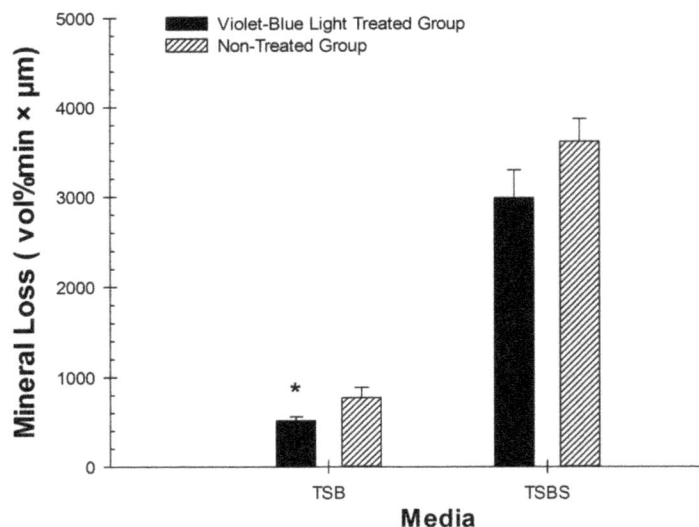

Figure 3. Comparison of the effect of violet-blue light on the mineral loss (TMR) produced by *S. mutans* biofilm on human enamel specimens in TSB and TSBS. Asterisks indicate statistical significance. Significance level was kept at $p < 0.05$.

3.5. pH Measurements

pH measurements of the supernatant or planktonic fluids at the beginning of the treatment on the first day were obtained. The violet-blue light treated group in TSB had a pH of 4.96 before treatment and the non-treated control groups had a pH of 4.99. The pH of planktonic or supernatant fluids in TSBS was 4.43 with violet-blue light treated groups and non-treated control groups had a pH of 4.45 on the first day before the treatment. On the final day of treatment, the pH values with TSB were 4.88 and 4.85 in the treated and in the non-treated groups, respectively. For TSBS, the pH values were 4.1 in both treated and non-treated groups.

4. Discussion

The current study demonstrated that violet-blue light had a statistically significant photoinhibitory effect on the number of CFUs of *S. mutans* after 5 days of treatment. Irrespective of the presence or absence of 1% sucrose, treatment with violet-blue light provided a reduction in the numbers of *S. mutans* biofilm cells. This effectiveness was based on a 13 h old biofilm, with two treatments on each of the first 4 days and one treatment on the final day of the treatment regimen. There was also a 6 h reincubation period in between the treatments with no reincubation on the final day of the treatment period. Previously we reported that metabolic activity of *S. mutans* biofilm at 0 h was reduced significantly compared to after 2 and 6 h of reincubation [21] (Gomez et al., *J. Oral Sci.*—in press). The baseline CFUs of *S. mutans* at 13 h were lower than the violet-blue light treated TSB and TSBS groups. These results demonstrated that, although violet-blue light was effective in reducing the numbers of the bacteria, there was regrowth of bacteria after photoinactivation. The findings correlate with the previous findings related to significant reduction in metabolic activity at 0 h compared to that activity following 2 and 6 h. It would be ideal to harvest bacterial cells after each time period to determine the temporal variation in bacterial viability with violet-blue light treatment. The supernatants containing planktonic bacteria above the biofilm were removed and used for pH measurements. Measuring the pH of biofilm would be an alternative option.

In relation to the QLF-D parameters, unlike the significant reduction of CFU numbers in the violet-blue light treated groups in TSB, there were no significant differences between the ΔF, ΔF_{max}, ΔQ, Area. Though there was slight reduction in all the QLF-D parameters, it was not statistically different from the non-treated groups. The results indicate that violet-blue light may inactivate the bacteria in a biofilm environment. Since the QLF-D parameters were not much different between the baseline and experimental groups, variations of the enamel surface would also have contributed to this finding. Another possible explanation is that violet-blue light affects the architecture and development of the extra polysaccharide matrix of the biofilm. *S. mutans* utilizes sucrose to form extracellular polysaccharides (EPS) and enmesh bacterial cells together to form microcolonies with acidic pockets [22,23]. A recent report found that blue light did not have an effect on the soluble EPS but had an increased effect on insoluble EPS, which is cariogenic. They also found that CFUs for *S. mutans* biofilm cells treated with blue light were significantly reduced, compared to the negative control 0.89% NaCl. However, viability was significantly reduced with 0.12% Chlorhexidine compared to treatment with light [13]. In the present study, with TSBS there was no significant difference in QLF-D parameters between the violet-blue light treated and non-treated control groups. There was a slight reduction in all the QLF-D parameters mentioned above in the violet-blue light treated groups compared to non-treated groups, with minimal deviation, but this was not statistically significant. The short-term biofilm model with two replenishments of fresh media on the undisturbed biofilm on the enamel specimen would have contributed to balanced bacterial metabolism, with less degradation of EPS causing reduced enamel demineralization [24]. The baseline values had lower QLF-D parameters and were significantly different than the violet-blue and non-treated groups.

The gold standard method for determining lesion depth is to section enamel specimens, process microradiography images, and analyze them. The present findings supported that baseline values for mineral loss and lesion depth were significantly lower compared to violet-blue light treated groups and non-treated control groups. In the absence of sucrose with TSB, lesion depth and mineral loss were significantly lower compared to the non-treated groups, however this was not found with TSBS-grown groups. Early caries detection devices such as QLF differ in sensitivity based on enamel or dentin. It has lower sensitivity with enamel compared to dentin. Artifacts on the surface of enamel such as sucrose-grown biofilm may have contributed to the above findings and might be one of the limitations of the study. Future studies directed at simulating in vivo carious lesions induced by *S. mutans*, in addition to saliva and pellicle formation, would provide in-depth results.

5. Conclusions

Colony-forming units (CFU), and lesion depth, measured as mineral loss or fluorescence loss, measured through QLF-D confirmed by the gold standard of transverse microradiography were compared between violet-blue light treated and non-treated groups in both TSB and TSBS at the end of the treatment period. Violet-blue light had an inhibitory effect on the bacterial viability of *S. mutans* biofilm in both TSB and TSBS. There was no statistically significant effect of violet-blue light on the mineral level of the tooth surface or the mineral loss obtained through QLF-D. There was a slight reduction in the amount of loss of fluorescence. Mineral loss obtained through TMR was statistically significant in the violet-blue light treated group; however, lesion depth was not statically significant. Violet-blue light has a more effective photoinhibitory effect at the bacterial level on the surface of the tooth than at the mineral level.

Acknowledgments: We would like to thank Anderson Hara for providing supplies for processing human dentin specimens. We thank Simone Duarte for critically reviewing the manuscript, and for helpful suggestions. Our sincere thanks to Jennifer Eder, Research Analyst for helping with the QLF-D Biluminator. We thank Nyi Nyi, Brian Ashmore, Adam Kelly, and Yuan for technical support. We also extend a special thank you to Sharon Gwinn and the staff of Oral Health Research Institute (OHRI), who assisted with this project.

Author Contributions: Grace Gomez Felix Gomez, PhD student in Dental Sciences, Indiana University School of Dentistry, conducted this translational study and collected data. Frank Lippert provided micro-radiographic image analysis, critical review of the paper and technical suggestions during the experiment. Masatoshi Ando contributed to conception of the idea and suggestions during the experiment, Andrea Ferreira Zandona contributed to the conceptualization and initiation of the project. George J. Eckert conducted statistical analysis, and interpretation of the analysis. Richard L. Gregory was the mentor for this project and is responsible for the review and approval of the paper.

References

1. Selwitz, R.H.; Ismail, A.I.; Pitts, N.B. Dental caries. *Lancet* **2007**, *369*, 51–59. [CrossRef]
2. Watt, R.G. Strategies and approaches in oral disease prevention and health promotion. *Bull. World Health Organ.* **2005**, *83*, 711–718. [PubMed]
3. Ten Cate, J.M.; Zaura, E. The numerous microbial species in oral biofilms: How could antibacterial therapy be effective? *Adv. Dent. Res.* **2012**, *24*, 108–111. [CrossRef] [PubMed]
4. Banas, J.A. Virulence properties of *Streptococcus mutans*. *Front. Biosci.* **2004**, *9*, 1267–1277. [CrossRef] [PubMed]
5. Soukos, N.S.; Goodson, J.M. Photodynamic therapy in the control of oral biofilms. *Periodontology 2000* **2011**, *55*, 143–166. [CrossRef] [PubMed]
6. Wood, S.; Metcalf, D.; Devine, D.; Robinson, C. Erythrosine is a potential photosensitizer for the photodynamic therapy of oral plaque biofilms. *J. Antimicrob. Chemother.* **2006**, *57*, 680–684. [CrossRef] [PubMed]
7. Zanin, I.C.; Lobo, M.M.; Rodrigues, L.K.; Pimenta, L.A.; Hofling, J.F.; Goncalves, R.B. Photosensitization of in vitro biofilms by toluidine blue O combined with a light-emitting diode. *Eur. J. Oral Sci.* **2006**, *114*, 64–69. [CrossRef] [PubMed]
8. Pereira, C.A.; Costa, A.C.; Carreira, C.M.; Junqueira, J.C.; Jorge, A.O. Photodynamic inactivation of *Streptococcus mutans* and *Streptococcus sanguinis* biofilms in vitro. *Lasers Med. Sci.* **2013**, *28*, 859–864. [CrossRef] [PubMed]

9. Rolim, J.P.; de-Melo, M.A.; Guedes, S.F.; Albuquerque-Filho, F.B.; de Souza, J.R.; Nogueira, N.A.; Zanin, I.C.; Rodrigues, L.K. The antimicrobial activity of photodynamic therapy against *Streptococcus mutans* using different photosensitizers. *J. Photochem. Photobiol. B* **2012**, *106*, 40–46. [CrossRef] [PubMed]

10. Feuerstein, O.; Moreinos, D.; Steinberg, D. Synergic antibacterial effect between visible light and hydrogen peroxide on *Streptococcus mutans*. *J. Antimicrob. Chemother.* **2006**, *57*, 872–876. [CrossRef] [PubMed]

11. Steinberg, D.; Moreinos, D.; Featherstone, J.; Shemesh, M.; Feuerstein, O. Genetic and physiological effects of noncoherent visible light combined with hydrogen peroxide on *Streptococcus mutans* in biofilm. *Antimicrob. Agents Chemother.* **2008**, *52*, 2626–2631. [CrossRef] [PubMed]

12. Chebath-Taub, D.; Steinberg, D.; Featherstone, J.D.B.; Feuerstein, O. Influence of blue light on *Streptococcus mutans* re-organization in biofilm. *J. Photochem. Photobiol. B Biol.* **2012**, *116*, 75–78. [CrossRef] [PubMed]

13. De Sousa, D.L.; Lima, R.A.; Zanin, I.C.; Klein, M.I.; Janal, M.N.; Duarte, S. Effect of Twice-Daily Blue Light Treatment on Matrix-Rich Biofilm Development. *PLoS ONE* **2015**, *10*, e0131941. [CrossRef] [PubMed]

14. Gomez, G.F.; Huang, R.; MacPherson, M.; Ferreira Zandona, A.G.; Gregory, R.L. Photo Inactivation of *Streptococcus mutans* Biofilm by Violet-Blue light. *Curr. Microbiol.* **2016**, *73*, 426–433. [CrossRef] [PubMed]

15. Huang, R.; Li, M.; Gregory, R.L. Effect of nicotine on growth and metabolism of *Streptococcus mutans*. *Eur. J. Oral Sci.* **2012**, *120*, 319–325. [CrossRef] [PubMed]

16. Lippert, F.; Juthani, K. Fluoride dose-response of human and bovine enamel artificial caries lesions under pH-cycling conditions. *Clin. Oral Investig.* **2015**, *19*, 1947–1954. [CrossRef] [PubMed]

17. Fontana, M.; Buller, T.L.; Dunipace, A.J.; Stookey, G.K.; Gregory, R.L. An In vitro microbial-caries model used to study the efficacy of antibodies to *Streptococcus mutans* surface proteins in preventing dental caries. *Clin. Diagn. Lab. Immunol.* **2000**, *7*, 49–54. [CrossRef] [PubMed]

18. Li, M.; Huang, R.; Zhou, X.; Qiu, W.; Xu, X.; Gregory, R.L. Effect of nicotine on cariogenic virulence of *Streptococcus mutans*. *Folia Microbiol.* **2016**, *61*, 505–512. [CrossRef] [PubMed]

19. Tagelsir, A.; Yassen, G.H.; Gomez, G.F.; Gregory, R.L. Effect of Antimicrobials Used in Regenerative Endodontic Procedures on 3-week-old *Enterococcus faecalis* Biofilm. *J. Endod.* **2016**, *42*, 258–262. [CrossRef] [PubMed]

20. Waller, E.; van Daelen, C.J.; van der Veen, M.H. *Application of QLF^{TM} for Diagnosis and Quality Assessment in Clinical Practice*; Inspektor Research Systems: Amsterdam, The Netherlands, 2012.

21. Gomez, G.F.; Huang, R.; Eckert, G.; Gregory, R.L. Effect of Phototherapy on the Metabolism of Streptococcus mutans Biofilm Based on Colorimetric Tetrazolium Assay. *J. Oral Sci.* **2017**, in press.

22. Xiao, J.; Koo, H. Structural organization and dynamics of exopolysaccharide matrix and microcolonies formation by *Streptococcus mutans* in biofilms. *J. Appl. Microbiol.* **2010**, *108*, 2103–2113. [PubMed]

23. Colby, S.M.; Russell, R.R.B. Sugar metabolism by *mutans streptococci*. *J. Appl. Microbiol.* **1997**, *83* (Suppl. S1), 80S–88S. [CrossRef] [PubMed]

24. Costa Oliveira, B.E.; Cury, J.A.; Ricomini Filho, A.P. Biofilm extracellular polysaccharides degradation during starvation and enamel demineralization. *PLoS ONE* **2017**, *12*, e0181168. [CrossRef] [PubMed]

16

Prioritizing the Risk Factors of Severe Early Childhood Caries

Noha Samir Kabil [1],* and Sherif Eltawil [2]

[1] Department of Pediatric Dentistry and Dental Public Health, Faculty of Dentistry, Ain Shams University, Cairo 11566, Egypt

[2] Department of Pediatric Dentistry and Dental Public Health, Faculty of Oral & Dental Medicine, Cairo University, Giza 12613, Egypt; Sherif.eltaweil@dentistry.cu.edu.eg

* Correspondence: pf.nohakabil@asfd.asu.edu.eg

Academic Editors: Barbara Cvikl and Katrin Bekes

Abstract: Severe early childhood caries remains the most common chronic disease affecting children. The multifactorial etiology of caries has established a controversy about which risk factors were more significant to its development. Therefore, our study aimed through meticulous statistical analysis to arrange the "well agreed upon" common risk factors in order of significance, to aid the clinician in tailoring an adequate preventive program. The study prioritized or reshuffled the risk factors contributing to severe early childhood caries and placed them in the order of their significance as follows: snacking of sugary food several times a day, increased number of siblings to three or more, night feeding, child self-employed brushing, mother's caries experience, two siblings, on demand feeding, once/day sugary food, sharing utensils, one sibling, male gender, father's education, late first dental visit, brushing time, mother's education, no dental visit, decreased brushing frequency, and no night brushing.

Keywords: severe early childhood caries; prioritizing risk factors

---

1. Introduction

Early childhood caries (ECC) remains a major unresolved dental public health problem in developing as well as developed countries, despite the continuous trials for implementation of preventive strategies [1,2]. The decline in the prevalence of ECC among children in developed countries cannot be denied but it continues to progress at epidemic proportions in low-middle income countries [3,4].

It has been established in the literature, that any child younger than six years of age presenting with at least one tooth which is decayed (cavitated or non-cavitated), missing (due to caries), or filled tooth surfaces in any primary tooth is suffering from ECC. When the child is younger the condition is more severe and hence the nomenclature "Severe early childhood caries (S-ECC)" [5].

Besides having a higher risk of developing new carious lesions at adolescence and adulthood, children with untreated and neglected S-ECC are prone to complications such as pain, absence from school days, compromised eating habits, and low self-esteem. These consequences will all adversely affect the children's well-being and their oral health-related quality of life (OHQoL) [6,7]. Moreover, the estimated treatment costs and expertise of highly skilled professionals required for treatment of the disease places pressure on the economy, which made it necessary to trace the contributing risk factors of early childhood caries in order to tailor a preventive economic approach to combat the deep-rooted disease [7].

Unfortunately, the risk indicators for the presence of dental caries in young children are far from a handful; in a systematic review, almost 90 risk factors were described [8]. This complex etiology of S-ECC has intrigued researchers to dig deeper into the various risk factors involved besides feeding [9] and oral hygiene practices [10]. Other contributing factors included, but were not limited to; *Streptococcus mutans* levels, active dental problems in parents/caregivers, socioeconomic status, and the onset of the first dental visit [11–13], which all apparently contributed to the risk of developing the disease [8].

Within the limitations of variations and confounders from different samples, as well as the study design itself, the statistical analysis techniques may also lead to different conclusions. As it would be impossible to ignore the multifactorial nature of ECC, and as far as our knowledge there was no study in the literature that places the risk factors in order of significance, our study therefore aimed through meticulous statistical analysis to arrange the "well agreed upon" common risk factors in order of significance in order to aid the clinician in tailoring an adequate preventive program for young children. We present it as an attempt to prioritize or reshuffle the risk factors contributing to severe early childhood caries and place them in the order of their significance.

2. Materials and Methods

2.1. Sampling and Sample Size

A minimal sample size of 108 was calculated using EpiCalc 2000 version 1.02 program (Brixton Health, USA) assuming a power of 80% and alpha = 0.05. It was based on the percentage of oral hygiene practices performed for children ('no brushing' and 'brushing three times/day' were 31.05% and 12.11%, respectively) [14].

We designed a cross-sectional study to analyze and prioritize the risk factors for ECC among preschool children. Prior to the main study, a pilot study was carried out in the Department of Pediatric Dentistry and Dental Public Health, Faculty of Dentistry, Ain Shams University, Cairo, on a group of 25 children. The preliminary study was carried out to evaluate the feasibility of conduct of a larger study and to aid in the calculation of sample size.

2.2. Study Design and Ethical Approval

In considering subject selection, in order to identify children for the study, Cairo was divided into four strata by administrative boundaries (four largest counties in Cairo). Subsequently, three immunization centers were selected in each stratum as primary sampling units and 13 subjects were selected randomly from each primary sampling unit. The project was submitted to and approved by the ethical committee of Ain Shams University. The study was conducted from November 2015 to April 2016. On the days assigned for examination patients attending the facility fulfilling the inclusion criteria were identified, then 13 were chosen with the aid of random tables for each day until the required sample size was reached.

2.3. Inclusion and Exclusion Criteria

Inclusion criteria were normal healthy children aged two to four years. Children with serious medical problems, those attending with a caregiver other than their mother whom the authors thought would not give accurate information in the process of interviewing, or children whose mothers declined to participate were excluded. Another exclusion criterion was previous fluoride varnish application as it could affect the bacterial *Streptococcus mutans* levels.

After their routine oral examination, the mothers were approached, the purpose of the interview was clearly explained; and they were assured that there were no possible side effects for the study on their children; after their verbal approval for participation, they were requested to sign the "Informed Consent" prior to enrollment. The final sample comprised 140 mothers and their preschoolers from the 12 assigned immunization centers.

All parents were motivated by offering preventive procedures such as fluoride application, and educational sessions on the proper oral hygiene measures and the needed dental treatment.

2.4. Data Collection

The study was divided into three stages: stage 1 included the intra-oral examination, stage 2 was the saliva sample collection, and stage 3 was a questionnaire survey.

2.4.1. Intra-Oral Examination

The children's teeth were examined by the principal investigator (N.S.K) who was unaware of the outcome of the mothers' interview by the co-author (S.E).

The intraoral examination was conducted in accordance with WHO (World Health Organization) standards in a well-lit natural light area with the use of disposable plain dental mirrors, gauze wipes, and wooden tongue depressors. Children were examined in a supine position on the examination beds present in the facility, except for those infants who were either required to be held on the lap of their caregiver, or required the "knee to knee" position for examination [3]. A child was considered to be suffering from ECC when he or she complied to the definition of the American Academy of Pediatric Dentistry (AAPD), which defined ECC as the presence of one or more decayed, missing, or filled tooth surface in any primary tooth in a child of 71 months of age or younger, while the term S-ECC is used to describe any sign of smooth surface caries in children younger than three years of age, also from ages three to five, one or more cavitated, missing due to caries, or filled smooth surfaces in primary maxillary anterior teeth or a decayed, missing, or filled score of ≥ 4 (age 3), ≥ 5 (age 4), or ≥ 6 (age 5) surfaces constitutes S-ECC. A white spot lesion or a filled tooth with recurrent caries was considered relevant [5].

2.4.2. Saliva Sample Collection and Estimation of *Streptococcus mutans* (S. *mutans*) Level

Saliva samples were obtained randomly from 25 children suffering from S-ECC, and 15 who were caries-free, as a representative sample for the rest of the population.

Whole saliva was collected between 9.30–11.30 a.m. with the aid of small disposable plastic syringes. The subjects were asked to refrain from eating for one hour before collection. Approximately 2 mL of saliva was collected in a sterile syringe and transported to the microbiology laboratory, then 1 mL aliquot of saliva was transferred to a labeled sterile tube containing 4 mL of broth (thioglycolate broth). The saliva sample was vortexed, to uniformly mix the saliva and the broth, using a cyclomixer.

Using an inoculation loop (4 mm inner diameter), 10 μL of the vortexed 1:5 dilution sample was streaked in duplicate on Mitis salivarius bacitracin agar (MSB) selective for *S. mutans*. The MSB agar plates were incubated anaerobically for 24 to 48 h at 37 °C in 5% CO_2 in nitrogen. After incubation, counts were done for the colonies with morphological characteristic for *S. mutans* on the MSB agar. Identification for *S. mutans* was confirmed by biochemical tests including manitol fermentation and gram staining catalyst test. Colony counting was done with a magnifying glass, and the count of *S. mutans* was expressed as the number of colony forming units per milliliter (CFU/mL) of saliva. The actual colony count was then multiplied by 1×103 on account of the saliva sample having been diluted one thousand times (1:5 dilution) [15–18].

2.4.3. Oral Health Questionnaire

The mothers were interviewed by the researcher (S.E) who was unaware of the outcome of the children's oral examination performed by the other researcher (N.S.K).

A structured questionnaire interview was designed after reviewing the literature, to choose from the most common, relevant, and significant risk factors of ECC [8,13,14,19,20]. It was pre-tested for validity, reliability, and clarity in the department, with the aid of 20 volunteer mothers of young children. During the trial, some questions were found to be confusing. These questions were revised and retested with other volunteering mothers. The responses were recorded through direct interviewing.

The questionnaire included four domains; sociodemographic and socioeconomic factors, oral hygiene measures, feeding practices, and dietary habits.

i   Sociodemographici

Questionnaires were administered to the mothers of participating children to obtain sociodemographic information such as name, gender, age, the number of siblings, level of education of the mothers and fathers, which were categorized into two levels: (a) school only, which included those who had their education limited to school or were school drop outs, and (b) University education or higher degrees. Mothers were asked about the presence of carious cavities or fillings in their mouth; if unsure they were examined for verification. To throw light on the child's oral health, the mother was asked about any previous dental visit, whether it was early, late, or whether there had not been a previous visit at all.

ii   Oral hygiene practice

In this domain, mothers were asked about their child's brushing frequency. Answers were categorized into 'no brushing', 'brushing once or twice/week', 'once/day', and 'twice/day'. They were specifically asked if brushing was performed at night or any random time. Finally, they were asked if brushing was self-implemented or performed by the mother.

iii   Feeding practice

Dietary and nutritional information involved questions about whether the child was breast or bottle fed. History of whether nighttime and on demand feedings was practiced. Weaning age of the child and whether the household shared the same utensils, specifically the spoon, was also investigated.

iv   Dietary Habits

Information was collected about consumption of food containing sugar, which was referred to as "sugary food", sweets, and drinks as well as fruit juices (answers were categorized into 'never', 'once a week', 'two or three times/week', 'once/day', 'two or three times/day', and 'several times/day').

2.5. Statistical Analysis

- Both the questionnaire and oral examination forms were manually checked for completion of the required information. Data was collected, recorded in a standardized form, and then entered into the SPSS software for statistical analysis.
- Chi-square test was performed for each categorical variable to assess whether significant differences were observed between the two groups (Figures 1–4).
- Spearman correlation was used to find the correlation between the different risk factors and the log streptococcal count (Table 1).
- A logistic regression model was used to identify risk factors for caries development among children by considering independent variables simultaneously (Table 2). A p-value < 0.05 was considered statistically significant.
- The odds ratio was calculated for all possible risk factors associated with the prevalence of EEC and arranged in descending order after omitting all the insignificant variables, which was the main idea of the study (Table 3).

3. Results

Chi-square was performed on variables in each of the four assigned domains (Figures 1–4).

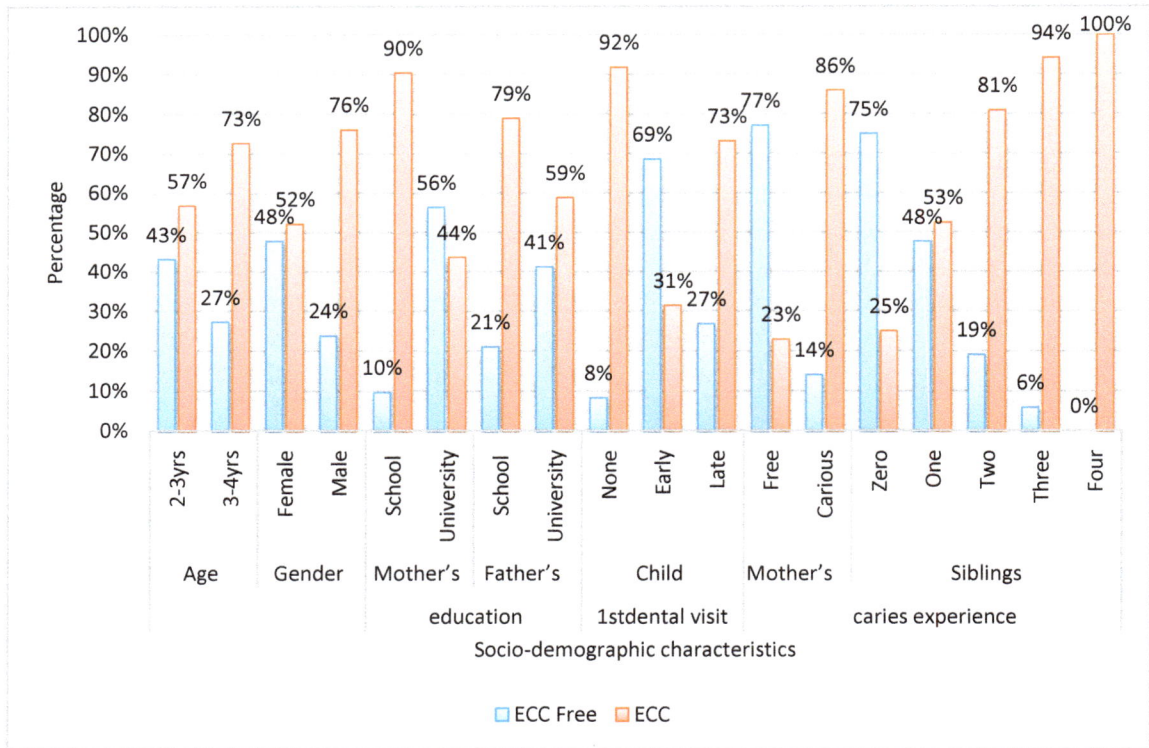

Figure 1. Bar chart comparing between early childhood caries (ECC)-free and children with ECC with regards to socio-demographic characteristics.

There were statistically significant differences among children with ECC and caries-free children in all socio-demographic data.

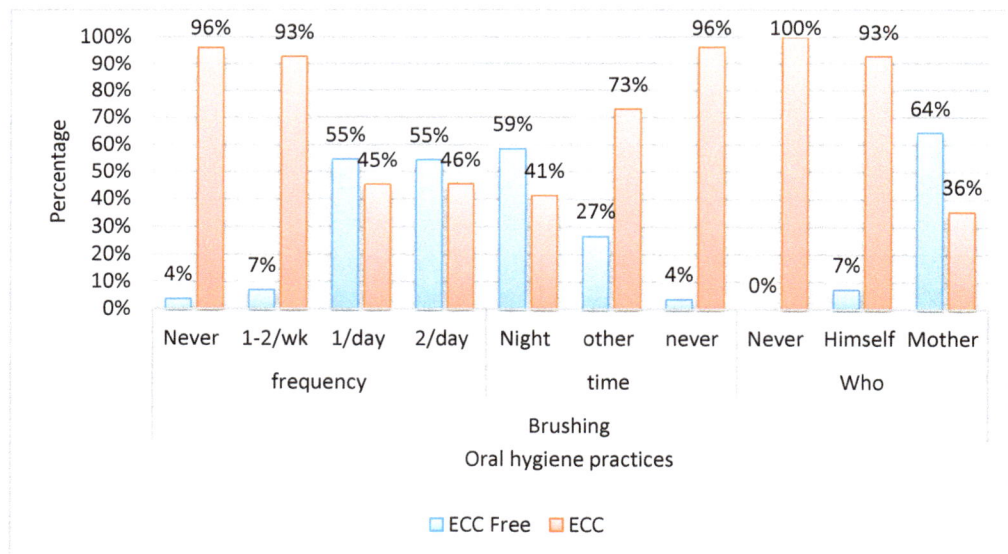

Figure 2. Bar chart comparing between children with ECC and ECC-free in regards to oral hygiene practice.

Regarding the oral hygiene practices, there was a highly significant statistical difference, between children with ECC and caries-free children in all the studied aspects. In ECC, the higher percentage of children either never brushed or employed self-brushing only once or twice a week.

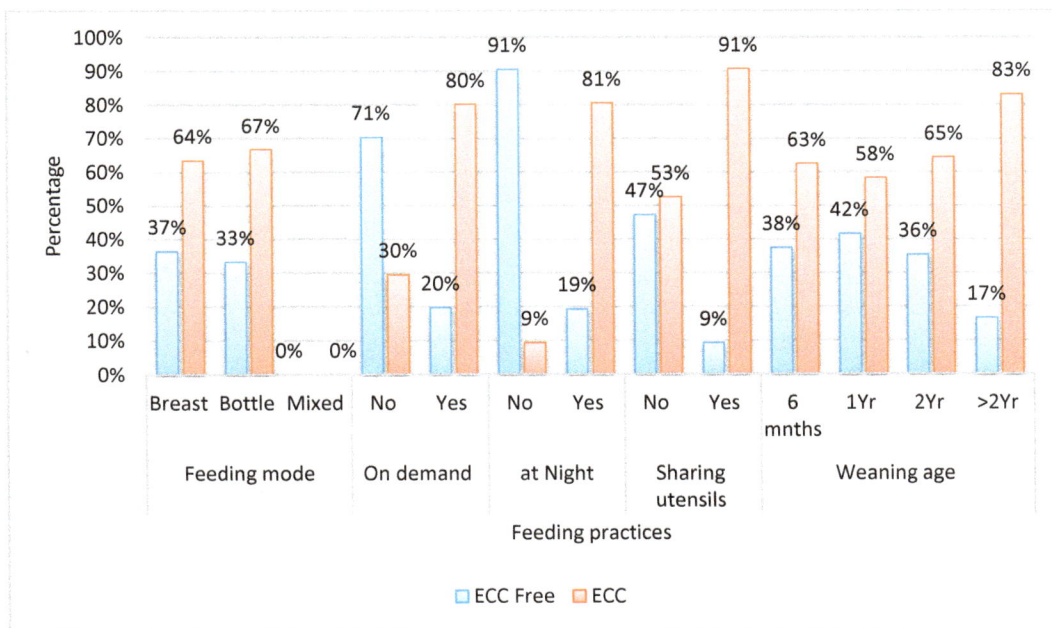

Figure 3. Bar chart comparing between children with ECC and ECC-free regards feeding practices.

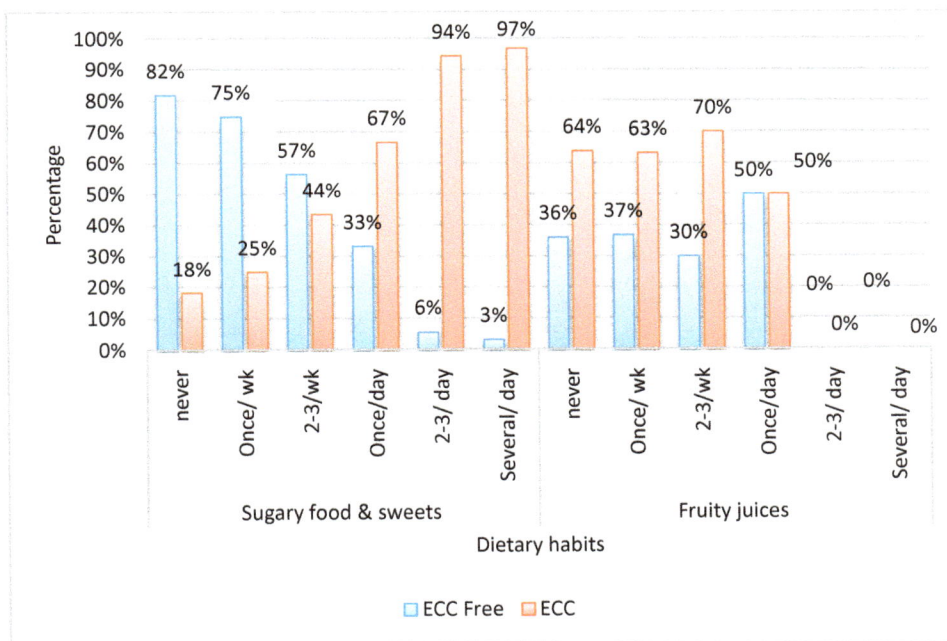

Figure 4. Bar chart comparing between children with ECC and ECC-free regards dietary practices.

Regarding the consumption of sugary food and sweets, a highly significant statistical difference existed between the two groups, while none was encountered regarding the consumption of fruit juices.

As displayed in Table 1, there were direct correlations between male gender, mother's current caries experience, the number of siblings, feeding on demand, night feeding, sharing utensils, sugary food intake frequency, and log. Streptococcal count in both groups.

While there was an inverse correlation between mother's and father's education, earlier child first visit, increased brushing frequency, night brushing, who brushes (mother), and log. Streptococcal count.

Table 1. Correlation between risk factors and log. Streptococcal count.

Risk Factors	Log. Streptococcal Count	
	Rho	p-Value
Age	−0.034	0.693
Male gender	0.287	0.001 **
Mother's education	−0.483	<0.001 **
Father's education	−0.198	0.019 *
Child's first dental visit	−0.364	<0.001 **
Mother's current caries experience	0.530	<0.001 **
Siblings	0.400	<0.001 **
Brushing frequency	−0.605	<0.001 **
Brushing time	−0.602	<0.001 **
Who brushes	−0.774	<0.001 **
Feeding on demand	0.452	<0.001 **
Night feeding	0.518	<0.001 **
Sharing utensils	0.420	<0.001 **
Sugary food intake frequency	0.584	<0.001 **

Spearman Correlations, ** HS = highly significant, <0.01 * S = significant. <0.05.

Table 2. Logistic regression analysis of the most predictable risk factors associated with prevalence of ECC.

Risk Factors		p-Value	Exp. (β)	95.0% C.I. for Exp. (β)
Night feeding	No	Ref.		
	Yes	0.012 *	44.48	2.32–853.99
Mothers' current caries experience	No	Ref.		
	Yes	<0.001 **	29.30	4.95–173.47
Gender	No	Ref.		
	Yes	0.017 *	11.54	1.56–85.54
Child's first dental visit	None	0.022 *	Ref.	
	Late	0.961	1.069	0.073–15.74
	Early	0.031 *	0.068	0.006–0.78
Brushing time	Never	0.294	Ref.	
	Others	0.183	0.070	0.001–3.50
	Night	0.117	0.048	0.001–2.15
Brushing frequency	Never	0.424	Ref.	
	1/day	0.194	11.02	0.30–409.85
	2/day	0.552	1.72	0.29–10.18
Mother's education	School	Ref.		
	University	0.175	0.094	0.003–2.87
Father's education	School	Ref.		
	University	0.274	6.27	0.23–168.34
On demand feeding	No	Ref.		
	Yes	0.177	4.08	0.53–31.44
Sharing utensils	No	Ref.		
	Yes	0.648	0.607	0.71–5.16

** HS = highly significant, <0.01 * S = significant. <0.05; Ref = Reference.

Possible risk factors of socio-demographic characteristics, feeding practices, and oral hygiene practices were adjusted into a regression model. Number of siblings, who brushes, and sugar consumption variables could not be entered into the regression since one cell of the table was empty.

After adjustment for the other possible risk factors, children who were night feeding, whose mothers had current caries experience, and with male gender predominance, will have a greater chance to develop ECC by 44.48, 29.30, and 11.54 times, respectively, than those who were not night feeding, had caries-free mothers, and a female gender predominance. Children who benefited from early dental visits had less chance to develop ECC than those who never visited the dentist by 93.2%.

To override the omitted variables, finally, the odds ratio was performed for all four domains then combined and arranged in one table (Table 3) in descending order (starting with the highest odds ratio) after omitting the non-significant variables. This table represents the core of the study or it is the "master table" as it displays the various risk factors in order of significance which gave us the opportunity to prioritize these factors instead of just counting them collectively.

Table 3. Odd's ratio of possible risk factors associated with prevalence of ECC (Master Table).

Risk Factor		ECC Free (n = 50)	ECC (n = 90)	OR	95% CI	p-Value
Frequency of Sugary Food Consumption	Never	18(81.8%)	4(18.2%)	Ref.		
	Several/Day	1(3.2%)	30(96.8%)	135.0	13.98–1303.95	<0.001 **
	Two to Three Times/Day	2(5.6%)	34(94.4%)	76.50	12.76–458.63	<0.001 **
Three Siblings	Zero	21(75.0%)	7(25.0%)	Ref.		
	Three	1(5.9%)	16(94.1%)	48.0	5.35–430.57	0.001 **
Night Feeding	No	29(90.6%)	3(9.4%)	Ref.		
	Yes	21(19.4%)	87(80.6%)	40.05	11.13–144.13	<0.001 **
Who Brushes	Mother	47(64.4%)	26(35.6%)	Ref.		
	Himself	3(7.3%)	38(92.7%)	22.90	6.43–81.48	<0.001 **
Mother's Caries Experience	Free	37(77.1%)	11(22.9%)	Ref.		
	Carious	13(14.1%)	79(85.9%)	20.44	8.37–49.92	<0.001 **
Two Siblings	Zero	21(75.0%)	7(25.0%)	Ref.		
	Two	9(19.1%)	38(80.9%)	12.67	4.12–38.91	<0.001 **
On Demand Feeding	No	31(70.5%)	13(29.5%)	Ref.		
	Yes	19(19.8%)	77(80.2%)	9.66	4.26–21.93	<0.001 **
Sugary Food Once/Day	Never	18(81.8%)	4(18.2%)	Ref.		
	Once/Day	4(33.3%)	8(66.7%)	9.0	1.79–45.34	0.008 **
Sharing Utensils	No	46(47.4%)	51(52.6%)	Ref.		
	Yes	4(9.3%)	39(90.7%)	8.79	2.92–26.51	<0.001 **
One Sibling	Zero	21(75.0%)	7(25.0%)	Ref.		
	One	19(47.5%)	21(52.5%)	3.32	1.15–9.54	0.026 *
Gender	Female	33(47.8%)	36(52.2%)	Ref.		
	Male	17(23.9%)	54(76.1%)	2.91	1.42–5.99	0.004 **
Father's Education	School	8(21.1%)	30(78.9%)	Ref.		
	University	42(41.2%)	60(58.8%)	0.381	0.16–0.91	0.030 *
Late First Child Dental Visit	None	4(8.3%)	44(91.7%)	Ref.		
	Late	11(26.8%)	30(73.2%)	0.248	0.072–0.852	<0.027 *
Brushing Time	Never	34(58.6%)	24(41.4%)	Ref.		
	Others	1(3.8%)	25(96.2%)	0.109	0.014–0.879	0.037 *
Mother's Education	School	6(9.7%)	56(90.3%)	Ref.		
	University	44(56.4%)	34(43.6%)	0.083	0.03–0.21	<0.001 **
Early First Child Dental Visit	None	4(8.3%)	44(91.7%)	Ref.		
	Early	35(68.6%)	16(31.4%)	0.042	0.013–0.136	<0.001 **
Brushing Frequency	Never	1(3.8%)	25(96.2%)	Ref.		
	Once/Day	29(54.7%)	24(45.3%)	0.033	0.004–0.263	0.001 **
	Twice/Day	18(54.5%)	15(45.5%)	0.033	0.004–0.276	0.002 **
Brushing Time	Never	34(58.6%)	24(41.4%)	Ref.		
	Night	15(26.8%)	41(73.2%)	0.028	0.004–0.223	0.001 **

** HS = highly significant <0.01 * S = significant <0.05, Ref = odds ratio reference.

Caries was found to develop more in children with one, two, and three siblings than those with zero siblings by a rate of 3.32, 12.67, and 48 times, respectively.

A higher risk of caries was found in children whose mothers had previous caries experience by 20.44 times more than those whose mothers were caries-free.

Children with male gender predominance had a greater chance of 2.91 times more than females to develop caries.

Children who had a late or early first dental visit had less chance to develop caries than those who never had dental visits by 75.2% and 95.8%, respectively. The children whose mothers and fathers had a university education had less chance to develop caries than those whose mother's and father's education was limited to school by 91.7% and 61.9%, respectively. Children with bushing frequency twice/day and once/day had less chance to develop ECC than those who never brushed by 96.7%.

Children who performed night brushing or no specified brushing time had less chance to develop ECC than those who never brushed by 97.2% and 89.1%, respectively. The children who were responsible for their own oral hygiene practices had a greater chance to develop ECC by 22.90 times more than those whose mothers were responsible for brushing.

Night feeding, feeding on demand, and sharing utensils was related to a higher chance of developing ECC by 40.05, 9.66, and 8.79 times, respectively, more than those not practicing these habits. Children with the frequency of sugary food intake once/day, two to three times/day, and several times/day had greater chance to develop ECC by 9.0, 76.50, and 135.0 times, respectively, more than those whose frequency of sugary food intake was never.

4. Discussion

Severe ECC remains a cause of both social and economic burden throughout the world. It has also been proven to affect the child's quality of life; therefore, it is mandatory for those interested in the improvement of public health to be cognizant of the deterioration in the level of oral health and increase in dental caries, and to direct their efforts towards the prevention of these problems [21,22].

A deeper insight into the risk factors of ECC is always of value to aid in its prevention and management. As previously mentioned, a systematic review stated that almost 90 risk factors were described for ECC; as such, the authors chose those that were agreed upon and repeated in most of the studies present in the review [8]. The findings of our study agreed with several others in most of the different variables in the tested domains, but our main aim was to prioritize the risk factors in an order of significance in order to shed light on the weight of each isolated variable as a caries risk indicator.

The collection of data on children's lifestyle factors and sociodemographic factors was performed by direct interviewing of parents rather than having them fill in a questionnaire by themselves in order to avoid misinterpretation of questions, which was noticed during the pilot study. Face to face questionnaires were assumed by some researchers to be "image enhancing" because subjects will attempt to say what they knew was right, rather than what they actually practiced [23], yet the low educational and socioeconomic level of many of the patients examined, made it impossible to conduct a self-administered questionnaire.

An age group of two to four years was chosen due to the difficulty of finding a caries-free cohort older than this age, as revealed from the results. The mean age of children with S-ECC was found to be higher than the caries free group. This finding was consistent with several studies that related this to the fact that older children have been exposed to cariogenic challenges for a longer time [8,10]. Further explanation to this can be attributed to the fact that as the age of the child increases the nature of food consumption differs (i.e., as children grow older especially at school age, they tend to consume more sweets).

Based on the clinical examination of children, the mean value of DMFT (dental caries index) in children with S-ECC was found to be 9.96 ± 3.86, which was close to other studies in developing countries [24,25].

In our study, boys have been reported to have a higher prevalence of caries compared to girls, with the results being highly significant ($p < 0.001$). This finding was consistent with some studies [10,26], which could suggest that the mothers, especially in low socioeconomic status countries such as Egypt, tend to prefer and indulge boys, therefore they parent them differently. This is interpreted by giving them more sweets and hence they have a higher tendency for caries development [27].

Interestingly, the number of siblings in the family was a strong significant risk factor in the present study. The more siblings the child has, the more his or her risk to develop S-ECC. This goes in agreement with several studies, especially in families having more than two children [28,29]. One explanation for this is that in large families, parents' attention towards their children's oral health is shared or divided between the larger number of siblings, thereby less care is provided for each child and chances to have oral problems increase. Also, horizontal transmission may play a role in this domain.

The maternal and paternal educational level was inversely proportional to the presence of S-ECC in children. The results were similar to another study that attributed this finding to the lack of information and education about oral health care for children of minimally educated or uneducated parents [30,31]. However, the effect of paternal education seemed to be stronger as it probably reflects the socioeconomic level of the family [28].

In the present study, mothers' current caries experience appeared to be an important factor in the development of S-ECC in children and the results were highly significant ($p < 0.001$). This was consistent with a study that reported evidence of maternal transmission of S. mutans in 41% of mother/child pairs [32]. A mother's continuous contact with their children was interpreted by higher influence on child's oral hygiene measures as compared to a father's whose employment status, and education did not affect their children.

Children who had a late first dental visit or no dental visits at all tend to be more liable to develop dental caries. A possible interpretation for this could be that early dental visits provide an excellent opportunity for educating parents on proper guidelines for promoting their child's oral health, especially among low socioeconomic groups where oral health is not considered a priority [33].

Regarding early feeding habits, the current study revealed no significant difference in caries experience between children who were breast or bottle fed. Our results were consistent with a systematic review revealing that the interaction of risk factors and intraoral bacterial load might carry a greater responsibility than the mode of feeding [28,34]. In addition, although children suffering from S-ECC were weaned at an older age than those in caries-free group, this difference was insignificant. Despite that, a significant association was detected in our research between overnight and on demand feeding and development of S-ECC. Night feeding decreases the clearance of liquid carbohydrates from the oral cavity due to decreased salivary flow at night. On the other hand, on demand feeding leads to increased amounts of fermentable carbohydrates in the mouth and early colonization by oral S. mutans [35]. Interestingly, this goes in line with a study attributing S-ECC mainly to the frequency of feeding rather than the age of weaning [36].

Considering other habits that could have a direct influence on bacterial transmission and caries incidence, sharing utensils was significantly more common in the S-ECC group as compared to the S-ECC free group. This explains why international guidelines for prevention of ECC [37] encourage parents to stop bacterial transmission to their children through sharing food, drinks, utensils, toothbrushes, and other items [32].

The sugary food intake frequency was higher among children with S-ECC than those who were caries-free. This was consistent with most of the literature which showed that caries incidence increases when the number of sugar containing snacks increased to more than four times a day [8]. Concerning the question regarding sugary snacks, it was explained to the caregivers to report any intake of sticky sweets as such as candies, marshmallows, and lollipops, etc. Although the nature of the food consumed played a role in the development of S-ECC, the scope of the study was not to categorize the sugar containing sweets, but rather to consider them as a single entity and prioritize how the frequency of their consumption ranked their weight as a risk factor for S-ECC. Children who consumed more sugary food, sweets, and sweetened beverages showed a significantly higher risk of developing S-ECC ($p = 0.001$) and this can be interpreted by the high sucrose content of confectionaries and sweetened beverages, since sucrose is considered the main carbohydrate responsible for the development of dental caries [33].

Among the beverages consumed that had a controversial relationship with the development of S-ECC in the literature were fruit juices [8]. In our study, there was a negative correlation between the consumption of 100% fruit juices and the presence of ECC ($p < 0.001$). On the other hand, artificially sweetened beverages most commonly contain sucrose or high fructose corn syrup, which are more effectively metabolized by Sm, while 100% juices contain fructose and glucose without sucrose [33].

From the results of this study it was shown that the ECC-free group adhered more to proper oral hygiene practices, especially the frequency of brushing ($p < 0.001$), regular brushing at night time ($p = 0.005$), as well as performance of the oral hygiene measures by the caregiver instead of the child himself ($p = 0.001$). Those results simulated a study, showing that parental training to brush their child's teeth and daily frequency of tooth brushing are major determinants in S-ECC [38]. Another study stated that S-ECC is more common among children who commenced brushing at an age older than 24 months [24] and hence oral hygiene measures should be implemented as early as the eruption of the first tooth.

5. Conclusions

This study prioritized the risk factors contributing to severe early childhood caries and placed them in the order of their significance as follows: snacking of sugary food several times a day, increased number of siblings to three or more, night feeding, child self-employed brushing, mother's caries experience, two siblings, on demand feeding, once/day sugary food, sharing utensils, one sibling, male gender, father's education, late first child dental visit, brushing time, mother's education, no dental visit, decreased brushing frequency, and no night brushing.

Acknowledgments: The authors would like to thank all the children and mothers who participated in this self-funded study. We have not received funds for covering the costs to publish in open access.

Author Contributions: Noha Samir Kabil conceived and designed the experiments; Noha Samir Kabil and Sherif Eltawil performed the experiments; Noha Samir Kabil analyzed the data; Noha Samir Kabil and Sherif Eltawil wrote the paper.

Conflicts of Interest: The authors declare no conflict of interest. The study was totally self-funded.

References

1.   Nobile, C.G.; Fortunato, L.; Bianco, A.; Pileggi, C.; Pavia, M. Pattern and severity of early childhood caries in Southern Italy: A preschool-based cross-sectional study. *BMC Public Health* **2014**, *14*. [CrossRef] [PubMed]

2.   Zhou, Y.; Lin, H.C.; Lo, E.C.M.; Wong, M.C.M. Risk indicators for early childhood caries in 2-year-old children in southern China. *Aust. Dent. J.* **2011**, *56*, 33–39. [CrossRef] [PubMed]

3.   Olatosi, O.; Inem, V.; Sofola, O.; Prakash, P.; Sote, E. The prevalence of early childhood caries and its associated risk factors among preschool children referred to a tertiary care institution. *Niger. J. Clin. Pract.* **2015**, *18*, 493–501. [CrossRef] [PubMed]

4.   Carino, K.M.; Shinada, K.; Kawaguchi, Y. Early childhood caries in Northern Philippines. *Community Dent. Oral Epidemiol.* **2003**, *3*, 81–89. [CrossRef]

5.   American Academy of Pediatric Dentistry (AAPD). *Definition of Early Childhood Caries (ECC)*; AAPD: Chicago, IL, USA, 2008; Volume 4, p. 15.

6.   Lee, G.H.; McGrath, C.; Yiu, C.K.; King, N.M. A comparison of a generic and oral health–specific measure in assessing the impact of early childhood caries on quality of life. *Community Dent. Oral Epidemiol.* **2010**, *38*, 333–339. [CrossRef] [PubMed]

7.   Casamassimo, P.S.; Thikkurissy, S.; Edelstein, B.L.; Maiorini, E. Beyond the dmft: The human and economic cost of early childhood caries. *J. Am. Dent. Assoc.* **2009**, *140*, 650–657. [CrossRef] [PubMed]

8.   Harris, R.; Nicoll, A.D.; Adair, P.M.; Pine, C.M. Risk factors for dental caries in young children: A systematic review of the literature. *Community Dent. Health* **2004**, *21*, 71–85. [PubMed]

9. Kolker, J.L.; Yuan, Y.; Burt, B.A.; Sandretto, A.M.; Sohn, W.; Lang, S.W.; Ismail, A.I. Dental caries and dietary patterns in low-income African-American children. *Paediatr. Dent.* **2007**, *29*, 257–264.

10. Gibson, S.; Williams, S. Dental caries in pre-school children: Associations with social class, toothbrushing habit and consumption of sugars and sugar-containing foods. *Caries Res.* **1999**, *33*, 101–113. [CrossRef] [PubMed]

11. Schroth, R.J.; Halchuk, S.; Star, L.A.C. Prevalence and risk factors of caregiver reported Severe Early Childhood Caries in Manitoba First Nations children: Results from the RHS Phase 2 (2008–2010). *Int. J. Circumpolar Health* **2013**, *72*, 1–10. [CrossRef] [PubMed]

12. Warren, J.J.; Weber-Gasparoni, K.; Marshall, T.A.; Drake, D.R.; Dehkordi-Vakil, F.; Dawson, D.V.; Tharp, K.M. A longitudinal study of dental caries risk among very young low SES children. *Community Dent. Oral Epidemiol.* **2009**, *37*, 116–122. [CrossRef] [PubMed]

13. Van Palenstein Helderman, W.H.; Soe, W.; Van't Hof, M.A. Risk factors of early childhood caries in a Southeast Asian population. *J. Dent. Res.* **2006**, *85*, 85–88. [CrossRef] [PubMed]

14. Hamila, N. Early Childhood Caries and Certain Risk Factors in a Sample of Children 1–3.5 Years in Tanta. *Dentistry* **2013**, *4*, 1–7. [CrossRef]

15. Nascimento Filho, E.; Mayer, M.P.; Pontes, P.; Pignatari, A.C.; Weckx, L.L. Caries prevalence, levels of mutans streptococci, and gingival and plaque indices in 3.0 to 5.0 old mouth breathing children. *Caries Res.* **2004**, *38*, 572–575. [CrossRef] [PubMed]

16. Axelsson, P. *Diagnosis and Risk Prediction of Dental Caries*; Quintessence Publishing Co. Inc.: Varmland, Sweden, 2000; Volume 2, pp. 156–168.

17. Jenen, B.; Brathall, D. A new method for the estimation of mutans streptococci in human saliva. *J. Dent. Res.* **1989**, *68*, 468–471. [CrossRef]

18. Pidamale, R.; Sowmya, B.; Thomas, A.; Jose, T.; Madhusudan, K.K.; Prasad, G. Association between early childhood caries, streptococcus mutans level and genetic sensitivity levels to the bitter taste of, 6-*N* propylthiouracil among the children below 71 months of age. *Dent. Res. J.* **2012**, *9*, 730–734.

19. Almushayt, A.S.; Sharaf, A.A.; El-Meligy, O.A.; Tallab, H.Y. Dietary and Feeding Habits in a Sample of Preschool Children in Severe Early Childhood Caries (S-ECC). *JKAU Med. Sci.* **2009**, *16*, 13–36. [CrossRef]

20. Mahesh, R.; Muthu, M.S.; Rodrigues, S.J.L. Risk factors for early childhood caries: A case–control study. *Eur. Arch. Paediatr. Dent.* **2013**, *14*, 331–337. [CrossRef] [PubMed]

21. Bagramian, R.A.; Garcia-Godoy, F.; Volpe, A.R. The global increase in dental caries. A pending public health crisis. *Am. J. Dent.* **2009**, *22*, 3–8. [PubMed]

22. Mani, S.; John, J.; Ping, W.; Ismail, N. *Early Childhood Caries: Parent's Knowledge, Attitude and Practice towards Its Prevention in Malaysia*; INTECH Open Access Publisher: Rijeka, Croatia, 2012; pp. 3–19.

23. El-Nadeef, M.I.; Hassab, H.; Al-Hosani, E. National survey of the oral health of 5-year-old children in the United Arab Emirates. *East. Mediterr. Health J.* **2010**, *16*, 51–55. [PubMed]

24. Farooki, F.A.; Khabeer, A.; Moheet, I.A.; Khan, S.Q.; Farooq, I.; ArRejaie, A.S. Prevalence of dental caries in primary and permanent teeth and its relation with tooth brushing habits among schoolchildren in eastern Saudi Arabia. *Saudi Med. J.* **2015**, *36*, 737–742. [CrossRef] [PubMed]

25. Schroth, R.J.; Cheba, V. Determining the Prevalence and Risk Factors for Early Childhood Caries in a Community Dental Health Clinic. *Pediatr. Dent.* **2007**, *5*, 387–396.

26. Maciel, S.; Marcenes, W.; Watt, R.; Sheiham, A. The relationship between sweetness preference and dental caries in mother/child pairs from Maringá-Pr, BraziLac. *Int. Dent. J.* **2001**, *51*, 83–88. [CrossRef] [PubMed]

27. Corrêa-Faria, P.; Martins-Júnior, P.A.; Vieira-Andrade, R.G.; Marques, L.S.; Ramos-Jorge, M.L.A.C. Factors associated with the development of early childhood caries among Brazilian preschoolers. *Braz. Oral Res.* **2013**, *27*, 356–362. [CrossRef] [PubMed]

28. Tiberia, M.; Milnes, A.R.; Feigal, R.; Morley, K.; Richardson, D.; Croft, W.; Cheung, W. Risk factors for early childhood caries in Canadian preschool children seeking care. *Pediatr. Dent.* **2007**, *29*, 201–208. [PubMed]

29. Manchanda, K.; Sampath, N.; De Sarkar, A. Evaluating the effectiveness of oral health education program among mothers with 6–18 months children in prevention of early childhood caries. *Contemp. Clin. Dent.* **2014**, *5*, 478–483. [CrossRef] [PubMed]

30. Plutzer, K.; Keirse, M.J.N.C. Influence of first-time mothers' early employment on severe early childhood caries in their child. *Int. J. Pediatr.* **2012**, *8*, 26–32. [CrossRef] [PubMed]

31. Stephen, C.; John, S. Maternal Transmission of Mutans Streptococci in Severe-Early Childhood Caries. *Pediatr. Dent.* **2009**, *29*, 997–1003.

32. Ghazal, T.; Levy, S.; Childers, N.; Broffitt, B.; Cutter, G.; Wiener, H.; Kempf, M.; Warren, J.; Cavanaugh, J. Factors associated with early childhood caries incidence among high caries-risk children. *Community Dent. Oral Epidemiol.* **2015**, *43*, 366–374. [CrossRef] [PubMed]

33. Perera, P.J.; Fernando, M.P.; Warnakulasooriya, T.D.; Ranathunga, N. Effect of feeding practices on dental caries among preschool children: A hospital-based analytical cross-sectional study. *Asia Pac. J. Clin. Nutr.* **2014**, *23*, 272–277. [PubMed]

34. Choi, E.; Lee, S.; Kim, Y. Quantitative real-time polymerase chain reaction for Streptococcus mutans and Streptococcus sobrinus in dental plaque samples and its association with early childhood caries. *Int. J. Paediatr. Dent.* **2009**, *19*, 141–147. [CrossRef] [PubMed]

35. Feldens, C.; Giugliani, E.; Vigo, A.; Vítolo, M. Early feeding practices and severe early childhood caries in four-year-old children from southern Brazil: A birth cohort study. *Caries Res.* **2010**, *44*, 445–452. [CrossRef] [PubMed]

36. American Academy of Pediatric Dentistry (AAPD). Guideline on Perinatal Oral Health Care. AAPD: Chicago, IL, USA, 2011; Volume 38, pp. 140–145.

37. Jiang, E.; Lo, E.; Chu, C.; Wong, M. Prevention of early childhood caries (ECC) through parental tooth brushing training and fluoride varnish application: A 24-month randomized controlled trial. *J. Dent.* **2014**, *42*, 1543–1550. [CrossRef] [PubMed]

38. Retnakumari, N.; Cyriac, G. Childhood caries as influenced by maternal and child characteristics in preschool children of Kerala-an epidemiological study. *Contemp. Clin. Dent.* **2012**, *3*, 2–8. [CrossRef] [PubMed]

17

Dental Attendance in Undocumented Immigrants before and after the Implementation of a Personal Assistance Program: A Cross-Sectional Observational Study

Martijn Lambert🆔

Department of Community Dentistry and Oral Epidemiology, Special Needs in Oral Health, Ghent University, 9000 Ghent, Belgium; Martijn.Lambert@UGent.be;

Abstract: Undocumented immigrants are a high-risk social group with low access to care. The present study aims to increase awareness and dental attendance in this subgroup, assisted by community health workers (CHW). Starting from 2015, two trained dentists volunteered to perform free oral health examinations and further dental care referral in a welfare organisation in Ghent, Belgium. In 2016 and 2017, a two-day oral health training was added, enabling social workers to operate as community oral health workers and to provide personal oral health advice and assistance. Over the three years, an oral health examination was performed on 204 clients from 1 to 69 years old, with a mean age of 36.7 (SD = 15.9), showing high levels of untreated caries (71.6%; $n = 146$) and a Dutch Periodontal Screening Index (DPSI) score of 3 or 4 in 62.2% of the sample ($n = 97$). Regarding dental attendance, the total number of missed appointments decreased significantly, with 40.9% in 2015, 11.9% in 2016 and 8.0% in 2017 ($p < 0.001$). Undocumented immigrants can be integrated into professional oral health care. Personal assistance by community health workers might be an effective method, although this requires further investigation.

Keywords: undocumented immigrants; oral health care; community health workers

1. Introduction

Undocumented immigrants are a very vulnerable social subgroup, consisting of a considerable number of people trying to remain undiscovered by local authorities. In contrast to asylum seekers and recognised refugees, they do not have a residence permit to stay legally in the country. Their estimated number varies between 7% and 13% of the total number of immigrants with an official residence permit [1]. In Belgium, there were 1,214,605 legal immigrants on the 1 January 2014, which means that the number of undocumented immigrants probably lies between 85,000 and 160,000, corresponding to approximately 1% of the total Belgian population [2].

Although epidemiological data on the oral health of undocumented immigrants are scarce, some authors previously described the oral health and oral health needs of refugees in general [3–5]. According to these publications, oral diseases are highly prevalent in refugees and care provision is impeded by several barriers. It can be assumed that the oral health conditions of undocumented immigrants and their access to care are comparable or even worse, because they cannot register for an official health care insurance. However, according to the United Nations International Bill of Human Rights (1966), every individual has the right to "urgent medical care", including dental care, whether he or she has a residence status or not. Belgium ratified this universal human right and integrated it into its legislation in 1996.

In Belgium, the medical assistance provided to undocumented immigrants is financed by the federal government and organised at city level, and care can be both preventive and curative. To apply for it, people have to meet three criteria: they have been living for longer than three months in the country without permission to stay, they live in the city in which they apply for help, and they do not have a substantial income. In addition, a registered doctor or dentist needs to confirm the need for medical treatment.

Since the organisation of urgent medical care occurs at city level, there are local differences in care provision between different cities. In Ghent, Belgium, undocumented immigrants can obtain a "medical card", allowing them to receive medical treatments for a three month period, which can be repeated for as long as the three previously mentioned conditions are met. The medical card covers every treatment which is reimbursed by Belgian Social Security. Regarding dentistry, the medical card has two main shortcomings: it does not cover tooth extractions for people under the age of 53, nor provision of a removable denture for people under the age of 50.

The present survey originates from a purely voluntary-based project in "De Tinten", an organisation providing material and social assistance to illegal immigrants in Ghent, Belgium. In 2015, the organisation started to refer its clients to local dental clinics, driven by the high demand for dental care. However, the initial rate of missed appointments was so high (9 out of 22) that further collaboration between the organisation and the local dentists was put at stake.

In order to improve the system of referral and to increase dental attendance, the organisation set up a collaboration with researchers from Ghent university in 2016. To reduce barriers between both care providers and care demanders, the involvement of community health workers (CHW) was proposed. The involvement of CHWs in primary care showed to be an efficient way to guide underprivileged individuals towards preventive care and social services, reducing resource utilisation and community costs [6]. CHWs can also play an active role in oral health care. Benzian et al. composed a global competency matrix for oral health, involving many health professionals and groups in society, including CHWs [7]. Since oral health care provision in Belgium is almost exclusively founded upon the shoulders of the dentist, a CHW can be a valuable intermediary in oral health promotion and referral to oral health care. Greenberg et al. demonstrated the positive impact of dental case managers on Medicaid beneficiaries' (low-income individuals) use of dental services and the number of dentists participating in the Medicaid program [8].

The present survey aims to describe the preliminary results of referring undocumented immigrants to the dental practitioner, assisted by community health workers (CHW). Apart from reporting the oral health status of the participants, the main hypothesis is the following: Is the proportion of undocumented immigrants missing their appointment with external dentists the same before and after providing personal assistance?

2. Materials and Methods

The present cross-sectional study, which was based on annual convenience samples, describes the evolution in the proportion of missed dental appointments in undocumented immigrants in Ghent, Belgium, from February 2015 to December 2017. The study was carried out in "De Tinten", an organisation providing material and social assistance to undocumented immigrants in the city of Ghent.

Starting from February 2015, two trained dentists volunteered to perform free oral health examinations and dental interviews on a two-weekly base in a separated room in the organisation building. After oral consent, clients were interviewed on age, nationality and smoking habits. Nationalities were grouped according to the world health organization WHO (world health organization) regions. Individual oral health parameters included D_3MFT, which is the total number of decayed (at cavitation level), missing (due to caries) and filled teeth [9]. Based on the D_3MFT scores, a restorative index ($RI = (FT/(D_3 + FT)) \times 100$) and treatment index ($TI = (M + FT)/(D_3 + M + FT) \times 100$) were calculated in order to gain insights regarding the level of care. Severity of untreated dental caries was assessed using PUFA index, counting the number of teeth with visible pulp exposure, ulcerations, fistula and abscesses [10]. The plaque index of Sillness and Löe was used to measure the amount of dental plaque [11]. Periodontal health was assessed by using the Dutch Periodontal Screening Index (DPSI) for participants older than 15 years old. This index describes the severity of periodontal disease (attachment loss around the teeth) and the need for further treatment on a scale from 0 to 4, after sounding the gums with a periodontal probe [12]. After the oral health examination, clients received a professional referral letter, as well as a dental goody bag, containing a toothbrush and toothpaste. Clients could apply for new toothpaste and a toothbrush every 8 weeks, even without oral health examination or referral. Before getting an appointment with an external dental clinic, all clients were required to obtain a "medical card" from the Ghent Social Welfare Organisation, confirming their undocumented status and allowing them to receive further medical care. Accordingly, only participants without a residence permit were included in the survey.

Starting from August 2016, the two-weekly oral health examinations remained unaltered, but the medical setting of the organisation changed, by training volunteers from the organisation to operate as community oral health workers. The training was held during a two-day program, and included provision of essential information on the normal development and anatomy of human dentition, oral diseases, preventive oral health, dental administration, motivational interviewing and case management. It was performed by two university researchers (one dentist and one psychologist), providing theoretical knowledge, clinical images, practical exercises and cases using an interactive PowerPoint presentation. In addition to the educational program, participants could consult and rehearse all information on a website (www.iedersmondgezond.be), which was specifically designed for the CHWs. As part of the website, a registration system was designed to follow up dental appointments. The information of this registration system was protected by a central log-in and password, and allowed the CHWs and the organisation to receive and send text messages when a client had a dental appointment in the upcoming 24 h.

The main task of the CHWs was to increase dental awareness and dental compliance among the undocumented immigrants, by completing all necessary administrative steps prior to the first dental visit, and by following up the further appointments. After the initial oral health examination, one of the CHWs called a local dentist to make an appointment in consultation with the client. When the appointment was made, it was registered in the digital registration system. Subsequently, the head of the organisation's medical service and the CHW considered whether the client needed personal assistance on the day of the appointment or not. The decision was made based on the linguistic capacities, personal competences and special needs of the individual client. In cases where doubt existed, or for first time visitors, personal assistance was always provided. When this personal assistance was required, the CHW received an expense allowance of €20 to cover transport and other direct costs.

At the end of the oral health examination, a referral letter was given to the client in case of need for further care. Clients were referred to the closest available dental office from their home address. When personal assistance was organised, a copy of the referral letter and the medical card of the client were given to the CHW in a closed envelope, in case the client lost or forgot it on the day of the appointment. If a second appointment was needed or the external dentist wanted to communicate directly with the organisation, the information was inserted in the closed envelope and returned to the organisation.

All external dentists were visited by the head of the medical service or contacted by phone before the first referral, in order to provide them with more information about the organisation and the involvement of CHWs. The dentists were informed and assured that the organisation would cover tooth extractions for people under the age of 53, which are not reimbursed by the government. Additionally, the dentists were allowed to apply for a "no show fee" in case of a missed appointment, which was also provided by the organisation.

The total number of appointments with external dentists was counted for 2015, 2016 and 2017. For each of these dental visits, the organisation registered whether the client was present or not. When an appointment was missed, the client was called by phone to ask for the reason for non-attendance. If the appointment was cancelled within the last 24 h, it was also considered as a missed appointment. Both the CHWs and the external dentists were asked to always contact the organisation in case of a missed appointment. When contacting the organisation, the external dentist could apply for a "no show fee" which was paid by the organisation. This fee ranged between €30 and €50, according to the dentist's standards.

Data analysis was carried in IBM SPSS Statistics V25.0 (SPSS Inc., Chicago, IL, USA). After explorative data analyses, differences in proportions were examined using crosstabs and Chi-square statistical tests. Alpha was set at 0.05.

The study was approved by the Ethics Committee of the University Hospital Ghent (B670201526486). All subjects gave their informed consent for inclusion before they participated in the study. They received a referral letter and were supported to visit a dentist when further care was needed. Clinical data were stored in a database specifically designed for the survey, using VTiger CRM system 7.1.0RC. The data, including personal data, were protected by an external hosting company and could not be consulted or modified by a third party. Before data analysis, all records were encrypted to ensure anonymity.

3. Results

Over the three years, an oral health examination was performed on 204 clients from 1 to 69 years old, with a mean age of 36.3 (Standard Deviation (SD) = 15.9). Baseline characteristics are indicated in Table 1. Untreated tooth caries were visible in 71.6% ($N = 146$) of the participants ($D_3 > 0$). From those with tooth decay, 46.7% had at least one tooth with visible pulpal exposure. The level of care was low, with an average restorative index of 30.3% (SD = 36.9) and a treatment index of 51.5% (SD = 37.9). Periodontal health was poor, with 62.2% ($N = 97$) of the clients having a DPSI score of 3 or 4.

Table 1. Characteristics of the examined sample.

Total Sample	$N = 204$		
	Mean	**SD**	**Missing**
Age	36.3	15.9	$N = 35$
Years in Belgium	4.6	4.7	$N = 0$
Plaque Index	1.4	0.8	$N = 18$
DPSI *	2.6	1.1	$N = 16$
D_3MFT	9.4	8.4	$N = 0$
PUFA	1.6	3.0	$N = 0$
Restorative Index	30.3	36.9	$N = 39$
Treatment Index	51.5	37.9	$N = 28$
Number of teeth with active caries per person	3.4	3.9	$N = 0$
Number of teeth with visual pulp exposure per person	1.3	2.5	$N = 0$
	Valid %	**N**	**Missing**
Origin (WHO region)	-	-	$N = 11$
African Region	11.9	23	-
Region of the Americas	1.0	2	-
South-East Asia Region	0.5	1	-
European Region	67.4	130	-
Eastern Mediterranean Region	37	19.2	-
Western Pacific Region	0.0	0	-
Smoker **	-	-	$N = 20$
Yes	46.2	60	-
No	52.3	68	-
Former smoker	1.5	2	-
Gender	-	-	$N = 10$
Male	44.3	108	-
Female	55.7	86	-
Active tooth decay	-	-	$N = 0$
Present	71.6	146	-
Not Present	28.4	58	-
Visible pulp Exposure	-	-	$N = 0$
Present	35.8	73	-
Not Present	64.2	131	-

* From those > 15 years old ($N = 143$); ** From those > 12 years old ($N = 150$).

Regarding dental attendance during the survey period, Figure 1 and Table 2 illustrate the number of external appointments provided to the target population for 2015, 2016 and 2017. The avoidable missed appointments without acceptable reason are indicated in red (Figure 1), the others in green. The orange bar indicates the number of missed appointments with legitimate reasons.

According to Table 2, the organisation registered 176 appointments with 16 different external dental practices in 2017, of which 89 were first dental visits. Physical assistance was provided for 87 appointments. Over the three years, the total number of missed appointments decreased significantly, with 40.9% in 2015, 11.9% in 2016 and 8.0% in 2017 ($p < 0.001$). The percentage of avoidable missed appointments dropped to 3.4%.

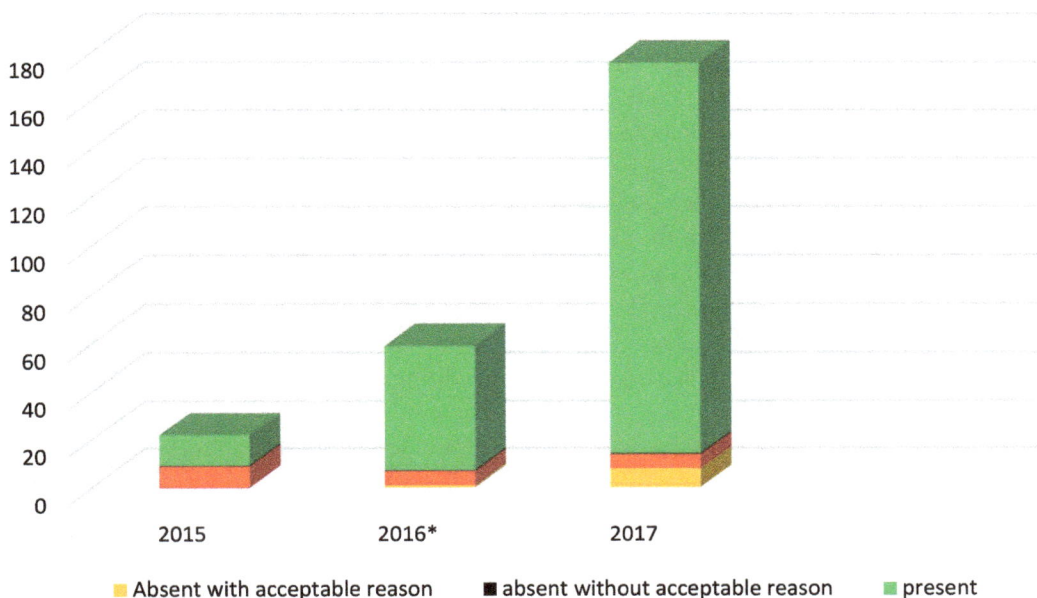

Figure 1. The number of appointments made with external dental practitioners and the proportion of missed appointments (y-axis) over the three study years (x-axis). *In August 2016, the personal assistance program was implemented.

Table 2. Total number of appointments for 2015, 2016 and 2017, and the proportion and explanation of missed appointments.

Appointments	2015	2016	2017
Total number of appointments	22 (100%)	59 (100%)	176 (100%)
Client present	13 (59.1%) *	52 (88.1%) *	162 (92.0%) *
Client absent	9 (40.9%)	7 (11.9%)	14 (8.0%)
Client absent without acceptable reason	9 (40.9%)	6 (10.2%)	6 (3.4%)
Client absent with acceptable reason	0 (0.0%)	1 (1.7%)	8 (4.5%)
Cancellation >24 h before appointment	-	-	4 (2.3%)
Unforeseen circumstances (arrestation, hospitalisation)	-	1 (1.7%)	2 (1.1%)
Error made by organisation or dentist			2 (1.1%)

* $p < 0.001$ according to chi-square test.

4. Discussion

The cross-sectional survey presented annual convenience samples within a Belgian organisation for undocumented immigrants. The participants were mainly young, with a mean age of 36.3. Their initial oral health care needs are considerable, as seen in Table 1. The presence of tooth decay was very high, with untreated decay at cavitation level ($D_3 > 0$) being present in 71.6% of the records, of which half had visible pulp exposure. Periodontal health was very poor, especially taking into account the mean age of 36.7, with 62.2% ($N = 97$) of participants having a DPSI score of 3 or 4. The bad periodontal condition can be partially explained by the high number of smokers (46.2%). Although the present oral health outcomes are alarming, they should be interpreted with caution. The present survey used a convenience sample, which means that the observed findings cannot be generalized for all undocumented immigrants, not even within the organisation. It can be assumed that people with high dental needs will be more likely to accept the offer of a dental screening and further referral, leading to selection bias and partially declaring the high level of tooth decay and periodontal disease in the initial examinations. No information was available from non-responders.

In contrast to the high dental need, the initial care level was almost negligible before the intervention. Although the present survey cannot draw conclusions on the causes of care avoidance, several determinants might play a role. First of all, the illegal character of the participants' residence forces them to hide from most official institutions. To get medical care, they need to present themselves to the local authorities. Although no one can ever be arrested while seeking help in one of these centres, officially registering for (oral) health care can still be a barrier. Furthermore, living in precarious conditions might also have an influence. As one of the most underprivileged groups in society, people without a residence permit suffer from the same social determinants which are mainly associated with deprived oral health: material deprivation, educational attainment, origin, professional status, and the lack of a social network. These factors are largely described in international literature as predictors of adverse oral health outcomes [13,14]. Since the average time of living in Belgium was almost five years in the presented sample, it is very likely that the adverse living conditions have played an important role in the oral health outcomes.

To support the target population, the intervention aimed to enable social workers, having a close relationship with the undocumented immigrants, to be involved in oral health care as community health workers. Since community health workers are people known by the target population, providing food and other assistance, they might have more authority and get more trust than an external caregiver. Acting as a contact person between care demander and care provider, the community oral health workers also consider the barriers perceived by the local dentists. Emphasis was put on adequate information and translation, and on the reduction of administrative burden and the number of missed appointments. Bedos et al. previously reported that frustrations expressed by dentists mainly concern missed appointments, difficulties in performing non-covered treatments and low government fees [15]. In our intervention, every dentist was called or visited personally by the head of the medical service of the organisation. During this conversation, the dentist could express his personal expectations and concerns, which were taken into account by the organisation and the CHWs. For example, when a dentist indicated not to speak French or English, the organisation only sent clients who were able to speak Dutch, or who were accompanied by a Dutch-speaking translator. The personal approach and mutual empathy resulted in a considerable network of 16 dentists accepting the undocumented immigrants in their dental practice. This can be considered a success, since the number of general dentists in Flanders is decreasing and dental practitioners are ageing. In 2017, the estimated number of qualified dentists was 1 per 1147 residents in Belgium and 1 per 1182 in Flanders (http://www.dekamer.be/QRVA/pdf/54/54K0138.pdf, p261). Furthermore, Belgium has until present no experience with dental hygienists as part of the professional dental team. When the number of dentists decreases, it can be assumed that the "law of demand and supply" will not be beneficial to vulnerable subgroups in society, such as undocumented immigrants.

Aiming to cope with the high unmet oral health needs and various user-side and supplier-side barriers, one of the major strengths of the present intervention was the creation of a safe and reliable partnership between the organisation and both the target population and the local dentists. Concerning the undocumented immigrants, the key elements of the intervention were outreach work, personal assistance and the involvement of existing networks. Indeed, oral health behaviour and oral health in general are largely affected by social networks and social support, defined as people's "social capital" [16].

Although the first results of the involvement of CHWs suggest a reduction in barriers towards dental care provision in both undocumented immigrants and local dentists, the effects might not be automatically applicable. Care provision strongly depends on national policy and health care budgets. According to a report of Cuadra, access to health care for undocumented immigrants varies between European countries [17]. Some countries, such as Belgium, only provide the minimum as set out by the UN Human Rights and specified by article 13.2 of the "Council of Europe Resolution 1509 (2006) on Human Rights of Irregular Migrants", whereas other countries provide more or sometimes less than this minimum access to care.

Even in Belgium, the results of the intervention might differ between cities. Since medical care for undocumented immigrants is organised at city level, inequalities in care provision between cities are probable, although this requires further investigation. The medical card in Ghent is an accessible instrument to help undocumented immigrants, but it does not exist in other cities such as Antwerp or Brussels, where decisions on reimbursement depend on each individual case. It is recommendable to obtain clear and equal legislation on a national scale, to avoid inequity and possible delocalisation of undocumented immigrants from one city to another. Medical care should not be determined by place of residence.

Although the medical card in Ghent might be an easy instrument to get access to dental care, the lack of coverage for tooth extractions for people under the age of 53 is a limitation, leading to high out-of-pocket costs. For 2017, the local organisation "De Tinten" spent €2311 of its own budget on no-show fees and uncovered basic treatment costs (excluding prosthodontic treatments), and paid €1616 for personal assistance by CHWs, yielding an average cost of €22.31 per appointment. Without external charity funding, this intervention could be compromised.

In order to reduce curative treatment costs in the future, the intervention did not focus exclusively on guiding clients to the dental office, but CHWs were trained during the educational program to pay attention to preventive oral health care and oral health behaviour. Furthermore, free dental goody bags were provided on a regular basis (every eight weeks). Budgets for preventive materials amounted to €2130 in 2017 and were also paid for by charity funding. It needs further research to investigate if this intervention can lead to a reduction of the overall costs in the long term due to improved oral health outcomes.

The present survey has some important limitations to report. Regarding the positive dental attendance rates in 2017, these results should be interpreted with caution. Increased dental attendance might not automatically imply increased dental awareness, better oral health behaviours or improved oral health outcomes, especially in the long term. Furthermore, the use of the words "urgent medical care" in legislation might also impede the mindset shift from curative care and falling from one oral health problem into the other, towards more cost saving preventive care. Although the law states that "urgent medical care" can be both curative and preventive, policy makers and stakeholders tend to consider preventive check-ups, supragingival scaling and small fillings as "non-urgent". Even some dental practitioners feel reluctant to sign the required form to confirm that their treatment was urgent. The author suggests that "necessary medical care" would be a better wording than "urgent medical care", avoiding semantic discussions and professional neglect of painless lesions.

Secondly, the survey could not link the external appointments to the original and individual characteristics of the clients, due to technical limitations. This makes it impossible to know if there were specific personal or oral health determinants, leading to more missed appointments. Furthermore, the present survey cannot provide information on responders and non-responders within the target population. The invitation to participate in the survey aimed to be as accessible as possible to undocumented immigrants. In order not to frighten them, it was impossible to make official lists and numbers of all undocumented immigrants who could possibly be involved. Furthermore, the recruitment process was carried out over several weeks during food distribution, making it impossible to count the total number of unique clients in this setting. Nevertheless, it is possible that the invitation attracted the most motivated clients, leading to higher rates of dental attendance.

As a final limitation, the present study is not a randomised controlled trial, exploring differences in outcomes between an intervention and control group over the same study period. Comparing different convenience samples before and after a program without the use of a proper control group inevitably leads to reporting bias. The absence of a control group was due to ethical reasons. The initial rates of missed appointments in 2015 (40.9%) negatively affected the reputation of undocumented immigrants among local dentists. Since there is no dental public health system in Belgium, all residents, legal and illegal, entirely depend on care from private dentists. If a control group was used, in which the number of missed appointments would remain high during some more years, it would be possible that local dentists would turn against all undocumented immigrants because of those in the control group. In real life circumstances, dealing with extremely vulnerable human beings, this was a risk nobody wanted to take.

Despite the clear scientific shortcomings of the survey, it is difficult to assume that the dramatic decrease in missed appointments over the two years would be due to factors other than the reported intervention. Even if this was due to other factors, the present survey shows that undocumented immigrants can be integrated into regular dental care and that high levels of dental attendance can be achieved in this population.

5. Conclusions

The present sample of undocumented immigrants shows very poor oral health, both in terms of tooth decay and periodontal disease. However, the decreasing proportions of missed appointments indicate that undocumented immigrants can be integrated into professional oral health care. Personal assistance by community health workers might be an effective method, although this requires further investigation.

Funding: This research received no external funding.

Acknowledgments: The author wants to acknowledge the indispensable support, dedication and innovative long term vision on oral and general health which is demonstrated by the medical and social service of "De Tinten", by providing high-quality assistance to undocumented immigrants on a voluntary basis.

References

1. Triandafyllidou, A. Clandestino Project—Final Report. Available online: http://clandestino.eliamep.gr/wp-content/uploads/2010/03/clandestino-final-report_-november-20091.pdf (accessed on 13 December 2018).

2. Baeyens, P.; Beys, M.; Bourguignon, M.; Büchler, A.; De Smet, F.; Dewulf, K.; Dutilleux, A.; Gaspart, G.; Lejeune, J.; Swankaert, J.; et al. Migration en droits et en chiffres 2015-Migratie in cijfers en in rechten 2015. Available online: https://www.myria.be/files/Migration-rapport_2015-LR.pdf (accessed on 13 December 2018).

3. Keboa, M.T.; Hiles, N.; Macdonald, M.E. The oral health of refugees and asylum seekers: A scoping review. *Glob. Health* **2016**, *12*, 59. [CrossRef]

4. Van Berlaer, G.; Bohle Carbonell, F.; Manantsoa, S.; De Béthune, X.; Buyl, R.; Debacker, M.; Hubloue, I. A refugee camp in the centre of Europe: Clinical characteristics of asylum seekers arriving in Brussels. *BMJ Open* **2016**, *6*, e013963. [CrossRef]

5. Riggs, E.; Rajan, S.; Casey, S.; Kilpatrick, N. Refugee child oral health. *Oral Dis.* **2017**, *23*, 292–299. [CrossRef] [PubMed]

6. Johnson, D.; Saavedra, P.; Sun, E.; Stageman, A.; Grovet, D.; Alfero, C.; Maynes, C.; Skipper, B.; Powell, W.; Kaufman, A. Community Health Workers and Medicaid Managed Care in New Mexico. *J Community Health* **2012**, *37*, 563–571. [CrossRef] [PubMed]

7. Benzian, H.; Greenspan, J.S.; Barrow, J.; Hutter, J.W.; Loomer, P.L.; Stauf, N.; Perry, D.A. A competency matrix for global oral health. *J. Dent. Educ.* **2015**, *79*, 353–361. [PubMed]

8.   Greenberg, B.J.S.; Kumar, J.V.; Stevenson, H. Dental case management—Increasing access to oral health care for families and children with low incomes. *JAMA* **2008**, *139*, 1114–1121.

9.   Klein, H.T.; Palmer, C.E.; Knutson, J.W. Studies on dental caries I dental status and dental needs of alimentary school children. *Public Health Rep.* **1938**, *53*, 751–765. [CrossRef]

10. Monse, B.; Heinrich-Weltzien, R.; Benzian, H.; Holmgren, C.; van Palenstein Helderman, W. PUFA—An index of clinical consequences of untreated dental caries. *Community Dent. Oral Epidemiol.* **2010**, *38*, 77–82. [CrossRef] [PubMed]

11. Silness, J.; Löe, H. Correlation between oral hygiene and periodontal condition. *Acta Odontol. Scand.* **1964**, *22*, 121–135. [CrossRef] [PubMed]

12. Van der Velden, U. The Dutch periodontal screening index validation and its application in The Netherlands. *J. Clin. Periodontol.* **2009**, *36*, 1018–1024. [CrossRef] [PubMed]

13. Sanders, A.E.; Slade, G.D.; Turrell, G.; Spencer, A.J.; Marcenes, W. The shape of the socio-economic-oral health gradient: Implications for theoretical explanations. *Community Dent. Oral Epidemiol.* **2006**, *34*, 310–319. [CrossRef] [PubMed]

14. Schwendicke, F.; Dörfer, C.E.; Schlattmann, P.; Page, L.F.; Thomson, W.M.; Paris, S. Socio-economic inequality and caries: A systematic review and meta-analysis. *J. Dent. Res.* **2015**, *94*, 10–18. [CrossRef] [PubMed]

15. Bedos, C.; Loignon, C.; Landry, A.; Richard, L.; Allison, P.J. Providing care to people on social assistance: How dentists in Montreal, Canada, respond to organisational, biomedical, and financial challenges. *BMC Health Serv. Res.* **2014**, *14*, 472. [CrossRef] [PubMed]

16. Rouxel, P.L.; Heilmann, A.; Aida, J.; Tsakos, G.; Watt, R.G. Social capital: Theory, evidence, and implications for oral health. *Community Dent. Oral Epidemiol.* **2015**, *43*, 97–105. [CrossRef] [PubMed]

17. Cuadra, C.B. Right of access to health care for undocumented migrants in EU: A comparative study of national policies. *Eur. J. Public Health* **2012**, *22*, 267–271. [CrossRef] [PubMed]

Permissions

All chapters in this book were first published in DJ, by MDPI; hereby published with permission under the Creative Commons Attribution License or equivalent. Every chapter published in this book has been scrutinized by our experts. Their significance has been extensively debated. The topics covered herein carry significant findings which will fuel the growth of the discipline. They may even be implemented as practical applications or may be referred to as a beginning point for another development.

The contributors of this book come from diverse backgrounds, making this book a truly international effort. This book will bring forth new frontiers with its revolutionizing research information and detailed analysis of the nascent developments around the world.

We would like to thank all the contributing authors for lending their expertise to make the book truly unique. They have played a crucial role in the development of this book. Without their invaluable contributions this book wouldn't have been possible. They have made vital efforts to compile up to date information on the varied aspects of this subject to make this book a valuable addition to the collection of many professionals and students.

This book was conceptualized with the vision of imparting up-to-date information and advanced data in this field. To ensure the same, a matchless editorial board was set up. Every individual on the board went through rigorous rounds of assessment to prove their worth. After which they invested a large part of their time researching and compiling the most relevant data for our readers.

The editorial board has been involved in producing this book since its inception. They have spent rigorous hours researching and exploring the diverse topics which have resulted in the successful publishing of this book. They have passed on their knowledge of decades through this book. To expedite this challenging task, the publisher supported the team at every step. A small team of assistant editors was also appointed to further simplify the editing procedure and attain best results for the readers.

Apart from the editorial board, the designing team has also invested a significant amount of their time in understanding the subject and creating the most relevant covers. They scrutinized every image to scout for the most suitable representation of the subject and create an appropriate cover for the book.

The publishing team has been an ardent support to the editorial, designing and production team. Their endless efforts to recruit the best for this project, has resulted in the accomplishment of this book. They are a veteran in the field of academics and their pool of knowledge is as vast as their experience in printing. Their expertise and guidance has proved useful at every step. Their uncompromising quality standards have made this book an exceptional effort. Their encouragement from time to time has been an inspiration for everyone.

The publisher and the editorial board hope that this book will prove to be a valuable piece of knowledge for researchers, students, practitioners and scholars across the globe.

List of Contributors

Tarek Mohamed A. Saoud
Department of Conservative Dentistry and Endodontics, Faculty of Dentistry, University of Benghazi, El Salmania, Abn Alathera Street No. 113, Benghazi 00218, Libya

Domenico Ricucci
Private practice, Piazza Calvario 7, 87022 Cetraro, Italy

Louis M. Lin
Department of Endodontics, College of Dentistry, New York University, 345 East 24th Street, New York, NY 10010, USA

Peter Gaengler
Department für Zahn-, Mund- und Kieferheikunde, Fakultät für Gesundheit, Universität Witten/Herdecke, Alfred-Herrhausen-Strabe 50, 58448Witten, Germany

Salma A. Bahannan
Oral and Maxillofacial Prosthodontics Department, Faculty of Dentistry, King Abdulaziz University, Jeddah 21589, Saudi Arabia

Somaya M. Eltelety
Dental Public Health Department, Faculty of Dentistry, Al Mansoura and King Abdulaziz Universities, Jeddah 21589, Saudi Arabia

Mona H. Hassan
Biostatistics Department, High Institute of Public Health, Alexandria University and Dental Public Health Department, Faculty of Dentistry, King Abdulaziz University, Jeddah 21589, Saudi Arabia

Suzan S. Ibrahim
Oral Diagnostic Sciences Department, Faculty of Dentistry, Ain Shams and King Abdulaziz Universities, Jeddah 21589, Saudi Arabia

Hala A. Amer
Dental Public Health Department, Faculty of Dentistry, Alexandria and King Abdulaziz Universities, Jeddah 21589, Saudi Arabia

Omar A. El Meligy
Pediatric Dentistry Department, Faculty of Dentistry, King Abdulaziz and Alexandria Universities, Jeddah 21589, Saudi Arabia

Khalid A. Al-Johani
Oral Diagnostic Sciences Department, Faculty of Dentistry, King Abdulaziz University, Jeddah 21589, Saudi Arabia

Rayyan A. Kayal
Periodontics Department, Faculty of Dentistry, King Abdulaziz University, Jeddah 21589, Saudi Arabia

Abeer A. Mokeem
Endodontics Department, Faculty of Dentistry, King Abdulaziz University, Jeddah 21589, Saudi Arabia

Akram F. Qutob
Dental Public Health Department, Faculty of Dentistry, King Abdulaziz University, Jeddah 21589, Saudi Arabia

Abdulghani I. Mira
Conservative Dentistry Department, Faculty of Dentistry, King Abdulaziz University, Jeddah 21589, Saudi Arabia

Dan Zhao and James Kit-Hon Tsoi
Dental Materials Science, Applied Oral Sciences, Faculty of Dentistry, the University of Hong Kong, Hong Kong SAR, China

Dan Zhao
School of Stomatology, Zhejiang Chinese Medical University, Hangzhou 310053, Zhejiang, China

Hai Ming Wong
Paediatric Dentistry, Faculty of Dentistry, the University of Hong Kong, Hong Kong SAR, China

Chun Hung Chu
Operative Dentistry, Faculty of Dentistry, the University of Hong Kong, Hong Kong SAR, China

Michael Crowe, Michael O' Sullivan and Oscar Cassetti
Division of Restorative Dentistry & Periodontology, Dublin Dental University Hospital, Trinity College Dublin, Dublin, Dublin 2, Ireland

Aifric O' Sullivan
UCD Institute of Food and Health, 2.05 Science Centre, South, UCD, Belfield, Dublin, Dublin 4, Ireland

Reem Naaman, Azza A. El-Housseiny and Najlaa Alamoudi
Pediatric Dentistry Department, Faculty of Dentistry, King Abdulaziz University, 21589 Jeddah, Saudi Arabia

Azza A. El-Housseiny
Pediatric Dentistry Department, Faculty of Dentistry, Alexandria University, 21526 Alexandria, Egypt

William Murray Thomson
Sir John Walsh Research Institute, Department of Oral Sciences, School of Dentistry, The University of Otago, Dunedin 9054, New Zealand

Amy Lynn Melok, Lee H. Lee and Siti Ayuni Mohamed Yussof ID
Department of Biology, Montclair State University, Montclair, NJ 07043, USA

Siti Ayuni Mohamed Yussof and Tinchun Chu
Department of Biological Sciences, Seton Hall University, South Orange, NJ 07079, USA

Sari A. Mahasneh
School of Dental Medicine, The University of Manchester, Manchester, M13 9PL, UK

Adel M. Mahasneh
Department of Biological Sciences, The University of Jordan, Amman 11942, Jordan

Tamara Abrams, Stephen Abrams and Koneswaran Sivagurunathan
Quantum Dental Technologies Inc., Toronto, ON M6B 1L3, Canada

Veronika Moravan and Koneswaran Sivagurunathan
VM Stats, Toronto, ON M5A 4R3, Canada

Warren Hellen and Gary Elman
Cliffcrest Dental Office, Toronto, ON M1M 1P1, Canada

Bennett Amaechi
Department of Comprehensive Dentistry, University of Texas Health Science Center, San Antonio, TX 78229-3900, USA

Andreas Mandelis
Center for Advanced Diffusion Wave and Photoacoustic Technologies (CADIPT), Department of Mechanical and Industrial Engineering, University of Toronto, Toronto, ON M5S 3G8, Canada

Ollie Yiru Yu, Irene Shuping Zhao, May Lei Mei, Edward Chin-Man Lo and Chun-Hung Chu
Faculty of Dentistry, The University of Hong Kong, Hong Kong SAR 999077, China

Charlotte Rombouts, Charlotte Jeanneau and Imad About
Aix Marseille Université, CNRS, ISM UMR 7287, 13288, Marseille, France

Athina Bakopoulou
Department of Fixed Prosthesis & Implant Prosthodontics, School of Dentistry, Aristotle University of Thessaloniki, GR-54124, Thessaloniki, Greece

Asmaa Alkhtib
Oral Health Division Operations, Primary Health Care Corporation, Doha 26555, Qatar

Abdul Morawala
Department of Dentistry, Primary Healthcare Corporation, Specialist Pediatric Dentist, Doha 26555, Qatar

Ollie Yiru Yu, Irene Shuping Zhao, May Lei Mei, Edward Chin-Man Lo and Chun-Hung Chu
Faculty of Dentistry, The University of Hong Kong, Hong Kong, China

LaQuia A. Vinson, Brian J. Sanders, James E. Jones and James A. Weddell
Department of Pediatric Dentistry Indiana University School of Dentistry, James Whitcomb Riley Hospital for Children Indianapolis, Indiana, IN 46202, USA

Matthew L. Rasche
Private Practice, Bloomington, IN 47401, USA

Mark A. Saxen
Department of Oral Pathology, Medicine, and Radiology, Indiana University School of Dentistry Indianapolis, Indiana, IN 46202, USA

Angela M. Tomlin
Department of Pediatrics Indiana University School of Medicine, James Whitcomb Riley Hospital for Children Indianapolis, Indiana, IN 46202, USA

Grace Gomez Felix Gomez and Richard L. Gregory
Department of Biomedical and Applied Sciences, Indiana University School of Dentistry, Indianapolis, IN 46202, USA

Frank Lippert and Masatoshi Ando
Department of Cariology, Operative Dentistry and Dental Public Health, Indiana University School of Dentistry, Indianapolis, IN 46202, USA

Andrea Ferreira Zandona
Department of Operative Dentistry, University of North Carolina, Chapel Hill, NC 27599, USA

George J. Eckert
Department of Biostatistics, Indiana University, Indianapolis, IN 46202, USA

Noha Samir Kabil
Department of Pediatric Dentistry and Dental Public Health, Faculty of Dentistry, Ain Shams University, Cairo 11566, Egypt

Sherif Eltawil
Department of Pediatric Dentistry and Dental Public Health, Faculty of Oral & Dental Medicine, Cairo University, Giza 12613, Egypt

Martijn Lambert
Department of Community Dentistry and Oral Epidemiology, Special Needs in Oral Health, Ghent University, 9000 Ghent, Belgium

Index

www.ingramcontent.com/pod-product-compliance
Lightning Source LLC
Chambersburg PA
CBHW050450200326
41458CB00014B/5129